Physician-Assisted Dying

Physician-Assisted Dying

The Case for Palliative Care and Patient Choice

Edited by

TIMOTHY E. QUILL, M.D.

Professor of Medicine, Psychiatry, and Medical Humanities,
Department of Medicine
Director, Center for Palliative Care and Clinical Ethics
University of Rochester School of Medicine and Dentistry
Rochester, New York

and

MARGARET P. BATTIN, Ph.D.

Distinguished Professor of Philosophy and
Adjunct Professor of Internal Medicine,
Division of Medical Ethics
University of Utah
Salt Lake City, Utah

The Johns Hopkins University Press
Baltimore and London

© 2004 The Johns Hopkins University Press
All rights reserved. Published 2004
Printed in the United States of America on acid-free paper
9 8 7 6 5 4 3 2 1

The Johns Hopkins University Press
2715 North Charles Street
Baltimore, Maryland 21218-4363
www.press.jhu.edu

Library of Congress Cataloging-in-Publication Data

Physician-assisted dying : the case for palliative care and patient choice / edited by Timothy E.
    Quill and Margaret P. Battin.
        p. ;   cm.
    Includes bibliographical references and index.
    ISBN 0-8018-8069-6 (hardcover : alk. paper) — ISBN 0-8018-8070-X (pbk. : alk. paper)
    1. Assisted suicide.   2. Right to die.   3. Palliative treatment.   4. Terminal care—Moral
and ethical aspects.   5. Patient satisfaction.   [DNLM: 1. Suicide, Assisted.   2. Euthanasia.
3. Palliative Care.   4. Right to Die. W 50 P5781 2004]   I. Quill, Timothy E.   II. Battin,
M. Pabst.
R726.P485   2004
179.7—dc22   2004010446

A catalog record for this book is available from the British Library.

For

Andrew Batavia
June 15, 1957 – January 6, 2003

Activist, Scholar, Teacher, Friend

Contents

Acknowledgments xi
List of Contributors xiii

Introduction False Dichotomy versus Genuine Choice:
The Argument over Physician-Assisted Dying 1
   Margaret P. Battin and *Timothy E. Quill*

PART ONE **Perspectives on Mercy, Nonabandonment,
Autonomy, and Choice**

1.   The Quality of Mercy 15
   Marcia Angell
2.   Nonabandonment: A Central Obligation for Physicians 24
   Timothy E. Quill and *Christine K. Cassel*
3.   The Role of Autonomy in Choosing Physician Aid in Dying 39
   Thomas Preston, Martin Gunderson, and *David J. Mayo*
4.   Disability and Physician-Assisted Dying 55
   Andrew I. Batavia
5.   When Suffering Patients Seek Death 75
   Eric J. Cassell

PART TWO **Clinical, Philosophical, and Religious
Issues about the Ending of Life**

6.   Why Do People Seek Physician-Assisted Death? 91
   Robert A. Pearlman and *Helene Starks*

7. Doctor-Patient Communication about
   Physician-Assisted Suicide   102
   Anthony L. Back

8. When Hastened Death Is Neither Killing Nor Letting Die   118
   Tom L. Beauchamp

9. Physician-Assisted Suicide as a Last-Resort Option
   at the End of Life   130
   Dan W. Brock

10. Death: A Friend to Be Welcomed,
    Not an Enemy to Be Defeated   150
    John Shelby Spong

PART THREE   Open Practice in a Legally
Tolerant Environment

11. The Oregon Experience   165
    Linda Ganzini

12. The Distortion of Cases in Oregon   184
    Peter Goodwin

13. A Model That Integrates Assisted Dying with Excellent
    End-of-Life Care   190
    Barbara Coombs Lee

14. Thirty Years' Experience with Euthanasia in the Netherlands:
    Focusing on the Patient as a Person   202
    Johannes J.M. van Delden, Jaap J.F. Visser, and *Els Borst-Eilers*

15. The Death of My Father   217
    Herman H. van der Kloot Meijburg

16. Assisted Death in the Netherlands: Physicians at the Bedside When
    Help Is Requested   221
    Gerrit K. Kimsma and *Evert van Leeuwen*

PART FOUR   Political and Legal Ferment

17. Political Strategy and Legal Change   245
    Eli D. Stutsman

18. Legal Advocacy to Improve Care and Expand Options at the
    End of Life   264
    Kathryn L. Tucker

19. Physician-Assisted Suicide: Shifting the Focus from
Means to Ends   282
Alan Meisel

20. Choice in Dying: A Political and Constitutional Context   300
Sylvia A. Law

21. Hastening Death: The Seven Deadly Sins of the Status Quo   309
Charles H. Baron

Conclusion   Excellent Palliative Care as the Standard,
Physician-Assisted Dying as a Last Resort   323
Timothy E. Quill and *Margaret P. Battin*

Index   335

Acknowledgments

It takes a team of dedicated people to create a multiauthored book such as this, and we gratefully acknowledge them here. The many chapter authors gave generously of their time, energy, and expertise, so that we could explore in depth the varied dimensions of this subject. Sadly, Andrew Batavia died shortly after completing his chapter, and we thank his brother Mitchell for helping us maintain Andrew's voice throughout the editing of his chapter. Maria Milella graciously and skillfully helped coordinate and assemble all the chapters, and maintained connection with the authors during the various stages of the book. Bette Crigger, who also worked on the counterpoint book, *The Case against Assisted Suicide: For the Right to End-of-Life Care* (Kathleen Foley and Herbert Hendin, volume editors), did a masterful job with the early editing, ensuring that the multiauthored chapters were coherent in style and content. Wendy Harris, senior editor at the Johns Hopkins University Press, has helped guide this project from conception to delivery, providing insight and oversight each step of the way. Finally, we thank the many people we have met, facing their own deaths or the deaths of loved ones, who have been so articulate in letting us know how important *both* palliative care *and* genuine choice can be at the end of life.

Contributors

Marcia Angell, M.D., Senior Lecturer, Department of Social Medicine, Harvard Medical School, Boston, Massachusetts; former Editor-in-Chief, *New England Journal of Medicine*

Anthony L. Back, M.D., Associate Professor, Department of Medicine, University of Washington, Seattle, Washington

Charles H. Baron, A.B., LL.B, Ph.D., Professor of Law, Boston College Law School, Newton, Massachusetts

Andrew I. Batavia, J.D., M.S. (deceased), Professor of Public Health, School of Policy and Management, Florida International University, Miami, Florida

Tom L. Beauchamp, Ph.D., Senior Research Scholar, Kennedy Institute of Ethics, and Professor, Philosophy Department, Georgetown University, Washington, D.C.

Els Borst-Eilers, M.D., Ph.D., former Dutch Minister of Health (1994–2002) and member of the Remmelink Committee on the medical practice of euthanasia (1991), Netherlands

Dan W. Brock, Ph.D., Charles Burgess McGrath Professor of Medical Ethics, Harvard University Medical School, Boston, Massachusetts

Christine K. Cassel, M.D., M.A.C.P., President, American Board of Internal Medicine, Philadelphia, Pennsylvania

Eric J. Cassell, M.D., M.A.C.P., Clinical Professor of Public Health, Weill Medical College of Cornell University, New York, New York

Barbara Coombs Lee, B.S.N., J.D., President and CEO, Compassion in Dying Federation, Portland, Oregon

Linda Ganzini, M.D., M.P.H., Professor of Psychiatry and Medicine, Oregon Health and Science University, Portland, Oregon

Peter Goodwin, M.B. Ch.B., F.R.C.S. Ed., Associate Professor Emeritus, Department of Family Medicine, Oregon Health and Science University, Portland, Oregon

Martin Gunderson, Ph.D., J.D., Professor, Department of Philosophy, Macalester College, St. Paul, Minnesota

Gerrit K. Kimsma, M.D., M.A., Associate Professor in Medical Philosophy, Center for Ethics and Philosophy, Vrije Universiteit, Amsterdam, Netherlands

Sylvia A. Law, J.D., Elizabeth K. Dollard Professor of Law, Medicine and Psychiatry, New York University School of Law, New York, New York

David J. Mayo, Ph.D., Professor, Department of Philosophy, University of Minnesota–Duluth, Duluth, Minnesota

Alan Meisel, J.D., Dickie, McCamey and Chilcote Professor of Bioethics and Professor of Law, School of Law and Center for Bioethics and Health Law, University of Pittsburgh, Pittsburgh, Pennsylvania

Herman H. van der Kloot Meijburg, D.Div., C.T., Health Care Ethicist and Consultant. Former General Secretary of the Standing Committee on Religious and Ethical Affairs of the Hospital Association of the Netherlands, Utrecht, Netherlands

Robert A. Pearlman, M.D., M.P.H., Professor of Medicine, Departments of Medicine, Medical History and Ethics, and Health Services, University of Washington, and Chief, Evaluation Service, National Center for Ethics in Health Care (Veterans Health Administration), Seattle, Washington

Thomas Preston, M.D., Professor, Department of Medicine, University of Washington, Seattle, Washington

John Shelby Spong, A.B., M.Div., Honorary D.D., D.H.L., Episcopal Bishop (retired), Diocese of Newark, Newark, New Jersey

Helene Starks, M.P.H., Ph.D., Research Manager, Department of Medical Education and Biomedical Informatics, University of Washington, Seattle, Washington

Eli D. Stutsman, J.D., Board Chairman, Death with Dignity National Center; Attorney at Law, Portland, Oregon

Kathryn L. Tucker, J.D., Director of Legal Affairs, Compassion in Dying Federation; Affiliate Professor of Law, University of Washington School of Law and Seattle University School of Law, Seattle, Washington

Johannes J.M. van Delden, M.D., Ph.D., Professor of Medical Ethics, Julius Center for Health Sciences, University Medical Center; Nursing Home Physician, Rosendael Nursing Home, Utrecht, Netherlands

Evert van Leeuwen, Ph.D., Professor in Philosophy and Medical Ethics, Center of Ethics and Philosophy, Vrije Universiteit Medical Center, Amsterdam, Netherlands

Jaap J.F. Visser, L.L.M., Department of Medical Ethics, Ministry of Health, Welfare and Sport of the Netherlands, Netherlands

Physician-Assisted Dying

False Dichotomy versus Genuine Choice

The Argument over Physician-Assisted Dying

Margaret P. Battin, Ph.D., and Timothy E. Quill, M.D.

D espite a growing consensus that palliative care should be a core part of the treatment offered to all severely ill patients who potentially face death,[1] challenging questions remain. How broad a choice should patients have in guiding the course of their own dying? What limitations should be placed on the physician's obligation to address patients' suffering? Physician-assisted death (also called physician-assisted suicide or physician aid in dying) has long been the focal point of ethical and political debate—a divisive, hot button issue in a domain in which there is otherwise considerable agreement.

At first glance, this focus on assisted death seems to miss the mark. If the question were posed, "What would you rather have, access to palliative care and hospice or access to physician-assisted death?" we would choose palliative care and hospice every time. To frame the question in this way, however, presents a false dichotomy. Palliative care should be part of the standard of care for all severely ill patients, even those who are continuing active, disease-directed treatment, and hospice should be the standard of care for all those who understand and accept that they are dying. We insist on a more inclusive question that fully addresses the needs, wishes, and realities of dying patients: "What would you prefer, access to excellent palliative care and hospice by themselves or access to excellent hospice and palliative care plus legal access to a physician-assisted death as a last resort if your suffering becomes intolerable and you wish an earlier, easier death?"

In this introduction and in the title of the book, we use the term *physician-assisted dying* because it is descriptively accurate and carries with it no misleading connotations. Other contributors to this volume prefer the synonymous term *physician-assisted suicide* because it is technically accurate, and still others prefer *physician aid in dying* because it is relatively neutral. Although suicide can be considered heroic or rational depending on setting and philosophical orientation, in much American writing it is conflated with mental illness, and the term suggests the tragic self-destruction of a person who is not thinking clearly or acting rationally. Although distortion from depression and other forms of mental illness must always be considered when a patient requests a physician-assisted death, patients who choose this option are not necessarily depressed but rather may be acting out of a need for self-preservation, to avoid being destroyed physically and deprived of meaning existentially by their illness and impending death. While in general we use the more neutral term *physician-assisted death* for this reason, we have allowed our authors—and ourselves—to use any of the three terms interchangeably.

Both proponents and opponents of legalization of physician-assisted death can join together in support of improving access to and delivery of comprehensive palliative care for all severely ill patients who wish it and to support expansion of hospice benefits to those whose prognosis is too uncertain to fall within the usual six-month time frame. Both sides can also acknowledge and bemoan inadequacies in access to and delivery of health care services in general in the United States, as well as end-of-life care in particular.[2]

Where we proponents of legalization part company with opponents is in our belief that it is not fair or justified to postpone legal access to physician-assisted death while we await the solution of these most difficult social problems. Relief of suffering—and with it the freedom to face dying as one wishes—must be available to suffering patients now. It is also our belief that legalization is a small but important part of the larger process of improving end-of-life options and care for many dying patients.

Opposing Claims about Physician-Assisted Dying

This book brings together classic and new work by a group of distinguished authors to present the case for legalization of physician-assisted death for terminally ill patients who voluntarily request it. Some of the impetus for compiling this book comes from *The Case against Assisted Suicide: For the Right to End-of-Life Care,* edited by Kathleen Foley and Herbert Hendin and also published by the Johns Hopkins University Press.[3] Indeed, the two might be considered complements. The contributors to the Foley and Hendin volume are articulate and thoughtful opponents of legalization of physician-assisted death. We congratulate that book: it is helpful to have the best arguments opposing the practice collected in one place.

We think it is also important to put the best arguments *for* the practice into a single collection, both to counter the false dichotomy that the Foley and Hendin book seems to presuppose as well as other misconceptions and misunderstandings in the opposition literature and, more important, to explore genuine differences in values. We agree with much of those authors' critique of health care in general and end-of-life care in particular in the United States. However, we disagree with many of their value assumptions, with how they construct arguments opposing physician-assisted death, and especially with their reliance on "slippery slope" arguments that predict wholesale abuse if physician-assisted suicide were to be legalized throughout the United States—a prediction that this volume will show is not supported by the data from either Oregon or the Netherlands. Our book provides a very different analysis of existing data. Where there are disagreements, it will be up to the reader to determine which interpretation is more objective, though it is not always clear that data will settle a debate that is often more moral, philosophical, and religious than empirical.[4] Nonetheless, for those who have an open mind on this question, these data are critical to understanding the practice and its implications for policy.

The voluminous literature opposing legalization makes a variety of points and argues in a number of characteristic ways. What follows is a quick summary of some of the most conspicuous of these points, since it is among the concerns of our book to show how these points can be addressed and refuted. In our estimation, thinkers who oppose legalization of physician-assisted death appear to rest their arguments on a number of problematic assumptions.

• *Physician-assisted suicide means that physicians will have control over who lives and who dies.* It isn't the physician who has control; it's the patient. Many contributors to our volume explore how patient autonomy is actualized in physician-assisted dying. For example, Herman van der Kloot Meijburg's account of his father's death, Pearlman and Starks' studies of patient motivation, and Back's examination of doctor-patient communication as patients seek an assisted death, all show how physicians participate reluctantly, out of a sense of commitment to their patients.

• *Already accepted methods of negotiating death, including withholding and withdrawal of treatment, treatment with high-dose opioids for severe terminal pain or shortness of breath, and the use of terminal sedation, are less morally problematic than actively assisting death, and so assisted death isn't warranted.* Although there is wide ethical and legal acceptance of such practices, even when they bring about the death of the patient, this is not to say they are less morally problematic than actively assisting death. They still bring about death, and they frequently offer fewer protections for the patient.[5] There are no systematic safeguards for patient voluntariness, transparency of action, or protection from pressures from family, clinicians, or health care institutions such as those in statutes or proposals for the legalization of physician-assisted death.

• *Because few patients would make use of physician-assisted death, it is not appropriate to make sweeping (and potentially dangerous) public policy for a small class of individuals, however compelling the stories of those individuals might be.* Three things are wrong with this claim: the assumption that if only a small proportion of dying people actually use it, the availability of physician assistance in dying isn't important to others who are facing death; the assumption that physician-assisted dying is dangerous; and the quite callous view that dismisses the rights and interests of those who would use it. The comfort provided by the possibility of an earlier, easier death, even if one never actually uses it, can be enormous. For those who do use it, the prospect of dying in a way of their own choosing rather than being gradually obliterated by disease can be of central importance in the meaning of their soon-to-be-completed lives.

• *Depression is endemic among those who are seriously ill, so such patients cannot make these decisions rationally.* The personal stories explored in this volume and, more important, the clinical data on patients in Oregon who actually received physician assistance at death, fail to show distorted thinking from depression.[6] Depression assessment can be tricky in any end-of-life decision,[7] a fact that argues for an open practice with careful clinical evaluation of all practices, legal or not, that might end in a patient's death. Society now allows patients to make other end-of-life decisions—for example, refusing further life-prolonging treatment such as dialysis[8]—that will also result in death, without assuming that the patient who makes such a choice is by definition depressed.

• *There is something wrong with patients who seek this kind of control.* All patients, like all people, eventually die. What patients sometimes seek is some control over the way in which their inevitable deaths come about. As a society, we admire those who use medicine to try to postpone their deaths, and we admire those who assume responsibility for the way they live their lives in other domains; there is no reason not to admire and assist them as they live the last portion of their lives.

• *Physician-assisted dying is an issue of life versus death.* This assumption, too, is in error. For a physician to assist in the death of a terminally ill patient does not make the difference between death and indefinitely continuing life;

rather, it makes the difference between an easier death now and a more difficult death a little later. The amount of life foreshortened is typically quite small.
Data from the Netherlands, where these practices are legal, show that patients
who choose physician-assisted dying forgo, on average, only a few weeks of life
and that in the vast majority of cases, assisted death is provided in the last
week or on the last day before death would otherwise have occurred.[9]

• *If physician-assisted suicide isn't legalized, it won't occur.* Nothing could be
further from the truth; every study of physician practice in the United States,
as well as studies in other countries, shows a measurable, fairly consistent incidence of physician-assisted suicide whether legal or not.[10] Therefore, the more
realistically posed question about legalization must focus on comparing an
open, legally regulated practice with a secret practice.

• *Jack Kevorkian is an example of what legalizing physician-assisted death would
bring.*[11] Neither Oregon's Death with Dignity Act nor any proposed statute for
legalization in the United States would permit providing physician-assisted
death for terminal patients without careful safeguards, including repeated oral
and written requests, waiting periods, confirmation of the diagnosis of termi-
nality, and provision for psychiatric evaluation if there is uncertainty about
voluntariness. Many of Dr. Kevorkian's cases would not meet these safeguards,
and he is probably more symptomatic of the dangers of a secretive, underground practice than representative of an open, publicly regulated practice of
physician-assisted death.

• *In Oregon and in the Netherlands, legalization has been accompanied by
real abuse, and patients are sometimes railroaded into choosing assisted death.*
Thanks to a series of three comprehensive studies of end-of-life decisions in
the Netherlands over a period of sixteen years (discussed in part 3 of this
book), Dutch practice is well understood. Data for the entire period of legalization in Oregon are also available. There is no evidence of abuse in Oregon,
and on close inspection the notorious "1,000 cases"[12] of life-terminating acts
without explicit request, said to represent serious abuse in the Netherlands,
prove not to do so. The Dutch do not defend everything that has happened in
their country regarding physician-assisted suicide, but they do not experience the serious, wholesale abuse of which opponents often accuse them. The
Netherlands has the lowest, not the highest, rate of ending life without the patient's explicit request compared to voluntary euthanasia with request of all six
European countries recently studied.[13] Furthermore, in both Oregon and the
Netherlands legalization has been associated with marked improvements in
palliative and end-of-life care.

• *Good palliative care, including that provided by hospice, is incompatible with physician-assisted death.* Of all the misconceptions and errors perpetrated by opponents of legalization, this is perhaps the most damaging in its departure from the truth. As Constance Putnam has argued, the choice between "hospice or hemlock" is not the issue.[14] Much of this volume explores the deep compatibility of excellent palliative care and physician-assisted death as a last resort. The majority of patients in Oregon who chose assisted death under the Death with Dignity Act were enrolled in hospice programs, and the majority of Oregon hospices have chosen to continue to care for those who are considering this choice. In addition, the Netherlands now has approximately one hundred inpatient hospices, and twenty-four-hour pain-control hotlines provide immediate advice for physicians. As several of the accounts of the practice in the Netherlands in part 3 of this volume show, better palliative care has been very much a goal of medical policy.

Our intent is not simply to rebut the claims of those who oppose physician-assisted death. This volume's principal objective is to make the positive case for the availability of physician-assisted death as a last resort, and to do so by presenting some of the strongest arguments put forward by respected philosophers, ethicists, lawyers, religious leaders, and clinicians. Some of our contributors make the case for the moral acceptability of physician-assisted dying; others primarily address the case for legalization; many are concerned with both. This volume thus makes the positive argument that the practice should have a small but critical role among the range of end-of-life possibilities available to patients.

Here, it is important to understand the shape of the argument over physician-assisted death.

Principal Arguments for Physician-Assisted Death	*Principal Arguments against Physician-Assisted Death*
• Patient autonomy • Mercy—the relief of pain and suffering • Nonabandonment—commitment to patient and family	• The wrongness of killing • The integrity of the physician • The risk of abuse (the slippery-slope argument)

Although many of these arguments are used by both sides, two philosophical concerns are central to the case for physician-assisted death: liberty, variously called freedom, self-determination, or (as philosophers put it) autonomy; and mercy, which asserts an individual's right to seek to be free from pain and suffering. These two basic principles, liberty and mercy (the right to live one's life as one sees fit, subject to the constraint that one not harm others, and the right to be free from pain and suffering, the obverse, one might say, of the right to the pursuit of happiness), are fundamental principles of the society in which we live. No one may be deprived of liberty, or be forced to suffer, without adequate cause. What is crucial to understand is that the burden of proof lies with those who object to these two cardinal points: they must show either that some still more basic principle trumps these claims or that honoring them would have seriously negative consequences. The third principle, nonabandonment, more precisely a norm of practice for physicians and other health care professionals, follows from the first two. There is an ethical requirement for physicians to try to respond to autonomous requests from their patients, especially when the requests revolve around extremes of suffering in those who are already dying.

Philosophers, ethicists, lawyers, religious leaders, and clinicians who oppose physician-assisted suicide appeal to principles as well. Quite plausibly, they assert that killing is intrinsically wrong—which, in the sense they have in mind, it is. Since physician-assisted dying does involve directly ending life, the accusation that it is killing and that killing is wrong might seem to have some purchase. However, physician aid in dying is certainly not "killing" in the pejorative sense of robbing someone of a life he or she values and that could otherwise continue; in physician-assisted death, the direct ending of life is an act of aid and reflects a deep concern for a person's well-being in the face of a death coming in any case—and thus the exact opposite of killing in the pejorative sense they have in mind. In a culture that accepts killing in self-defense, in war, and (more controversially) in capital punishment, it is hard to see why we should prohibit assisting a person who earnestly wants help in ending his or her own life, when that person's illness is terminal, the person is suffering, and life is ending anyway.

Opponents of physician-assisted dying claim that the consequences of legalizing physician-assisted suicide would be bad in two further respects: legalization would corrupt physicians and thus undermine the integrity of the medical profession, and it would fuel a slide down the slippery slope from a few sympathetic cases to widespread abuse. Yet there is no evidence for these claims, and there is substantial evidence to the contrary. The opposition must show that the principles of liberty and freedom from suffering, basic to an open, liberal, democratic society, should be overridden. This we believe they cannot do.

Since people of good will and considerable clinical, policy, and legal experience differ significantly on many of the issues underlying physician-assisted dying, those wanting to deeply explore both sides of this complex issue will want to read both the Foley and Hendin volume and this book. However, the present volume stands on its own in presenting the strongest arguments supporting ethical acceptance and legalization of the practice of physician-assisted dying. Here the practice is seen not as an alternative to excellent palliative care but as a last resort for those relatively infrequent cases in which palliative care becomes ineffective or unacceptable to dying patients whose conception of dying well includes some measure of control over the circumstances of death.

Brief Introduction to the Chapters

The contributors to part 1 examine the critical values of autonomy and mercy, the anchor points of the case for assisted dying, both of which are essential foundations for physician involvement in these activities. Autonomy in this context focuses on the values and wishes of the particular patient who finds himself or herself in an untenable situation. Patient autonomy is clearly a central point in considerations of assisted death, since it is the patient's life and death that are at stake in these decisions. However, assistance in dying, if it is also to involve physicians, cannot be solely a matter of patient choice; it must also be a response to medical distress, to actual or imminent suffering. The nature of the patient's suffering and why it is intolerable to the patient must be understood by the physician, who must then try to respond as a matter of mercy and in fulfillment of his commitment not to abandon the patient. Thus autonomy, mercy, and nonabandonment go hand in hand: for the physician to participate in assistance in dying, it must both be the patient's choice and help the patient avoid suffering that is intolerable or about to become so.

Marcia Angell, a distinguished physician and editor-in-chief emerita of the *New England Journal of Medicine,* explores the concept of mercy, drawing from her personal experience as the daughter of a man who took his life violently to avoid further indignity from his terminal illness. Timothy Quill and Christine Cassel, also physicians, use their experience in geriatrics, primary care, and palliative care to explore the central value of nonabandonment: the obligation of the physician who assumes care of a patient not to desert the patient at the end of his or her life; given the not infrequent tendency of physicians to distance themselves from their patients when nothing more can be done, this obligation is of particular weight. Tom Preston, Martin Gunderson, and David Mayo—

a physician, a lawyer, and a philosopher—provide a sustained examination of the concept of autonomy and its centrality in physician-assisted death. Drew Batavia, a law professor who lived with a severe disability until his death in 2003, looks at the issue from the viewpoint of a disabled person and offers a broader analysis of this community's views about choice and about the possibility of an assisted death than is ordinarily presented. In the final chapter of part 1, physician Eric Cassell draws on his considerable clinical experience and philosophical background to understand human suffering and the real threat that terminal illness poses to the integration of the person, exploring in particular the interface of illness, suffering, and control.

The chapters in part 2 explore some of the clinical, philosophical, and religious issues that underlie end-of-life practices. Robert Pearlman and Helene Starks, a physician and a researcher, using an extended series of in-depth interviews with patients and their families, explore the question why a dying patient seeks physician-assisted death. The answer is not simply avoidance of pain and suffering but also the wish to retain some measure of control over the circumstances of one's dying. The physician Tony Back extends this clinical picture by examining the complex, delicate interaction among doctor, patient, and family as they communicate concerning the decision to seek assisted death. Tom Beauchamp, a philosopher, critically explores the often-used distinction between killing and letting die, and Dan Brock, also a philosopher, examines conceptual and practical distinctions among two already accepted methods of hastening death—voluntary cessation of eating and drinking and terminal sedation—and the more controversial physician-assisted suicide. Finally, Bishop John Shelby Spong explores some of the religious implications of physician-assisted death, showing how it is compatible—even when it is called "suicide"—with a deep understanding of Christianity.

Contributors to part 3 turn their attention to the empirical data about patterns of practice in those places where physician-assisted death has been legalized, especially Oregon and the Netherlands. Linda Ganzini, a physician researcher at Oregon Health and Science University, reviews cumulative data from the Oregon Health Division reports on the practice of physician-assisted suicide under Oregon law and additional research conducted since legalization. Peter Goodwin, an Oregon physician who has been active in the referendum movement as well as both the *Glucksberg* and *Quill* Supreme Court cases, corrects common misrepresentations of two controversial cases in Oregon, drawing on his experience as a clinician at the bedside and in the care of these patients. Barbara Coombs Lee, a nurse and lawyer and the executive director of the Compassion in Dying Federation, an organization dedicated to improving end-of-life care and expanding choice at the end of life, presents her experience in assessing and working with patients who desire a hastened death.

From the Netherlands, a number of well-respected authorities provide a comprehensive picture of legalized voluntary active euthanasia and physician-assisted suicide there. Hans van Delden, Jaap Visser, and Els Borst-Eilers (who was Minister of Health in the Netherlands for many of the years under study) review thirty years' experience in the Netherlands, including three major nationwide studies and an account of the distortion of this data by Herbert Hendin and other American authors. Herman van der Kloot Meijburg, the former director of bioethics for the Dutch Hospital Association, provides a vivid personal account of his father's death in a country in which active voluntary euthanasia and physician assistance in suicide are legal. Gerrit Kimsma, a physician, and Evert van Leeuwen, a philosopher, both on the faculty of the Free University in Amsterdam, offer a perspective from the bedside. The comprehensive picture these three chapters paint is illustrated in an anonymous offhand remark one of us heard in the Netherlands some years ago: "We Dutch have to fear dying less than you Americans do."

In part 4, some of the legal and political turmoil that has surrounded questions of physician-assisted death is examined. Eli Stutsman, an Oregon attorney who has been active in defending the state's Death with Dignity Act and in working to pass similar legislation in other states, discusses some of the politics of legal change in Oregon and other parts of the country. Kathryn Tucker, well known for her role as the lead lawyer along with Lawrence Tribe in the two cases contesting this issue before the United States Supreme Court, *Glucksberg v. Washington* and *Vacco v. Quill* (decided jointly in 1997), and as an important litigator on behalf of Compassion in Dying in improving accountability for inadequate pain treatment, provides an overview of these two cases and developments in their wake.

Alan Meisel, a professor of law, provides an analysis of the legal implications of the distinction between actively and passively hastening death that have been central to the thinking of many ethicists. Of particular importance in this analysis is the distinction between negative and positive rights, a distinction missed by opponents who believe that a "right" to physician-assisted death would obligate physicians to perform it. Sylvia Law, also a law professor, explores the political and constitutional issues raised by the movement for legalization of physician-assisted death and puts it into context with other liberation movements over the past forty years. Finally, law professor Charles Baron traces the legal risks of maintaining the current policy of passive legal prohibition outside of Oregon.

The brief concluding essay presents our answer to the dilemmas presented in this book and in the counterpart volume edited by Foley and Hendin. We firmly believe that physician-assisted death should be one—not the only one, but one—of the last-resort options available to a patient facing a hard death. We agree that these options should include high-dose pain medication if needed, cessation of life-sustaining therapy, voluntary cessation of eating and drinking, and terminal sedation. We also believe, however, that physician-assisted dying, whether it is called physician-assisted death or physician aid in dying or physician-assisted suicide, should be among the options available to patients at the end of life. Clinical assessments required before accessing any of these last-resort options are more similar than they are different. We believe that physician-assisted dying, as one among them, should be safe and legal—and relatively rare.[15] Most important, like all the other options, it should be a matter of open choice for patients, since different people who are dying have different ideas and values about what would be, for them, the "least worst" death.[16] An open practice that includes frank conversation, a broad search for alternatives, second opinions by those with expertise in palliative care, and clear documentation is better for patients, families, and society than the current secret practice, which discourages open discussion, often has patients and families acting on their own, is not documented, and encourages altering the truth about actions and motivations. We invite readers to look at the arguments and data and make up their own minds, for the deeper the understanding we all have of the underlying issues, the better able we will be to develop sensible policies that are both responsive to and protective of patients and their families.

Notes

1. M.J. Field and C.K. Cassel, eds., *Approaching Death: Improving Care at the End of Life* (Washington, D.C.: National Academy Press, 1997).

2. T.E. Quill, D.E. Meier, S.D. Block, and J.A. Billings, "The Debate over Physician-Assisted Suicide: Empirical Data and Convergent Views," *Annals of Internal Medicine* 128 (1998): 552–58.

3. K. Foley and H. Hendin, eds., *The Case against Assisted Suicide: For the Right to End-of-Life Care* (Baltimore: Johns Hopkins University Press, 2002).

4. M. Angell, "Euthanasia in the Netherlands—Good News or Bad?" editorial, *New England Journal of Medicine* 335 (1996): 1676–78.

5. T.E. Quill, B. Lo, and D.W. Brock, "Palliative Options of Last Resort: A Comparison of Voluntarily Stopping Eating and Drinking, Terminal Sedation, Physician-Assisted Suicide, and Voluntary Active Euthanasia," *Journal of the American Medical Association* 278 (1998): 2099–104.

6. L. Ganzini, H.D. Nelson, T.A. Schmidt, D.F. Kraemer, M.A. Delorit, and M.A. Lee, "Physicians' Experiences with the Oregon Death with Dignity Act," *New England Journal of Medicine* 342 (2000): 557–63; L. Ganzini, T.A. Harvath, A. Jackson, E.R. Goy, L.L. Miller, and M.A. Delorit, "Experiences of Oregon Nurses and Social Workers with Hospice Patients Who Requested Assistance with Suicide," *New England Journal of Medicine* 347 (2002): 582–88; L. Ganzini, personal communication about clinical interviews with inpatients being evaluated for possible physician-assisted suicide, July 6, 2004.

7. S.D. Block, "Assessing and Managing Depression in the Terminally Ill Patient," *Annals of Internal Medicine* 132 (2000): 209–18.

8. L.M. Cohen, J.D. McCue, M. Germain, and C.M. Kjellstrand, "Dialysis Discontinuation: A 'Good' Death?" *Archives of Internal Medicine* 155 (1995): 43–47.

9. E.J. Emanuel and M.P. Battin, "What Are the Potential Cost Savings from Legalizing Physician-Assisted Suicide?" *New England Journal of Medicine* 339 (1998): 167–72.

10. D.E. Meier, C.A. Emmons, S. Wallenstein, T.E. Quill, R.S. Morrison, and C.K. Cassel, "A National Survey of Physician-Assisted Suicide and Euthanasia in the United States," *New England Journal of Medicine* 338 (1998): 1193–1201; E.J. Emanuel, E.R. Daniels, D.L. Fairclough, and B.R. Clarridge, "The Practice of Euthanasia and Physician-Assisted Suicide in the United States: Adherence to Proposed Safeguards and Effects on Physicians," *Journal of the American Medical Association* 280 (1998): 507–13.

11. D. Callahan, "Reason, Self-Determination, and Physician-Assisted Suicide," in *The Case against Assisted Suicide: For the Right to End-of-Life Care,* edited by K. Foley and H. Hendin (Baltimore: Johns Hopkins University Press, 2002), 52–68.

12. L. Pijnenborg, P.J. van der Maas, J.J.M. van Delden, and C.W.N. Looman, "Life Terminating Acts without Explicit Request of Patient," *The Lancet* 341 (1993): 1196–99.

13. A. van der Heide, L. Deliens, K. Faisst, T. Nilstun, M. Norup, E. Paci, G. van der Wal, and P.J. van der Maas, on behalf of the EURELD consortium, "End-of-Life Decision-Making in Six European Countries: Descriptive Study," *The Lancet* 362 (2003): 345–50.

14. C.E. Putnam, *Hospice or Hemlock: Searching for Heroic Compassion* (Westport, Conn.: Praeger, 2002).

15. M.P. Battin, "Physician-Assisted Suicide: Safe, Legal, Rare?" in *Physician-Assisted Suicide: Expanding the Debate,* edited by M.P. Battin, R. Rhodes, and A. Silvers (New York: Routledge, 1998), 63–72.

16. M.P. Battin, *The Least Worst Death: Essays in Bioethics on the End of Life* (New York: Oxford University Press, 1994).

PART ONE

Perspectives on Mercy, Nonabandonment, Autonomy, and Choice

1

The Quality of Mercy

Marcia Angell, M.D.

Death is not fair and it is often cruel. Some die young, others in extreme old age. Some die quickly, others slowly but peacefully. Some find personal or religious meaning in the process, as well as an opportunity for a final reconciliation with loved ones. Others, especially those with cancer, AIDS, or progressive neurologic disorders, die by inches and in great anguish. Good palliative care usually can help in these cases, but not always and often not enough. The problem is not just pain, although that can be devastating. Other symptoms, such as breathlessness and nausea, can be worse and even harder to relieve. There are no good treatments for weakness, loss of bodily functions, and helplessness—probably the most important reasons for despair in those who are dying slowly, along with the knowledge that it can only grow worse.

Just as dying differs, so too do people's hopes and fears about their own deaths. Most people probably hope for a sudden death—in old age during sleep—but not everyone. Some would prefer a slower death, to have time to prepare and to take leave of loved ones. For some, the ultimate terror is loss of their mental faculties. For others, it is intractable pain, and for still others, it is immobility, dependence, and a loss of control over the circumstances of their lives. Experience in Oregon in the six years since its Death with Dignity Act came into effect is illuminating. Under this act, patients with terminal illness may request physicians to help them hasten death by providing a prescription for a lethal dose of sleeping pills.[1] Physicians may legally do so, if they choose, and the state has kept careful records of the practice. Those records show that fear of loss of control is a powerful motive for those who request help in ending their lives—or, more properly, in ending their protracted dying.[2]

Like other healthy, young people, I knew little about death when I went to medical school forty years ago. If I thought about it at all, it was in a stylized way, gleaned from death scenes from operas or movies or novels—for example, the poignant but peaceful farewell of Mimi in the opera *La Bohème*. Medical school did not help much. In those days, physicians and their instructors paid little formal attention to the dying process. I do not remember a single mention of it in the medical school curriculum. It was as though dying were a medical failure and thus too shameful to be discussed. As doctors, we were to succeed, not fail, and success was measured by our ability to stave off death. Our failures were kept hidden.

Sooner or later, of course, my classmates and I did come into contact with death—not the peaceful death of our fantasies but death as it really happened, over and over again, in the hospitals where we worked. Some deaths were peaceful, but we also saw patients in virtually unrelieved agony, often because pain medication was given in doses too small and too far apart. We saw patients isolated as they died—by their doctors because we thought there was nothing more we could do for them and by their families because we conspired with them to withhold the truth from dying patients. On morning hospital rounds, we simply avoided dying patients—this despite the fact that most of us went to medical school at least in part because we wanted to relieve suffering. Sometimes doctors—particularly the older, experienced ones—would hasten the deaths of suffering patients by administering large doses of morphine, but the practice was rarely explicitly acknowledged. All of this we young doctors were left to absorb silently. It had no place in the curriculum or in the discourse of the medical profession at large. We just did not talk about it.

The Importance of Treating Pain

I broke my own silence on the subject in 1982, a few years after I had joined the editorial staff of the *New England Journal of Medicine*. In an editorial entitled, like this chapter, "The Quality of Mercy," I criticized the systematic failure to treat pain adequately in dying patients:

> One consideration that limits the use of narcotics is the possibility of a
> variety of side effects, including drowsiness, constipation, urinary retention,
> and most serious, respiratory depression. A more important factor is a dis-
> proportionate, sometimes irrational fear on the part of the medical pro-
> fession and the public alike that patients will become addicted. The desire

to protect patients from becoming insidiously drawn into a state of addiction distorts both our sense of priorities and our scientific judgment. A survey of medical house officers in two New York teaching hospitals documented the strong tendency to exaggerate the dangers of narcotics, as well as a curious belief that very low doses were effective against severe pain, and higher doses would provide no added relief.

These attitudes and misconceptions have led to a rather ritualized and parsimonious use of narcotics for the relief of pain. The drugs are given in doses that are often inadequate, at time intervals that are often too long, according to a pro re nata (prn) regimen [doses given no more often than every four hours and only if requested by the patient] that requires the patient to wait out the time interval, no matter how severe the pain. Even the inadequate amounts of narcotics ordered may not in fact be received by the patient. The prn regimen, by placing the onus on the patient to request the drug, introduces considerations other than whether or not he is in pain. Patients may be inhibited by a desire to please the medical staff and not be a nuisance. Those who do decide to ask for pain relief must keep track of both the time and the drug schedule and have the strength and endurance to summon a nurse if one is not nearby. The extent to which nurses share the common concerns about addiction may influence their readiness to respond. Thus, in practice, the average daily dose of narcotics received is even smaller than the amounts ordered, and uncorrelated with the degree of persistent pain.

We are left, then, with the image of a patient who can anticipate severe pain toward the end of each three- or four-hour period, who counts the minutes until the end of the interval, and desperately hopes that a nurse will be nearby and promptly give him his dose of narcotics when it is time. To such a patient, the medical profession's attention to pain must seem confined to limiting relief from it. To doctors and nurses, on the other hand, the patient's anxiety and clock watching may seem to indicate growing dependence on the drug, not inadequate relief of pain. I believe there is a tendency for an adversarial relationship to develop in which the doctor or nurse ascribes to the patient the motivations and impulsions of an addict. He is seen to be obsessed with drugs—not pain—and too weak to stop himself.

What are the facts? Addiction among patients who receive narcotics for pain is exceedingly unlikely; the incidence is probably no more than 0.1 percent. Even those who develop tolerance and physical dependence are unlikely to become addicted, and withdrawal can be accomplished easily if the painful stimulus is no longer present. The purpose of the drugs for these patients is, after all, the relief of pain; "street" addicts, in contrast, take drugs for quite different purposes. The incidence of serious respiratory depression in patients who receive narcotics for pain is similarly low. As tolerance develops to the analgesic effects of narcotics, so it does to the respiratory effects. No more than 1 percent of patients who receive narcotics for pain develop serious respiratory depression.

It is instructive to contrast the very low incidence of important side effects with the very high incidence of inadequate pain relief. I can't think of any other area in medicine in which such an extravagant concern for side effects so drastically limits treatment. We are used to a closer balance between risks and benefits. The relative weighting we give to risks and benefits in relieving pain should, of course, depend on the patient's medical condition and preferences. The patient with transient pain from benign disease may be unwilling to accept and should not experience more than minimal side effects. At the other extreme, concerns about addiction in the patient with terminal cancer are irrelevant, and those about respiratory depression should be secondary to relief of pain.

Given a commitment to pain relief, how is this best accomplished? The prn regimen for dispensing narcotics has been strongly criticized. Many authorities believe that it is not only punishing but inimical to the efficient use of narcotics, since the dose required to abolish pain is larger than the dose required to prevent its re-emergence. The usual alternative to the prn regimen is to give the drug at fixed intervals, to prevent pain rather than to treat it. This is the regimen used at St Christopher's Hospice in London. Both these approaches to pain relief have advantages and drawbacks, which have been well described by Beaver. I would like to suggest an intermediate approach. A prn order for a range of doses could be written, but the patient asked at each specified interval whether he needs relief from pain and, if so, whether he needs a relatively small or large dose. This system would give the patient a great deal of control over his symptom relief and also allow for fluctuations in the intensity of pain. Thus, it is more flexible than the fixed schedule. More important, it has the advantage over the prn regimen that the patient is never placed in the demoralizing position of a supplicant who must hunt down his help every three or four hours. It goes without saying that the doses and frequency of administration must be fully adequate for analgesia.

I ended the editorial with an appeal to doctors: "Pain is soul destroying. No patient should have to endure intense pain unnecessarily. The quality of mercy is essential to the practice of medicine; here, of all places, it should not be strained."[3]

Since then, largely stimulated by the hospice movement that began in London and found widespread acceptance in the United States in the 1980s, attitudes toward the treatment of pain at the end of life have improved greatly. The use of patient-regulated intravenous pain relief is now common, providing the flexibility and control I advocated more than twenty years ago. New methods of treating pain have been devised, and pain clinics have been established in many medical centers and large hospitals. In addition, the whole spectrum of symptoms of dying patients is now receiving professional attention. Hospice care is widely available, and palliative medicine is a recognized specialty. Despite all this progress, however, pain relief is still generally inadequate, particularly for children and other vulnerable patients, and there are still exaggerated concerns about "drug-seeking" patients and the side effects of opiates.

Existential Suffering

Symptoms of terminal illness other than pain are often harder to manage. That is particularly true of existential suffering—the sense of the utter pointlessness of a protracted death. If tomorrow will be worse than today, one day after another until the end, why not die today? Why continue to disintegrate, to lose bodily functions, to grow ever more helpless and dependent? I believe it was largely because of such feelings that a movement arose to legalize physician-assisted suicide as a choice for the dying, even as the palliative care movement also grew in importance.

Over time I became convinced that physician-assisted suicide should be an option for dying patients when palliative care has failed. I further came to believe that the judgment as to whether palliation had failed could be made only by each patient individually, since suffering is entirely subjective.[4] My growing conviction was reinforced by my father's death in 1988. I told his story in an amicus brief on behalf of Oregon in *Oregon v. Ashcroft* (the U.S. attorney general's ongoing attempt to nullify the Oregon Death with Dignity Act)[5] and in the *Washington Post*. Here is that story:

On March 15, 1988, my father, Lester W. Angell, then 81 years old, took a pistol from his bedside table and shot himself through the head. He died instantly. About seven years earlier he had been diagnosed with prostate cancer. For a few years, he did reasonably well with treatment. Four months before his death, however, the cancer began to spread throughout his body, and he required radiation for excruciating back pain. Although the pain was lessened, he suffered from nausea and vomiting as a result of the radiation and from side-effects of his various medications. He knew he had nothing to look forward to except further decline and a protracted death. Worst of all for him was the prospect of losing his independence.

My father was a man of great dignity for whom independence was enormously important. He saw it as his responsibility to take care of his family, not the other way around. He had a successful career as a civil engineer, first with the Tennessee Valley Authority, then the Army Corps of Engineers, and eventually as Chief Design Engineer of the St. Lawrence Seaway. In World War II, despite being in his late thirties, he volunteered and served as a Seabee in the South Pacific. (He had a lot in common with the fictional Mr. Roberts.) He later became a Lt. Colonel in the U.S. Army Reserves. All his life he was a conservative Republican who believed in patriotism and the duties of citizenship. But he also believed in the right to self-determination. To my knowledge, he never suffered from depression.

At the time my father killed himself, he and my mother were living near Orlando, Florida. My mother was a housewife who had always been dependent on him. Now it was the other way around. The day before his death, he fell while walking to his bed from the bathroom. My mother was unable to lift him, so she called the emergency medical technicians. They lifted him to the bed and said they would return the next day to take him to the hospital to make certain he had not fractured a bone. I believe he decided to kill himself that night because it might be his last chance to do it. He had always kept a pistol in his bedside table. If he went to the hospital the next day, he would be without it and he might never again have the option of ending his own life.

My mother was sleeping in the next room, and had to bear the shock of finding his body. If he had told her his intentions, she would have stopped him, as she later told me. So he did not tell her. Later, I could see from the trajectory of the bullet that he had turned in such a way that the bullet could not have gone through the wall and harmed her. I believe he had planned on the possibility of taking his own life for some time, since he had left his affairs in perfect order, including a long letter to my mother, with copies to my brother and me, instructing her on exactly what needed to be done. My father also did not tell me of his intentions, even though I am a physician and he confided in me about other aspects of his illness. Although I do not know for certain why he did not tell me or ask for my help, I suspect he did not want to compromise me in any way.

If physician-assisted suicide had been available to my father, as it is to the people of Oregon, I have no doubt that he would have chosen a less violent and lonely death. My mother could have been brought around to accepting his decision, death could have been peaceful, and his family could have been with him. If he knew he had the option to get help in ending his life at any time in the future, he probably also would have chosen to live longer. That night would not have been his last chance.

My father's situation was hardly unique or even unusual. Many people with terminal illness face the same dilemma. It is not a choice between life and death. It is a choice between a slow, agonizing death and a quick, merciful one. Many people—not just my father—would choose the latter if they could. What was unusual about my father was not his choice, but his courage and resolve in achieving it. The Oregon Death with Dignity Act makes that choice much easier for patients and their families. But it does not preclude people from making a different choice. People who prefer a longer life to an easier death are not prevented from choosing that. It seems to me that Oregon has chosen a path that gives dying patients the opportunity to exercise the greatest possible self-determination with the full support of their families and communities. I cannot imagine why anyone would want to prevent that.[6]

Trusting Dying Patients

Ironically, some of the people who *do* want to prevent that are closely associated with the move to improve palliative care, including advocates of good hospice care. An unfortunate schism has opened up between people who have in common the overarching desire to mitigate suffering at the end of life. In a recent book, *The Case against Assisted Suicide,* edited by Kathleen Foley and Herbert Hendin, some of the most prominent opponents of physician-assisted suicide argue their case.[7] The arguments vary. For some, it is a moral matter, although it is hard for me to imagine anything morally uplifting about requiring helpless people to endure protracted agony. Kass states, "Doctors must not kill."[8] But physician-assisted suicide is not about "killing"; rather, it is about helping patients to hasten their own deaths. And surely there is something off point in Kass's focus on doctors, not patients. Other essayists emphasize medical considerations rather than moral ones. To them, assisted suicide is not necessary. They believe that all suffering can be relieved if caregivers are sufficiently skillful and compassionate. They fear that permitting physician-assisted suicide would deflect attention from providing good palliative care.

I have no doubt that if expert palliative care were available to everyone who needed it, there would be few requests for assisted suicide. I also have no doubt that even under the best of circumstances, there will always be a few patients whose suffering simply cannot be adequately alleviated; and there will be some who would prefer suicide to other measures to deal with unremitting suffering, such as heavy sedation without fluids and food until death. I would certainly like to be proved wrong about this. I would welcome all attempts to show that palliative care can be so effective that no one wants physician-assisted suicide. That outcome could only be achieved, however, by preserving the choice, not closing it off. It would require trust that dying patients know what they want. If physician-assisted suicide is illegal, there will be no way of knowing whether what Cicely Saunders calls "the hospice and palliative care movement"[9] has been successful—whether it has won its point and physician-assisted suicide is truly unnecessary. We cannot simply assume that good palliative care is always effective.

I am also concerned that the hospice and palliative care movement, as it has grown in importance and influence, has developed a mindset typical of many specialized disciplines: a professional pride that borders on hubris and rigidity. Proponents have in some respects devised a picture of a good death that is no less stylized than the one I brought to medical school. In this picture, patients see the dying process as a time of "growth," during which they come to realize deeper meanings in their lives and relationships and eventually achieve a peaceful acceptance of death. Suffering is to some extent overcome by this acceptance. As Saunders puts it, "People need time to evaluate their lives, repair their relationships, and plan for others. They may also find new depth of enjoyment in a transient world."[10]

This ideal of the good death does not leave much room for patients for whom control and independence are highly important—people like my father, people who dread dying more than they fear death. I have even heard such people disparaged as overly controlling—as though they should somehow get with the program and die right. But it is wrong to assume that all people will approach death the same way. Some will, indeed, become ideal hospice patients, but others will rail against the dying process until the end, and they will want that end to come sooner. They too are human. We should be careful not to impose our views of a good death on others.

Long before my father's death, I believed that physician-assisted suicide ought to be permissible under some circumstances, but his death strengthened my conviction that it is simply a part of good medical care, something to be provided reluctantly and sadly, as a last resort, but provided nonetheless. There should be safeguards to ensure that the decision is well considered and consistent, but these should not be so daunting or so violate privacy that they become obstacles instead of protections. In particular, they should be directed not toward reviewing the reasons for an autonomous decision but only toward ensuring that the decision is indeed autonomous.

There is no right way to die, and there should be no schism between advocates for better palliative care and advocates for making the choice of assisted suicide available. Surely every effort should be made to improve palliative care, as I argued in 1982. When those efforts are unavailing and suffering patients desperately long to end their lives, they should have the choice to do so. The argument that permitting physician-assisted suicide would deflect us from redoubling our commitment to good palliative care asks these patients to pay the penalty for our failings. It is also illogical. Good palliative care and the availability of physician-assisted suicide are no more mutually exclusive than good cardiologic care and the availability of heart transplantation. To require dying patients to endure unrelievable suffering, regardless of their wishes, is callous and unseemly. Death is hard enough without being bullied. Like the relief of pain, this too is a matter of mercy.

Notes

1. Oregon Death with Dignity Act, *Oregon Revised Statutes,* secs. 127-800–127.995 (1995), www.ohd.hr.state.us/chs/pas/pas.cfm (accessed December 12, 2003).

2. A.D. Sullivan, K. Hedberg, and D.W. Fleming, "Legalized Physician-Assisted Suicide in Oregon—The Second Year," *New England Journal of Medicine* 342 (2000): 598–604.

3. M. Angell, "The Quality of Mercy," editorial, *New England Journal of Medicine* 306 (1982): 98–99.

4. M. Angell, "The Supreme Court and Physician-Assisted Suicide—The Ultimate Right," editorial, *New England Journal of Medicine* 336 (1997): 50–53.

5. R. Steinbrook, "Physician-Assisted Death in Oregon—An Uncertain Future," Health Policy Report, *New England Journal of Medicine* 346 (2002): 460–64.

6. M. Angell, "No Choice But to Die Alone," *Washington Post,* February 24, 2002, 137.

7. K. Foley and H. Hendin, eds., *The Case against Assisted Suicide: For the Right to End-of-Life Care* (Baltimore: Johns Hopkins University Press, 2002).

8. L.R. Kass, "'I Will Give No Deadly Drug': Why Doctors Must Not Kill," in *The Case against Assisted Suicide: For the Right to End-of-Life Care,* edited by K. Foley and H. Hendin (Baltimore: Johns Hopkins University Press, 2002), 17–40.

9. C.A. Saunders, "A Hospice Perspective," in *The Case against Assisted Suicide: For the Right to End-of-Life Care,* edited by K. Foley and H. Hendin (Baltimore: Johns Hopkins University Press, 2002), 288.

10. Ibid.

2

Nonabandonment

A Central Obligation for Physicians

Timothy E. Quill, M.D., and Christine K. Cassel, M.D., M.A.C.P.

The secret of the care of the patient is caring for the patient.
Francis Peabody, 1927

The principle of nonabandonment represents a continuous caring partnership between physician and patient. This relationship may begin in health or in sickness, may last through potential recovery or adjustment to chronic illness, and often continues until a patient dies.[1] Nonabandonment acknowledges and reinforces the centrality of an ongoing personal commitment to caring and problem solving between physician and patient. It also captures the essential qualities whereby physicians and patients commit to mutual decision making over time, even when the course is uncertain. Many dimensions of this covenant are articulated in the virtues of caring, fidelity, altruism, and devotion,[2] yet none of them captures the particular importance of a long-term, engaged presence that continues until the patient dies or recovers.

Nonabandonment suggests a human relationship with an open-ended commitment over time. It is particularly mandated by three challenging aspects of modern medicine: One is the changing health care environment and its growing emphasis on managed care systems and competitive market approaches to cost containment. These forces may limit a patient's choice of physicians, disrupt the continuity of a physician-patient relationship by requiring frequent changes in exclusive provider organizations, and create perverse physician incentives that may cast doubt on his or her role as a patient advocate.[3] The growing prevalence of chronic illness and the aging of the population are the second challenges that bring the centrality of nonabandonment into focus. For these populations, the evaluation of clinical performance must move beyond episodic decision making about diagnostic or therapeutic options to establish a relationship grounded in continuity, realistic expectations, and a shared understanding of goals and values.

Medicine's extraordinary success in prolonging life, as well as its simultaneous ability to increase suffering and prolong dying if used indiscriminately, reinforces the importance of long-term, committed medical relationships. Finding the proper balance between palliative and life-prolonging treatments is increasingly complex in this context, and understanding that such interventions may at times be complementary rather than mutually exclusive is crucial.[4] Severely ill patients need physicians who will help them understand medicine's potential, taking into account where they are in their lives' trajectory, and work with them through to their deaths to achieve the best possible quality and meaning in their lives. In this environment, making nonabandonment an essential obligation of all physicians seems vitally important. These complex challenges are much easier when faced by partners who know and trust one another than by strangers. Sometimes, however, strangers must come together when a patient is in crisis and must learn to trust and commit to one another as quickly and as deeply as possible. We focus our presentation with two clinical experiences.

Cynthia

Cynthia was a thirty-seven-year-old graduate student in psychology.[5] A practicing Buddhist, she considered quality, human connection, and spirituality to be central to her life. She developed dyspeptic symptoms, and in three days what was initially thought to be an easily treated stress-induced gastritis turned out to be terminal metastatic gastric adenocarcinoma.

Cynthia was devastated by her diagnosis. When her physicians recommended hospice care and promised to keep her free from pain until her death, she felt abandoned. She found no hope in their offer and needed to find a way to fight her illness. Although her prognosis was poor, she believed she could beat the odds. For Cynthia, accepting her prognosis without a medical fight would have meant giving in to hopelessness and despair.

As Cynthia explored experimental therapy, she needed assurance that she could stop the treatment at any time if it became too harsh or was not working. She also needed to inquire about what dying might be like. She feared severe physical pain, lingering on the verge of death without quality of life, and being kept alive without sufficient consciousness. Because death in her religious tradition was a form of rebirth, she hoped that her physician would help her find death peacefully if her condition evolved in that direction, as extremes of suffering before death seemed more terrifying to her than death itself.

It was in this context that Cynthia first became my patient. To a physician with a belief in palliative care and negative feelings about the futile, medically invasive treatment of dying patients, Cynthia's request for an aggressive medical approach initially posed a significant challenge. Cynthia needed the slim hope that experimental medical intervention provided, but she also needed honesty about the odds and the potential toxic effects of such treatment. Armed with assurance that I would not abandon her no matter what her clinical course, Cynthia eventually chose experimental therapy, despite its potential risks and burdens.

Not surprisingly, treatment was harsh and ineffective against the relentless progression of the cancer. As the burdens of her illness and its treatment increased over the next month, hospice care began to take on a different meaning for her. The promise of exclusive attention to symptom relief, without adding to her suffering with aggressive treatment of her disease, now seemed more sensible and meaningful to Cynthia than continuing to futilely fight her disease. She sadly accepted that she was dying, and all efforts were subsequently directed to maximizing the quality of the time that remained to her. Because the tumor had invaded her entire abdomen, she depended on intravenous fluids and nutrition, which she chose to continue. A continuous intravenous morphine drip helped relieve her pain.

Cynthia left the hospital with the support of her family and a home hospice program. She tried to find meaning in each day and simultaneously prepared for death. She married her long-time boyfriend, and her parents moved to town to be near her. The local Buddhist community regularly had group meditations at her home. She gave away many of her favorite possessions as she prepared for death. It was an intensely sad and unforgettably meaningful time for all who had the privilege of being with her.

After several weeks, Cynthia's quality of life deteriorated despite everyone's best efforts. She required increasing doses of morphine and had to make hourly trade-offs between pain and sedation. She experienced nausea and vomiting that could not be relieved, and her wounds and ostomies created an unpleasant smell that she found inescapable and humiliating. Cynthia sadly accepted her inevitable death and said good-bye to the important people in her life. At this point, no viable avenues were available to recapture quality in her life, and further disintegration and suffering were larger enemies than death itself.

Because I had made a commitment not to abandon Cynthia at this critical moment, my obligation as her physician was to help her meet death on her own terms as much as possible. For Cynthia, this meant discontinuing central hyperalimentation treatment and accepting the sedation that came with escalating doses of the intravenous narcotics that were used to control her pain. She was prepared to die but did not want to be perceived as committing suicide. She and her family were reassured that this method was fully compatible with widely accepted ethical principles.

Cynthia gradually became more sedated, went into a coma, and died relatively peacefully several days later, with her husband, parents, and friends in attendance.

Mrs. K.

Mrs. K. was a ninety-three-year-old woman who had survived the Nazi death camps in which most of her family perished.[6] She began a new life in the United States, raised a son in her second marriage, and outlived her husband by twenty years. She lived alone in a small apartment, and her social contacts were increasingly limited because of her own physical infirmities and the deaths of many friends.

Mrs. K. was healthy until the age of eighty-five, when a painful neuropathy developed in her left leg. It was eventually diagnosed as reflex sympathetic dystrophy. Seeking pain relief and a way to stem its associated loss of strength, she saw an unending series of consultants. Trials of antidepressants, antiepileptics, nonsteroidal and narcotic analgesics, orthotics, and physical therapy were ineffective and often had unacceptable side effects.

She valued only two medications: flurazepam (Dalmane) for inducing sleep and diazepam (Valium) for treating the "aggravation" of chronic pain. Although she insisted that these medications were helpful to her, Mrs. K. was repeatedly told by a series of physicians that these were the wrong medications because of their long half-lives, sedative side effects, absence of analgesic properties, and potential for addiction. Mrs. K. determinedly expressed her concerns, attributions, and experience to each physician she saw; she would dismiss most medical suggestions other than these two medications as unworkable and then proceed with her litany of problems—pain, sleeplessness, loneliness, and frustration with old age and infirmity. Strong willed and opinionated, she traveled from physician to physician—to the mutual frustration of all involved.

After initially repeating this unproductive pattern of intervention and rejection, I eventually realized that what Mrs. K. most needed was to be cared about and listened to. She did not expect medical answers to all of her problems. She wanted a confidante and adviser, someone who knew the whole picture and could interpret what was happening to her and find value in her personhood. I began to listen intently to her descriptions of the suffering and frustration of her daily life. Hearing about her past suffering and losses in the death camps, and about how she had survived, I came to understand how lonely it could be to outlive one's family and friends. Mrs. K. became more complex to me as a person, which allowed me to empathize more meaningfully with her plight. I helped her with bouts of constipation, guided her through cataract surgery, conservatively evaluated her chest pain of uncertain cause, and allowed her to openly explore whether life was worth living in the face of loneliness and loss. I also reinitiated therapy with flurazepam and diazepam without constantly questioning her need or their efficacy, accepting the small risk that she could be secretly stockpiling them in case she decided to end her life.

Over the next two years, Mrs. K. suffered two vertebral crush fractures and as a consequence experienced severe pain that limited her physical activity. Because of this and generalized frailty, she decided to move to an assisted living facility. As feisty as she was, this was not an easy decision, and she vacillated, sometimes saying, "I would be better off dead." She had been living in the same apartment for thirty years and had no family available to help her with this transition, so the staff at the geriatrics clinic functioned as surrogate family. Medicare, of course, doesn't pay for these services, but the team understood this role as central to the principle of nonabandonment. Shortly after she had moved, a fall caused a hip fracture. She refused surgical intervention, telling us that she wanted to keep her wits about her for the time she had left but that she was ready to "say good-bye." She was enrolled in hospice, where she experienced the human interaction that meant so much to her. She elected to refuse antibiotics for a bronchopneumonia that developed secondary to her immobility and died without suffering.

Mrs. K. did not have to die alone. She was able to talk with her physician and the hospice workers about the meaning of her life as it ended on her own terms, with respect and dignity.

The Obligation of Nonabandonment

As the cases of Cynthia and Mrs. K. show, the quality of medical care can be substantially enhanced when it is provided in the context of a caring, continuous, committed physician-patient relationship. The mutual decision making described in these two case presentations can never be adequately covered in formal "practice guidelines," treatment algorithms, or rigidly defined contracts. Standardized approaches cannot possibly attend adequately to the distinct and profound specificity of the patient and physician as persons or the shared experiences and meanings that develop between them over time. Medical care can be both humanized and individualized in such relationships. Respect for and curiosity about the person are essential, as is the desire to actively involve patients in their own care and empower them to the greatest extent possible.[7] Although patients often become more dependent and vulnerable when ill, a caring, committed relationship can respect and explore that vulnerability while simultaneously allowing as much choice and control as possible given the patient's circumstance and personality. Relationships between physicians and patients can be both personal and professional, and empathy and personal connection can enrich the task of facing the reality of the patient's condition together.[8] Intuition and emotion supplement the intellect, and there is a flow between sharing information and making decisions about the patient's condition while simultaneously exploring any associated feelings and reactions.

The obligation of nonabandonment emphasizes the longitudinal nature of a caring and problem-solving commitment between physician and patient.[9] Principle-based ethical analyses of clinical actions sometimes focus on one moment in time and seek generalizable rules or answers. Patients and their families and physicians, however, do not have the luxury of existing in such isolation. Clinical decisions involve a series of choices over time, and the consequences of one decision may immediately and inevitably lead to a series of subsequent new dilemmas, each with its own cascade of consequences.

Furthermore, the meaning and critical nature of any particular medical act cannot be understood or judged by isolating it into rules that do not acknowledge the personal histories, values, motivations, and intentions of the persons involved.[10] Cynthia's choice to discontinue life-sustaining treatment at the end of her life had wide moral acceptance even though it resulted in a desired death (she was "allowed to die" of her underlying disease). Easing her suffering under these circumstances might be viewed as fulfilling a final commitment not to abandon her to further personal disintegration, which she had begun to view as worse than death. However, if that decision had stemmed in part from undertreated pain or from her physician's personal frustration with the difficulty of her dying, then such "allowing to die," though legally permissible, could be the worst form of abandonment. No act can be fully understood or judged by putting it into an abstract category without considering the values, intentions, and circumstances of the actors.

Promising to face the future together is a central obligation of the physician-patient relationship.[11] This commitment is open ended, for neither person knows what the future will hold or what might be asked for or required. The American Medical Association's Council on Ethical and Judicial Affairs has stated a minimal expectation: "Once having undertaken a case, the physician should not neglect the patient, nor withdraw from the case without giving notice to the patient, the relatives, or responsible friends sufficiently long in advance of withdrawal to permit another medical attendant to be secured."[12] The depth and specificity of this obligation may vary from patient to patient depending both on the patient's requests and clinical circumstances and on what the physician can and is willing to commit to. For Dr. Quill and Cynthia, nonabandonment initially meant promising to work with Cynthia in a desperate fight against her disease but later evolved to mean helping her find meaning, choice, and symptom relief as she faced death. For Dr. Cassel and Mrs. K., nonabandonment meant a willingness to share the patient's loneliness and suffering, acceptance of the limits of medicine, prescribing medications that Mrs. K. was adamant were helping without constantly questioning her need or their effectiveness, and staying alert for those opportunities when medical advice might improve Mrs. K.'s function, mood, or most recent crisis. For both of us, nonabandonment meant being there for our patient through the end of her life, no matter what the clinical path.

The specific methods that such commitments eventually require cannot be known in advance. Most physicians and patients commit to working together through an unknown future. The physician is committed to responding to the patient's clinical situation and requests in a medically skilled and open-minded way but is not obligated to violate his or her own values and beliefs in the process. When such conflict arises, the physician and patient should make every effort to find common ground and shared meaning. Mrs. K. and her physician eventually worked together in a way that allowed her to share her loneliness, report symptoms without constantly submitting to testing, and procure an adequate amount of benzodiazepines without having to constantly justify her need. The meaning and morality of any clinical actions largely depend on the quality of mutual decision making, the depth of the interpersonal relationship, and the shared meaning that these both reflect.

Nonabandonment reinforces several obligations for physicians when they encounter vulnerable persons and populations. At a societal level, physicians as professionals and as persons must help solve the problems caused by a lack of basic health care services and a coherent primary care system for significant disempowered segments of our community.[13] The continuity of care that we are committed to preserve in health care reform has never been widely available to the poor and uninsured. Many such persons are being abandoned to impersonal and episodic care until their medical or psychosocial problems become so overwhelming that the medical system has no choice but to accept them.

Nonabandonment also reflects an obligation to respond to vulnerable persons whom we contact in our daily clinical work. Just as we must commit to working with those who are dying or chronically ill for whom cure is impossible, we must learn how to work with persons with overwhelming psychosocial and medical problems. This commitment does not imply an ability to resolve all such problems, but it does require that a physician be willing to care about, advocate for, and ultimately not desert such persons. For many disadvantaged persons, a physician may be the only caring contact and advocate that they have.

Key Illustrations of Nonabandonment in End-of-Life Care

Although nonabandonment can be demonstrated at many points in a severely ill patient's clinical course, two moments are particularly important and illustrative: first, when circumstances prompt the patient to contemplate the future and second, if and when suffering becomes extreme.

Reassurance about the Future

A person who has been diagnosed with a potentially life-threatening illness, or one whose clinical course has taken a turn for the worse, will begin to contemplate the future, including what dying and death might be like. Sometimes, particularly late at night when usual distractions disappear, this imaginative journey will take patients to the deaths they have known or seen. For a person who has witnessed harsh death, or death in which physicians had not been adequately responsive, frightening experiences will certainly come to mind.

According to Cynthia's Buddhist beliefs, her psychological and spiritual state as a person at the moment of death would have a strong bearing on how she would be reborn in the next life. Dying at peace bodes well, whereas dying in agony might have devastating implications. For Cynthia, dying in peace meant being in control of her mental faculties, preserving alertness and the ability to connect with others, and being free from extremes of physical suffering. Mrs. K., on the other hand, had survived the horrors of the Holocaust. How these memories influenced her search for responses to chronic pain and loneliness is not certain, but it is likely that memories of past suffering returned after she was diagnosed with a terminal illness.

Fortunately, patients will talk about their fears and experiences with death and suffering if health care providers have the courage to ask about them. Questions such as "How have other people died in your family?" or "What are your biggest fears about the future?" will often yield important information about a patient's prior experiences. When a patient reports having witnessed a painful death in which the patient was given insufficient pain medication, physicians should promise no such reluctance on their part. If the patient has observed severe shortness of breath or agitated delirium before death, it may not be easy for physicians to simply reassure. Most patients and families want their health care providers to be willing to face the unknown together with them, and to address any extremes of suffering that may arise. Most are less concerned with the methods of assistance than the willingness to work together until the patient's death. This commitment by one's physician and health care team is at the core of nonabandonment and should be explicitly articulated whenever a patient's clinical course deteriorates significantly. Those patients and families who have this reassurance are freer to spend their precious energy on other matters. Fears about extremes of future suffering and potential abandonment by one's physician probably underlie a significant part of the public support for more open access to physician-assisted suicide.

Responding to Extremes of Suffering

At times in their illnesses, patients who receive state-of-the-art palliative care delivered by a committed multidisciplinary team may develop symptoms that challenge their caregivers' skills, but most will not experience extremes of unrelieved suffering. Therefore, the physician's initial commitment will usually be satisfied by standard palliative care protocols and procedures. Even in Oregon, where palliative care is generally good, hospice is readily available, and physician-assisted suicide is legal, physician-assisted suicide accounts for far less than 1 percent of deaths.[14]

Yet like Cynthia, some patients have generally good relief of symptoms and make excellent progress toward psychological and spiritual closure at the end of life only to experience extreme suffering as death approaches. Fulfilling one's commitment to remain responsive and not abandon the patient is critical at this juncture and is not adequately solved by referring the patient to hospice. (In fact, most of the patients who died under the Oregon Death with Dignity Act were simultaneously hospice enrollees.) While Cynthia clearly benefited from the comprehensive palliative care service she received in hospice, her quality of life eventually deteriorated to the point at which she was ready to die. We then had to consider how best to help her. Once the team was assured that no opportunities for better palliation were being missed, the challenge became how to help Cynthia meet death in the least harmful way possible. (The methods by which this might be accomplished are presented in chapter 9 of this volume.) Cynthia was allowed to stop intravenous fluids and accept the sedation that would most likely come with higher doses of analgesia. Fortunately, both of these interventions have widespread clinical, ethical, and legal support, so the process of easing her death was conducted out in the open with consensus building, consultation, documentation, and support.

In Oregon, cases in which physician-assisted suicide is being considered as a last resort can be addressed with this same kind of open consultation and consensus building. Contrast this with the rest of the country, where physician-assisted suicide is separated out from other last-resort options and conducted in secret without any formal consultation or documentation. In our opinion, the differences between the methods chosen in these circumstances are less critical than the careful clinical assessments, assurance of adequate palliative care, respect for the patient's values, and the commitment not to abandon.[15]

Limits of Nonabandonment

The central commitment of nonabandonment as an obligation of physicians must be balanced by other ethical considerations.[16] Although physicians should try to respond to the needs and requests of their patients over time, they must not violate their own values in the process. A creative tension should exist between respect for the values and choices of unique human beings, on the one hand, and respect for societal traditions, precedents, and more general implications, on the other. There should be a dynamic interplay between patient and physician, individuals and society, traditional and personal values, subjective interpretations and objective analysis, and emotion and intellect. Grappling with these inherent tensions adds depth and complexity to the process of moral decision making and thus more accurately reflects the reality of the human condition.

Nonabandonment as an obligation has inherent limitations. Beyond the provision of some form of continuity as suggested by the American Medical Association, the depth and nature of this commitment may vary for both physician and patient. The relationship is partly defined and explicit but partly open ended and implicit; it is more a covenant than a contract.[17] Although the focus of this chapter has primarily been on the obligations of physicians, these relationships are ultimately reciprocal, although not equal or symmetrical. Often, the rewards for physicians who make these commitments far exceed what is required of them, but the extent of caring and the level of personal responsibility will ultimately depend on a mutual give-and-take with the patient over time. Sometimes, as in Dr. Quill's relationship with Cynthia, the pace of coming to know each other is accelerated by a severe illness. At other times, as in Dr. Cassel's relationship with Mrs. K., trust and genuine caring develop slowly, after considerable testing and working through adversity. Still other times, the depth of a relationship is limited by either party's reluctance or inability to trust or to address major medical issues (for example, substance abuse or dementia). Through shared experience over time, a comfortable and effective level of interaction that ranges from superficial to intense can usually be established.

Although many clinicians choose the profession of medicine because of their need to serve and care, they must also lead balanced, healthy lives.[18] Many clinicians are more skilled at recognizing and responding to the needs of others than to their own needs.[19] If we ask clinicians to provide a more caring, long-term commitment to their patients, we must also reinforce their need to set limits and take care of themselves. For physicians, these limits might be expressed by limiting practice size or encouraging group practice for the built-in support system and potential of shared coverage. Although fully committed relationships are ideal, given the complexity and diversity of patients and doctors, the possibility of limited relationships under some circumstances, or even explicit termination when a mutually satisfactory relationship cannot be established, must be allowed. There is sometimes an irresolvable tension in medicine between commitment to the care of others and self-care.

We must also try to ensure that our ethical precepts and our health care system reinforce rather than undermine clinicians' willingness to engage with patients when their problems seem insoluble or are not clearly resolved through current ethical thinking. The principle of nonabandonment is paramount and may allow clinicians to take some risks on behalf of patients who have no good alternatives. However, taking physician-assisted suicide as an example, clinicians should not be expected to violate their own fundamental values simply because a patient requests a certain kind of assistance. Clinicians' personal values should be explored and challenged but ultimately respected. They should make every effort to find common ground with such patients and to find alternative ways of responding to the patient's dilemma that both can live with. Such analyses often require intense self-examination and consultation with trusted colleagues. We must try both to challenge ourselves and to respect our limitations.

Final Thoughts

The principle of nonabandonment is fundamental to the long-term physician-patient relationship, as well as to other relationships between clinicians and their patients. Patients seek clinicians who will make a commitment to care about them and know them as persons and to be guides and partners in sickness and health until their deaths. In this context, clinicians and patients can learn to judiciously use the power of medicine and expand the concept of healing to include working with persons with severe chronic illness and disability and those who are dying. A commitment not to abandon supplements a caring relationship because it requires that the clinician and patient work together over time, even when the path is unclear. Clinical and moral challenges must be met and engaged with the patient, not shied away from by recourse to falsely bright lines or unbending rules. There is a world of difference between facing an uncertain future alone and having a medically skilled, caring partner who will be present no matter what happens.

Such commitments between clinicians and patients are at the core of the medical profession, so they must be explicitly represented in the discourse of medical ethics. Physicians who find that their work with patients has lost its excitement and meaning would do well to consider whether they are engaged in these types of relationships. Health planners, legislators, risk managers, medical educators, and ethicists should carefully examine whether their contributions to health care tend to reinforce or to obstruct such commitments. Clinical medicine is ultimately a humbling and exhilarating profession, filled with joy, sorrow, and an overabundance of uncertainty that comes with establishing a genuine long-term connection with patients. To practice medicine with a commitment to caring and being present and responsive no matter what the future holds is to experience the richness of the human condition and to know one has made a difference. If the obligation of nonabandonment is better incorporated into medical ethics, medicine may become more humanized and more responsive to the real problems faced every day by physicians and patients.

Notes

This chapter is adapted from T.E. Quill and C.K. Cassel, "Nonabandonment: A Central Obligation for Physicians," *Annals of Internal Medicine* 122 (1995): 368–74.

1. F.W. Peabody, "The Care of the Patient," *New England Journal of Medicine* 88 (1927): 877–82; E.J. Cassell, *The Nature of Suffering and the Goals of Medicine* (New York: Oxford University Press, 1991); V.E. Frankl, *Man's Search for Meaning* (Boston: Beacon, 1959); M. Buber, *I and Thou* (New York: Scribner's Sons, 1937); T.E. Quill, *Death and Dignity: Making Choices and Taking Charge* (New York: Norton, 1993); "Evaluation of Humanistic Qualities in the Internist," *Annals of Internal Medicine* 99 (1983): 720–24; D.H. Novack, "Therapeutic Aspects of the Clinical Encounter," *Journal of General Internal Medicine* 2 (1987): 346–55; C.R. Rogers, *On Becoming a Person: A Therapist's View of Psychotherapy* (Boston: Houghton Mifflin, 1961); D.A. Matthews, A.L. Suchman, and W.J. Branch Jr., "Making 'Connexions': Enhancing the Therapeutic Potential of Patient-Clinician Relationships," *Annals of Internal Medicine* 118 (1993): 973–77.

2. A.D. Sullivan, K. Hedberg, and D.W. Fleming, "Legalized Physician-Assisted Suicide in Oregon—The Second Year," *New England Journal of Medicine* 342 (2000): 598–604; A. MacIntyre, *After Virtue* (Notre Dame: University of Notre Dame Press, 1984); W.F. May, *The Physician's Covenant: Images of the Healer in Medical Ethics* (Philadelphia: Westminster, 1983); P. Ramsey, *The Patient as Person: Explorations in Medical Ethics* (New Haven: Yale University Press, 1970).

3. E.J. Emanuel and A.S. Brett, "Managed Competition and the Patient-Physician Relationship," *New England Journal of Medicine* 329 (1993): 879–82.

4. M.J. Field and C.K. Cassel, eds., *Approaching Death: Improving Care at the End of Life* (Washington, D.C.: National Academy Press, 1997).

5. Cynthia was a patient of Dr. Timothy Quill. Her story is presented in greater detail in T.E. Quill, *A Midwife through the Dying Process: Stories of Healing and Hard Choices at the End of Life* (Baltimore: Johns Hopkins University Press, 1996), chap. 1.

6. Mrs. K. was cared for by Dr. Christine Cassel.

7. Peabody, "Care of the Patient"; Rogers, *On Becoming a Person*; Novack, "Therapeutic Aspects of the Clinical Encounter."

8. W. Zinn, "The Empathic Physician," *Archives of Internal Medicine* 153 (1993): 306–12; Matthews, Suchman, and Branch, "Making 'Connexions'"; C.W. Lidz, P.S. Appelbaum, and A. Meisel, "Two Models of Implementing Informed Consent," *Archives of Internal Medicine* 148 (1988): 1385–89; J. Katz, "Duty and Caring in the Age of Informed

Consent and Medical Science: Unlocking Peabody's Secret," *Humane Medicine* 8 (1992): 187–97; T.E. Quill and P. Townsend, "Bad News: Delivery, Dialogue, and Dilemmas," *Archives of Internal Medicine* 151 (1991): 463–68.

9. Peabody, "Care of the Patient"; Cassell, *Nature of Suffering and the Goals of Medicine;* Quill, *Death and Dignity;* "Evaluation of Humanistic Qualities in the Internist"; Matthews, Suchman, and Branch, "Making 'Connexions.'"

10. MacIntyre, *After Virtue;* A.D. Sullivan, K. Hedberg, and D. Hopkins, "Legalized Physician-Assisted Suicide in Oregon, 1998–2000," *New England Journal of Medicine* 344 (2001): 605–7; A.R. Jonsen, M. Siegler, and W.J. Winslade, *Clinical Ethics: A Practical Approach to Ethical Decisions in Clinical Medicine,* 2d ed. (New York: Macmillan, 1986); S. Toulmin, "The Tyranny of Principles," *Hastings Center Report* 11, no. 6 (1981): 31–39; J.M. Gustafson, "Moral Discourse about Medicine: A Variety of Forms," *Journal of Medicine and Philosophy* 15 (1990): 125–42; A.R. Jonsen and S. Toulmin, *The Abuse of Casuistry: A History of Moral Reasoning* (Berkeley: University of California Press, 1988); R.M. Zaner, *The Way of Phenomenology* (New York: Bobbs-Merrill, 1970); S. Sherwin, *No Longer Patient: Feminist Ethics and Health Care* (Philadelphia: Temple University Press, 1992).

11. Peabody, "The Care of the Patient;" Cassell, *Nature of Suffering and the Goals of Medicine;* Frankl, *Man's Search for Meaning;* Buber, *I and Thou;* Quill, *Death and Dignity: Making Choices and Taking Charge;* "Evaluation of Humanistic Qualities in the Internist"; Novack, "Therapeutic Aspects of the Clinical Encounter"; Rogers, *On Becoming a Person;* Matthews, Suchman, and Branch, "Making 'Connexions.'"

12. American Medical Association, Council on Ethical and Judicial Affairs, *Current Opinions—1986* (Chicago: American Medical Association, 1986), 8–10.

13. J. Noble, G.H. de Friese, F.D. Pichard, and A.R. Meyers, "Concepts of Health and Disease," in *Textbook of General Medicine and Primary Care,* edited by J. Noble (Boston: Little, Brown, 1987), 3–13; A.M. Kraut, "Healers and Strangers: Immigrant Attitudes toward the Physician in America—A Relationship in Historical Perspective," *Journal of the American Medical Association* 263 (1990): 1807–11.

14. Sullivan, Hedberg, and Fleming, "Legalized Physician-Assisted Suicide in Oregon— The Second Year"; Sullivan, Hedberg, and Fleming, "Legalized Physician-Assisted Suicide in Oregon, 1998–2000"; A.E. Chin, K. Hedberg, G.K. Higginson, and D.W. Fleming, "Legalized Physician-Assisted Suicide in Oregon—The First Year's Experience," *New England Journal of Medicine* 340 (1999): 577–83.

15. Interested readers can refer to our original article (Quill and Cassel, "Nonabandonment") for a discussion of the relation of nonabandonment to traditional ethical principles and then a brief exploration of its relation to newer ethical paradigms such as casuistry, phenomenology, and feminist, cross-cultural, and narrative frameworks that consider issues of relationship more centrally.

16. E.D. Pellegrino, "Compassion Needs Reason Too," *Journal of the American Medical Association* 270 (1993): 874–75.

17. May, *Physician's Covenant;* T.E. Quill, "Partnerships in Patient Care: A Contractual Approach," *Annals of Internal Medicine* 98 (1993): 228–34; E.J. Emanuel and L.L.

Emanuel, "Four Models of the Physician-Patient Relationship," *Journal of the American Medical Association* 267 (1992): 2221–26.

18. T.E. Quill and P. Williamson, "Healthy Approaches to Physician Stress," *Archives of Internal Medicine* 150 (1990): 1857–61.

19. A. Miller, *Prisoners of Childhood: The Trauma of the Gifted Child and the Search for the True Self* (New York: Basic, 1981).

3

The Role of Autonomy in Choosing Physician Aid in Dying

*Thomas Preston, M.D., Martin Gunderson, Ph.D., J.D.,
and David J. Mayo, Ph.D*

A fundamental argument in support of physician aid in dying appeals to
the principle of respect for autonomy: Whenever possible, people should
be free to determine their fates by their own autonomous choices, especially
in connection with private matters, such as health, that primarily involve one's
own welfare.[1] Our control over our own deaths is limited by biology and a host
of external influences; absent compelling considerations to the contrary, it
should not be further limited by the state. This constitutes what we call the autonomy argument for physician aid in dying.

Whereas earlier critics of physician aid in dying argued that there are compelling considerations to the contrary, more recent critics have directly attacked
the autonomy argument itself. Among these latter criticisms there are three distinct but overlapping threads. First, critics claim that most who would choose
physician aid in dying are incapable of doing so autonomously, and hence their
requests would not fall within the range of the principle of respect for autonomy. Second, it is claimed that the argument presumes excessive independence,
control, and self-centeredness. Third, some critics argue that the autonomy argument for physician aid in dying is self-defeating. Each of these criticisms
relies on some important misinterpretation of the principle of respect for autonomy, and we find them unpersuasive.

The Principle of Respect for Autonomy

Autonomous choice is an ideal. It posits a fully informed individual who
makes a reasoned and intentional choice among available options in light of

that information, on the basis of his or her "true" or "authentic" values and in the absence of either internal or external coercive influences.[2] The principle of respect for autonomy demands that others take an individual's autonomous choices seriously. It requires that autonomous choices be respected unless there is compelling reason not to do so.

Although there is much debate about how to translate this ideal into practice, four points need to be noted for present purposes. First, a person influenced by others can still act autonomously, as long as the influence falls short of coercion. Second, persons who must depend on others in order to act on their choices can still act autonomously.[3] Third, choices may be more or less autonomous, depending on whether they are more or less fully informed or more or less subject to coercive influences. Fourth, choices may be more or less important to the person making them.

These points are mirrored by important features of the principle of respect for autonomy. The principle does not require that one entirely avoid dependency or act without influence. In addition, how much weight it carries depends on the importance of the choice and on the extent to which the choice is autonomous.[4] We routinely (if grudgingly) tolerate violations of autonomy when the choice at issue is unimportant but not when important choices are at stake.

Thus the principle of respect for autonomy demands that moral consideration be given to an individual's autonomous choices in proportion to both the degree to which those choices are autonomous and the importance (to the individual) of the values on which they are based. The principle imposes a burden that is primarily negative—a burden of noninterference. It does not by itself require us to assist others in carrying out their autonomous choices. In the case of physician aid in dying, almost no one claims that physicians have a duty to engage in the practice or that they should be required to perform aid in dying.[5] After all, the principle protects the autonomous choices of physicians as well as patients, neither of whom should be compelled to participate in activities they find objectionable.[6] Finally, it should be noted that respect for an individual's autonomy may be outweighed by competing considerations, such as the rights of others. Although we respect the autonomy of travelers to wander where they choose, for example, travelers may not violate the property rights of landowners by trespassing.

Given this background, the autonomy argument for physician aid in dying can be stated more fully as follows: There is a moral reason to respect others' autonomous choices, and this reason gains strength as the importance of the choice under consideration increases. An autonomous decision to hasten one's death is a profoundly important decision for a terminally ill person that involves his or her most significant values. There is therefore an extraordinarily strong moral reason not to restrict such a decision. This reason becomes even stronger when provisions are in place to ensure that the choice is indeed highly autonomous and not coerced.

The autonomy argument does not logically preclude the possibility that there may be even more compelling reasons *not* to permit an individual to act on his or her autonomous choice. However, when both principled moral disagreement and unresolved empirical issues about risks are present, as is the case in the debate over physician aid in dying, it is crucial to remember where the burden of proof falls. Current public policy and moral discussion typically assume that the burden is on those who advocate physician aid in dying. However, the autonomy argument reminds us that the burden falls on those who would *restrict* autonomy, and that this burden is very heavy indeed.

Concerns about Decision-Making Capacity

One of the most common objections to the autonomy argument for aid in dying is that terminally ill patients cannot possibly choose physician aid in dying autonomously because virtually every requirement for fully autonomous decision making—knowledge and understanding of the situation, the ability to reason, a sense of one's authentic values, and freedom from coercion—tends to be compromised in the terminally ill patient.

A variety of factors influence patients' decision-making capacity. The patient's physical condition may directly limit the possibility of autonomous choice.[7] Physical distress resulting directly from illness can compromise autonomy, as terminally ill patients "may be experiencing too much pain, discomfort, or depression to make independent and truly voluntary decisions."[8] Treatment with a mechanical ventilator or powerful drugs such as narcotics may also diminish capacity for autonomous decision making.

Patients' dependence on caregivers may also limit autonomy. The desire of many patients to have their physicians make treatment decisions for them is said to compromise patient autonomy. As Kass stresses, dying patients are profoundly dependent on health professionals—particularly physicians—for the information they need to make decisions. The ability to make reasoned, informed decisions is eroded if physicians do not fully inform patients of all the options available to them; and as Kass notes, "Physicians are masters at framing the options to guarantee a particular outcome."[9] Terminally ill patients are subject to the coercive influences of family and friends as well as those of caregivers.[10] Those whom the patient has named as beneficiaries may subtly encourage a frightened and dependent individual to give up prematurely.[11] A patient's vulnerability may be exacerbated by the desire not to be a burden on caregivers, a sentiment expressed by many dying patients.[12] Some critics also contend that health care economics and the growth of managed care organizations may lead caregivers to interact with patients in ways that further compromise the patient's capacity for autonomous decision making.[13] Treatments that might help sustain a patient's will to live may not be made available if they are costly. Patients may not receive the attention and care that would enable them to deal with their illness.

In short, opponents contend, just when they must make the most important end-of-life decisions, the capacity of many patients for autonomous decision making is impaired. Because true autonomy is unattainable in this context, critics conclude, even the principle of respect for autonomy cannot justify physician aid in dying.[14]

These arguments apply much more broadly than their advocates realize, however. Nearly all of these challenges to capacity for autonomous decision making could apply equally to any seriously ill patient. Consider a patient facing emergency surgery, for example: Can she possibly understand the arcane technical arguments for and against a particular operation for her condition? Will the physician, or perhaps family or loved ones, subtly manipulate her in a time of crisis? All terminally ill patients who seek hospice care, or who ask not to be resuscitated or to have life-sustaining therapy withdrawn, may be influenced by the same autonomy-compromising factors that critics assert undermine the decision-making capacity of patients who request physician aid in dying—patterns of medical practices, insurance coverage, arguments by advocacy groups, and often the urgings of friends, loved ones, and attorney or pastor. Patients facing lingering deaths who might consider physician aid in dying will typically be capable of decisions at least as autonomous as those of most critically ill patients. In short, this criticism of the autonomy argument for physician aid in dying would seem to entail calling for a return to medical paternalism generally.

Those who criticize the autonomy argument for physician aid in dying on these grounds lose sight of the fact that autonomy is an ideal. They selectively set the bar for measuring actual human decisions impossibly high for physician aid in dying. They demand that choices for aid in dying be "completely" or "fully" autonomous in the sense that there be complete understanding and complete freedom from outside influences and then say that terminally ill patients do not meet this standard. However, the standard is one that is virtually never met in clinical medicine. As Kass himself, a staunch opponent of physician aid in dying, puts it, "Truth to tell, the ideal of rational autonomy . . . rarely obtains in actual medical practice."[15]

The ideal autonomy that critics require for aid in dying is unreasonable because it is unattainable in any medical interaction. Yet all of us understand our circumstances more or less, and all of us are routinely subject to influences that are more or less controlling. We believe it reasonable to set the bar for patients who would opt for physician aid in dying at what is currently required for informed consent by patients who refuse life-sustaining medical treatment or ask that such treatment be withdrawn. That is, roughly, the patient must understand those facts that would be likely to influence a reasonable person. The decision must also be free from coercion and mental illness that undermines choice. None of this requires that the decision be made with perfect understanding of all possible details or that it be completely free from all potentially coercive influences. Indeed, autonomous choosers might well want to consult friends and family members and expect to be influenced by their concerns and their counsel.

Concerns about Extreme Individualism

In contrast to those who contend that persons electing physician aid in dying would be insufficiently free of external influences in their decision making, other critics hold that the autonomy argument for physician aid in dying is objectionable because it glorifies a distorted understanding of autonomy. This refers to unfettered autonomy in the sense of extreme independence, unhealthy desire for control over one's life, or self-centered individualism.

Autonomy as Extreme Independence

Some critics have claimed that in appealing as strongly as it does to the principle of respect for autonomy, the autonomy argument for physician aid in dying encourages extreme independence. They find this objectionable for several reasons.[16] It may lead people to undervalue relationships and various community goods—for instance, efforts to help the less fortunate. It may also lead to a general stigmatizing of dependency on others. As a result, those who are independent might come to see the lives of those who are dependent as less valuable, while at the same time terminally ill patients who need help might opt for physician aid in dying rather than accept dependence.[17] In this way, critics claim, the autonomy defense might ultimately function to push into seeking physician aid in dying people who otherwise might accept dependence gracefully.

These critics misunderstand the principle of respect for autonomy in two crucial ways. First, they confuse respect for autonomy with the value of independence. It is true that "autonomous" can mean "independent" and that some forms of dependency limit the capacity for autonomous choice. A person with severe disabilities, for instance, may be dependent on others in ways that limit autonomy. However, this is not relevant to the autonomy argument for physician aid in dying, which simply holds that autonomous choices should be respected. Second, the critics mistake respect for autonomy for the claim that autonomy is a value that should be maximized. The principle of respect for autonomy is not, however, a maximizing principle. In fact, there is often good reason to autonomously choose to accept dependency or limit one's autonomy in other ways—for instance, by signing an exclusive contract or joining the military. The principle of respect for autonomy holds merely that the choice to do so should be respected.

Autonomy as Need for Control

Other critics have objected that invoking the value of self-determination to legitimate physician aid in dying glorifies an unhealthy desire for control of one's circumstances. Callahan, for instance, argues that euthanasia and assisted suicide represent an unrealistic drive for "a final and total control of human life: autonomy triumphant." He views those who want the option of assisted suicide as having a "sickly preoccupation" with control that he finds "both subtly demeaning and socially troubling."[18] He claims that the autonomy argument for physician aid in dying is embedded in a broader ideology of control that advocates a duty to try to control all aspects of human life and death.

This criticism, like the preceding, misunderstands the principle of respect for autonomy. The principle holds that there is reason to respect the self-governance of individuals, but it does not specify in what this self-governance should consist. Although it might be used to exert tight control over one's life (and death), it need not be used in this way. Again, the principle of respect for autonomy does not dictate what one ought to choose; it even allows individuals to choose to surrender some degree of control over their lives or to delegate all decision making to others. Callahan has a point in cautioning against attempting to control every aspect of one's life, insofar as doing so may exclude the needs or wishes of others. In deriding those who want the option of assisted suicide as having a "sickly preoccupation" with control, however, he is using the means (autonomy) to attack the end (assisted suicide) that he opposes. Legitimate use of autonomy depends on whether a decision to take a particular action is truly autonomous, not on a value judgment of the action taken.

Still, the positive value of being in control of one's life should not be underestimated. In fact, being an autonomous individual and acting autonomously require a high degree of self-control.[19] This is part of what it means to be free from internal constraints. We encourage people to try to control their future health and longevity with healthy diet and exercise. We encourage control over pregnancy. Many patients choose hospice for the specific purpose of self-control. With the Patient Self-Determination Act, even the federal government encourages people to take control over end-of-life decisions by completing advance directives.[20]

Self-Centeredness and Indifference to Others

These strands of extreme individualism and drive for control intermingle in a third critique. Critics of the autonomy argument often worry that patients might ignore the interests of others in opting for physician aid in dying. According to this third line of argument, the "extreme" exercise of autonomy represented by aid in dying engenders a moral attitude of self-centeredness that fails to take account of the interests of others. Zylicz claims that patients who are control oriented "frequently do not see that other people around them are suffering."[21] Nuland echoes the concern that those who advocate physician aid in dying are abandoning the old method of "compassionate caring to the end" in favor of something new: "self-determination, the *cri de guerre* that drowns out the protestations of friends and relatives whose lives are affected by decisions made in the name of an autonomous will, without regard for the needs of those left behind."[22]

There are several general points to be made in reply to this criticism. First, the possibility that self-centered patients will make important health care decisions that adversely affect others is not unique to physician aid in dying. It is already implicit in the doctrine of informed consent. An elderly patient with pneumonia, for example, could refuse antibiotics in order to hasten her death in callous disregard for the needs of others. No one argues this is a reason for the state to police health care decisions that are selfish.

Second, this sword cuts both ways in connection with end-of-life decisions. The autonomy critics of physician aid in dying offer no reason for thinking that self-centered disregard for the interests of others would be more likely to play out one way rather than another. Terminally ill patients who are deeply loving take account of the impact their lingering deaths would have on loved ones; depending on circumstances, this might prompt them to try either to hasten or to delay their death. Conversely, selfish patients might show no regard for the interests of loved ones in deciding either to hasten death or to delay it. Furthermore, patients who desire physician aid in dying may be thwarted by the selfish whims or desires of others. This objection to physician aid in dying, then, seems diametrically opposed to the concern that terminally ill patients might be pressured into opting for it because loved ones have made their wishes known.

This brings us to a third reply: Although as a general rule people should be respectful of the feelings of those close to them, in the final analysis the choice is that of the individual. Individual freedom to marry, worship, or live where one chooses—and indeed, even refuse life-prolonging therapies as one sees fit—all are personal freedoms that may be exercised in ways that show selfish disregard for the feelings and concerns of others. Yet it would never occur to us to characterize our institutionalized respect for these freedoms as the abandonment of "compassionate caring to the end" or as a battle cry that drowns out the protestations of friends and relatives who may be affected. Rather, these are basic freedoms that we encourage people to exercise responsibly—with the full realization that sometimes they will fail to do so.

Concerns That Physician Aid in Dying Would Undercut Individual Autonomy

Two final clusters of criticisms hold that the autonomy argument for physician aid in dying is flawed because it overlooks ways in which permitting the practice would actually compromise autonomy. The first few of these criticisms are rather abstract in that they focus on an alleged loss of autonomy the patient would suffer independent of the specifics of the patient-physician relationship. The rest focus on ways in which legalizing physician aid in dying would "medicalize" suicide and be destructive of autonomy within the context of the patient-physician relationship.

Suicide as Termination of Autonomy

Some opponents ridicule the presumed use of autonomy as a moral justification for assisted suicide by pointing out that anyone opting for aid in dying thereby terminates any capacity for future autonomous choice. Safranek provides a version of this argument when he states, "Acts of assisted suicide committed in the name of autonomy annihilate the very basis of individual autonomy."[23] According to this criticism, there is an inherent tension or contradiction between the principle of respect for autonomy and the acceptance of physician aid in dying.

Our reply was anticipated earlier: There is nothing about the principle of respect for autonomy as such that precludes choosing options that foreclose future autonomous choices. Again, the principle demands respect for autonomous choices but says nothing about what those choices should be. Marriage, employment agreements, military service, and refusal of life-prolonging therapies are all options that limit future autonomy. On our view, respect for the principle of autonomy requires respect for autonomous choices, including, sometimes, decisions that limit one's autonomy. The principle of respect for autonomy does not hold that autonomy should be maximized, only that it should be respected.

The Principle of Respect for Autonomy as Self-Defeating

Safranek also raises the possibility of a more profound inconsistency. He claims that liberal proponents of autonomy need some way in which they can "distinguish opprobrious from acceptable autonomous acts."[24] Some autonomous acts—robbery and assault, for example—should not be tolerated because they are clearly immoral and pose the risk of grave harm. Safranek claims that liberal proponents of autonomy typically argue that these cases can be delineated by relying on some version of John Stuart Mill's harm principle, according to which society is justified in restricting the liberty of one of its members when it is necessary to prevent harm to others. The problem with this strategy, according to Safranek, is that to determine what constitutes a harm, proponents of autonomy and the harm principle must presuppose some theory of the good. At this point the liberal's autonomy principle smuggles in a view of the good and thus no longer has the sort of value neutrality that liberals claim for it as they invoke it to create a sphere of liberty in which people pursue their own vision of the good without interference from others. Safranek thus claims that the principle of respect for autonomy is inconsistent because its application will require appeal to some specific theory of the good that will license some individuals to act in ways that restrict the autonomy of others.[25]

Safranek's critique is effective against principles that articulate an absolute right to autonomy. For any such principle to be plausible there must be some way of restricting its scope so that it does not encompass obviously immoral acts, and Safranek's argument that this requires a theory of the good is plausible.

The principle of respect for autonomy should not be understood in this way, however. Nor does it articulate an absolute right or require rejecting a substantive notion of the good. Instead, the principle of respect for autonomy demands tolerance of another's autonomy, not submission to it. It creates a burden of proof for those who would restrict autonomous acts. In the case of obviously immoral acts, this burden can easily be met by citing various competing values and principles. The case of physician aid in dying differs in important ways, however. Given that a person considering physician aid in dying bases that decision on values important to him or her, and given safeguards that ensure that those who choose physician aid in dying are in fact choosing autonomously, this burden becomes very heavy indeed. Again, the principle of respect for autonomy does not provide a conclusive reason for adopting physician aid in dying but merely shifts a heavy burden of proof to those who would oppose it. Our concern here is not to argue that this burden cannot possibly be met; it is rather to evaluate criticisms of the autonomy argument for physician aid in dying itself.

Concerns That Physician Aid in Dying Would Compromise Autonomy within the Patient-Physician Relationship

Another cluster of criticisms raises concerns about the impact physician aid in dying would have on the practice of medicine—specifically, on the autonomy of patients or physicians. Although some of these criticisms overlap one another, we find enough unique in each to justify discussing them separately.

Autonomy-Reducing Regulations

Some critics argue that physician aid in dying would inevitably involve guidelines and restrictions that would be an affront to patient autonomy. Salem writes that "requiring that the patient submit to medical surveillance is, in itself, an outrage to autonomy as this value is classically defined."[26] But surely it is non-sense to suggest that greater respect is shown for someone's autonomy by pro-hibiting a practice entirely than by placing restrictions on it, especially when those restrictions are designed to ensure autonomous choice. Requiring that those about to undergo surgery read a consent form and discuss safety con-cerns and alternatives with their surgeon is less of an infringement on auton-omy than banning the surgery outright. Physicians do at times subject patients to assessments of their decision-making capacity when they make high-risk decisions or decisions contrary to medical advice. Aid in dying falls outside the "traditional" range of professional obligations and raises the stakes for patients and clinicians, but the restrictions typically recommended are of the same nature as for other procedures, although they call for greater scrutiny of the decision-making process to ensure autonomous choice.

Medicalized Suicide as a Restriction of Patient Autonomy

Closely related to the concern that patient autonomy would be reduced through regulation of physician aid in dying is a concern that physician aid in dying would tend to "medicalize" suicide and death in general, diminishing patients' autonomy by ceding even more power to physicians.[27] Salem extends the pre-vious criticism by claiming that physician aid in dying would transform suicide from a private act into a medical event that would become the exclusive pre-rogative of physicians. This, according to Salem, would require medical proto-cols, and bureaucratic oversight and regulation, with the physician becoming the ultimate arbiter of whether a patient was actually making a rational choice.[28]

Pellegrino echoes Salem's concern about the physician's new role as gate-keeper. Current proposals for physician aid in dying inevitably make the deci-sion to die a joint decision between patients and physicians, since the physician must acquiesce in the patient's decision and provide a lethal prescription. Ac-cording to Pellegrino, physicians will agree to assisted suicide only when they believe that compassion requires it. The physician's decision to participate is made on the basis of what the physician believes to be the good of the patient. Hence the physician is positioned to exercise a paternalistic veto over the pa-tient's choice to engage in physician aid in dying.[29]

We agree with Salem and Pellegrino on several points. Physician aid in dying would medicalize the suicides of terminally ill patients in some important re-spects. Safeguards to ensure the autonomy of a patient's decision would become institutionalized as part of medical practice, and the availability of lethal medicines for physician aid in dying for a particular patient would be subject to gate-keeping by a particular physician, who might refuse to participate on the basis of a personal judgment about the patient's situation. The decision to engage in physician aid in dying would in fact need to be made jointly with a physician—who, one hopes, would be motivated by compassionate concern for the patient's best interest. Finally, the acceptance of physician aid in dying might even serve to legitimate suicide by autonomous persons at the ends of their lives, in much the same way that new reproductive technologies, for instance, have legitimated the birth of children sired by friends to women whose partners are sterile.

Nothing in Salem's argument, however, suggests that this medicalization would conflict with the principle of respect for autonomy. If patients and physicians are given new options—even options that are restricted, and even if one party becomes the gatekeeper to ensure that the restrictions are observed—no one's autonomy is thereby further restricted. At worst, some now have only the same options they had before. Again, the restrictions are explicitly tailored to ensure that physician aid in dying is made available only to patients who choose it autonomously.

Even if physicians agree to participate only when they feel compassion so dictates, the physician is not thereby violating the principle of respect for autonomy. The principle does not require that one assist others to do what he or she believes is unwise or immoral. Rather, respect for autonomy requires that one not interfere with agreements reached between the patient and the physician.

The case of new reproductive technologies is instructive. First, there is no doubt that such technologies have medicalized reproduction for patients who choose them. Second, although many of these technologies are controversial on independent grounds, the main argument given in their defense is that they provide previously sterile couples with new options. Third, physicians are involved in mutual decision making and are free to refuse sophisticated procedures only when they believe such procedures are not in their patients' best interests. Most criticism has called for more stringent regulation (for example, on surrogacy contracts), not less. It would be absurd to object that the availability of the new options, however regulated, yields a net reduction in reproductive autonomy.

There is a final flaw in the argument. Insofar as medicalization of death means dying under the supervision of a physician or other health care professional with appropriate safeguards (for example, an advance directive) to protect choice, death is already highly medicalized in our culture. Approximately three-quarters of all Americans die in medical institutions and hence under medical supervision.[30] Death in an intensive care unit is highly medicalized. Withdrawal of life-supporting therapy is certainly a medicalization of death, with physicians (not patients) performing the necessary procedures that eventuate in death. Even many hospice deaths at home are under the control of a medical team. If, however, medicalization of death means the use of extraordinary medical treatment, such as ventilators and feeding tubes, then physician aid in dying should be seen as a way to avoid a highly medicalized death. The terminally ill patient who swallows lethal medication at home avoids this sort of highly medicalized death.

Medicalized Suicide as a Restriction of Physician Autonomy

While Salem, Pellegrino, and others worry that the medicalization of suicide would compromise patient autonomy by giving too much authority to medicine and physician judgment, others fear that it will compromise physician autonomy by giving too much authority to patients. Callahan, for example, worries that the medicalization of physician aid in dying would mean that "the desires and wishes of patients alone legitimate a doctor's skills," with physicians reduced to the role of "artisans in the fashioning of a patient's life and death."[31] Similarly, Kass states that physicians would be bound to kill out of deference to autonomy.[32] There has, of course, been a shift in the balance of power from the days of medical paternalism, when physicians routinely withheld information and options from patients, to today's acceptance of the doctrine of informed consent. It is unclear why the legalization of physician aid in dying would represent any more dramatic a breakthrough in this regard than was the legalization of any other procedure that was controversial on independent grounds (for example, abortion or artificial insemination of single women) or than occurs now when patients go to their physicians seeking specific surgical procedures. The doctrine of informed consent does not imply that a patient has the right to dictate treatment any more than the principle of respect for autonomy generally implies a right to require the assistance of others in carrying out one's autonomous choices.

The Burden of Proof

The principle of respect for autonomy has played an important role in medical practice. It justifies the requirement of informed consent in both therapeutic and research contexts. It also forms the basis of the autonomy argument for physician aid in dying. While critics of this argument have offered a range of objections, they make several characteristic mistakes. Some confuse the ideal of autonomous choice with the operational standard of autonomous choice that is incorporated in workable health care policies. Some confuse the principle of respect for autonomy with a particular substantive view of the good that places a premium on rugged individualism. Some critics mistakenly assume that the principle requires maximizing autonomy; rather, it provides reason to respect autonomous choice even when someone chooses to limit his or her own autonomy. Some critics mistakenly interpret the principle as stating an absolute right; on this interpretation, the principle is clearly unacceptable. On our interpretation, however, the principle imposes a burden of proof on those who would restrict autonomous choice. It does this in a way that takes account of context, and the burden it imposes may be more or less heavy. Advocates of physician aid in dying believe that in the particular context of terminally ill patients autonomously choosing on the basis of deeply held values, the heavy burden on those who would prohibit physician aid in dying cannot be met.

Notes

1. See, for example, R. Dworkin, *Life's Dominion* (New York: Knopf, 1993), and D. Brock, "Voluntary Active Euthanasia," in *Life and Death*, edited by D. Brock (Cambridge: Cambridge University Press, 1993), 202–32, esp. 205–6.

2. This fits with the way autonomy is described in bioethics textbooks; T.A. Mappes and D. DeGrazia, *Biomedical Ethics*, 5th ed. (Boston: McGraw-Hill, 2001), 39. See also T.L. Beauchamp and J.F. Childress, *Principles of Biomedical Ethics*, 5th ed. (New York: Oxford University Press, 2001), 59. Beauchamp and Childress do not include an autonomy condition in their description.

3. Barbara Secker emphasizes that one can act autonomously even while dependent and influenced by others. See B. Secker, "The Appearance of Kant's Deontology in Contemporary Kantianism: Concepts of Patient Autonomy in Bioethics," *Journal of Medicine and Philosophy* 24 (1999): 43–66, 60. Secker considers this a special sort of autonomy, but her insights can be accommodated by the core concept of autonomy typically used by bioethicists.

4. These are not the only variables. It also depends, for instance, on the relationship between the two parties. Our focus, however, is solely on those variables relevant to the autonomy argument for physician aid in dying.

5. Rhodes is an exception. She argues that physicians have a responsibility based on beneficence, as well as patient autonomy and patients' rights, to engage in physician aid in dying. See R. Rhodes, "Physicians, Assisted Suicide, and the Right to Live or Die," in

Physician-Assisted Suicide: Expanding the Debate, edited by M.P. Battin, R. Rhodes, and A. Silvers (New York: Routledge, 1998), 165–76.

6. Along these lines, Dworkin (*Life's Dominion,* 259 n. 23) claims that "we have a right not to act in ways that we believe deny our sense of the moral importance of someone else, even if he would prefer that we do."

7. Secker, "Appearance of Kant's Deontology in Contemporary Kantianism," 49.

8. S.W. Wolf, "Pragmatism in the Face of Death: The Role of Facts in the Assisted Suicide Debate," *Minnesota Law Review* 82 (1998): 1063–1101, 1077.

9. L.R. Kass, "'I Will Give No Deadly Drug': Why Doctors Must Not Kill," in *The Case against Assisted Suicide: For the Right to End-of-Life Care,* edited by K. Foley and H. Hendin (Baltimore: Johns Hopkins University Press, 2002), 17–40, 24–25.

10. Secker, "Appearance of Kant's Deontology in Contemporary Kantianism," 49.

11. Kass, "'I Will Give No Deadly Drug,'" 24.

12. Oregon Department of Human Services, *Sixth Annual Report on Oregon's Death with Dignity Act,* March 10, 2004, table 4, www.ohd.hr.state.or.us/chs/pas.ar.htm (last accessed May 23, 2003). See also A.L. Back, J.I. Wallace, H.E. Starks, and R.A. Pearlman, "Physician-Assisted Suicide and Euthanasia in Washington State: Patient Requests and Physician Responses," *Journal of the American Medical Association* 275 (1996): 919–25, esp. 921–22.

13. See, for example, M.A. Rodwin, *Medicine, Money, and Morals: Physicians' Conflicts of Interest* (New York: Oxford University Press, 1993), chap. 5.

14. Kass, "'I Will Give No Deadly Drug,'" 25.

15. Ibid., 24.

16. Secker, "Appearance of Kant's Deontology in Contemporary Kantianism," 50.

17. Ibid., citing G. Agich, "Reassessing Autonomy in Long-Term Care," *Hastings Center Report* 20, no. 6 (1990): 12–17, 12–13.

18. D. Callahan, *The Troubled Dream of Life* (New York: Simon and Schuster, 1993), 17–18, 71.

19. For an extended discussion of the nature of self-control and its relation to autonomy, see A.R. Mele, *Autonomous Agents: From Self-Control to Autonomy* (New York: Oxford University Press, 1995).

20. Patient Self-Determination Act of 1990, *U.S. Code* 42, secs. 1395cc–1396a.

21. Z. Zylicz, "Palliative Care and Euthanasia in the Netherlands: Observations of a Dutch Physician," in *The Case against Assisted Suicide: For the Right to End-of-Life Care,* edited by K. Foley and H. Hendin (Baltimore: Johns Hopkins University Press, 2002), 122–43, 134.

22. S. Nuland, "The Principle of Hope," *New Republic* 226, no. 19 (2002): 25–29, 26.

23. J.P. Safranek, "Autonomy and Assisted Suicide: The Execution of Freedom," *Hastings Center Report* 28, no. 4 (1998): 32–36, 35.

24. Ibid., 33.

25. Ibid.

26. T. Salem, "Physician-Assisted Suicide: Promoting Autonomy—or Medicalizing Suicide?" *Hastings Center Report* 19, no. 3 (1999): 30–38, 33.

27. L.R. Kass, "Why Doctors Must Not Kill," *Commonweal* 118, Suppl. no. 14 (1991): 8–12, 9–10; E.D. Pellegrino, "Compassion Is Not Enough," in *The Case against Assisted Suicide: For the Right to End-of-Life Care,* edited by K. Foley and H. Hendin (Baltimore: Johns Hopkins University Press, 2002), 41–51, 48. See Salem, "Physician-Assisted Suicide," 30–33; M. White and D. Callahan, "Oregon's First Year: The Medicalization of Control," *Psychology, Public Policy and Law* 6 (2000): 331–41, 337.

28. Salem, "Physician-Assisted Suicide," 30–33.

29. Pellegrino, "Compassion Is Not Enough"; M.J. Field and C.K. Cassel, eds., *Approaching Death: Improving Care at the End of Life* (Washington, D.C.: National Academy Press, 1997), 39.

30. Field and Cassel, *Approaching Death.*

31. D. Callahan, "Reason, Self-Determination, and Physician-Assisted Suicide," in *The Case against Assisted Suicide: For the Right to End-of-Life Care,* edited by K. Foley and H. Hendin (Baltimore: Johns Hopkins University Press, 2002), 52–68, 58.

32. Kass, "'I Will Give No Deadly Drug,'" 18.

4

Disability and Physician-Assisted Dying

Andrew I. Batavia, J.D., M.S.

The ongoing debate in this country over assisted dying, often portrayed in the media as assisted suicide or physician-assisted suicide, examines the desire of some people with terminal illnesses (and some with nonterminal conditions) to seek the assistance of another person in ending their lives. The legal, political, religious, and ethical issues concern whether such individuals should have a right to obtain assistance from another person and, if so, under what circumstances. Although virtually anyone with certain basic physical and mental capabilities could provide aid in dying, physicians have been the focus of the debate because they are deemed to have the technical expertise to offer competent assistance.

Typically, in a case of aid in dying, the physician prescribes a lethal dose of pharmaceuticals, and the patient independently takes the drugs to induce death. Depending on the specific law authorizing assisted dying, a variety of regulatory safeguards apply to ensure that only those who are authorized to obtain such assistance may do so and that a person's decision to obtain assistance is entirely voluntary, not subject to coercion or other abusive practices.

Self-administration by the individual ending his or her life is considered a defining characteristic of assisted suicide. If the physician or another person were to administer the lethal drugs, the act would be characterized as euthanasia, which is considered murder—and thus prohibited—in every jurisdiction in the United States. (The Netherlands is the one country that allows such active, voluntary euthanasia; it requires adherence to an extensive protocol with safeguards against abuses.) To date, the only U.S. jurisdiction to authorize physician-assisted dying, in the form of assisted suicide, is Oregon, although several other states have contemplated enacting such statutes.

Almost every aspect of the debate over assisted dying has been covered by the national media. However, one key aspect has received short shrift: the debate within the disability community over assisted dying and disability rights. The few general newspaper articles that have addressed these issues do so mostly in a superficial manner that does not do justice to the complexity and sophistication of the debate. In-depth treatments of these issues have been published by a couple of medical and legal journals, but these reach limited, albeit important, audiences. Only the specialized disability press, consisting of a few magazines and newspapers, have attempted to address these issues comprehensively for a national audience, but that audience again is limited—to those who are likely to read a disability-oriented publication.

Although disability issues may seem relatively obscure, this "debate within the debate" has served as an important subtext that has had a dramatic impact on the broader debate on assisted dying. This is because the legal rights accorded people with disabilities under the U.S. Constitution and laws such as the Americans with Disabilities Act of 1990 can be applied to resolve the issue of whether assisted dying can and should be legal. Advocates on all sides of the debate have contended that disability rights support their position; some have argued that their position is required by the disability rights laws. This chapter examines those positions and the rights that are being demanded.

A Community Divided

The views of people with disabilities on whether people with terminal illnesses should be allowed to end their lives with the assistance of their physicians appear to be sharply divided.[1] A vocal group of people with disabilities, including several prominent disability leaders, have indicated publicly that they are strongly against recognition of a right to physician-assisted suicide. Taking their name from a skit by the British comedy group Monty Python, the members of Not Dead Yet have used a variety of aggressive and often melodramatic strategies and tactics, including protests, vigils, lobbying efforts, and legal actions, in an effort to dominate the assisted-dying debate. They have made a broad array of arguments that people with disabilities will be harmed by a right to assisted dying and have claimed that all or most people with disabilities oppose legalization of any form of assisted dying.

Not Dead Yet got its start in the early 1990s, opposing the so-called right to die, and has been very successful. Part of that success derives from the organization's ability to convince leaders in other general disability organizations, such as United Cerebral Palsy and the American Paralysis Association, to take an organizational position against physician-assisted dying and the right to die generally. Once the general disability organizations adopted the position promoted by Not Dead Yet, it proved difficult to get them to abandon their position, much as it takes an enormous effort to change the course of an ocean liner once it has started moving. Thus far, these organizations have been reluctant even to become neutral, despite strong indications that a substantial majority of people with disabilities actually support a right to assisted dying—suggesting that a substantial majority of their members are likely also to support such a right.

I am often asked whether Not Dead Yet is really just a mouthpiece of the right-to-life movement and religious conservatives generally. Based on my limited knowledge of their leadership and membership, my response is always that this is not the case. My general impression is that the people involved in Not Dead Yet are primarily on the other end of the political spectrum—liberals and radicals. To the extent that this is so, this is a case of some very strange political bedfellows. Support of a right to physician-assisted dying is traditionally considered a liberal position, much like support of the right to an abortion. (Interestingly, both rights are characterized by supporters as "the right to choose.")

Why would liberals, like some members of Not Dead Yet, oppose a right to assisted dying? My hypothesis is that many of those in the opposition have congenital disabilities (that is, disabilities from birth or from very early childhood) and were told that their physicians had recommended that health care interventions be terminated. People who feel that their doctors wanted to kill them might be predisposed to distrust doctors and would, I suggest, tend to oppose physician-assisted dying. This hypothesis should be tested by examining the experiences of people with disabilities who oppose or support the right.

Although I strongly believe that Not Dead Yet is neither a creation nor a puppet of the religious Right, this does not mean that none of the disability opposition to a right to assisted dying is associated with religious conservatism. An organization called the National Right to Life Committee has actively supported this cause, including filing a brief in support of Attorney General John Ashcroft.[2] This group appears to consist of people with and without disabilities who are fundamentalist Christians. They file briefs that are entirely separate from those filed by Not Dead Yet.

AUTONOMY, Inc.

Not Dead Yet convinced many disability organizations that virtually all people with disabilities opposed a right to physician-assisted dying, leading organizations to solidify their positions in opposition to such a right. Yet there is evidence to suggest that in fact a substantial majority of people with disabilities do support physician-assisted dying.[3] In April 2002 I and other prominent members of the disability community established AUTONOMY, Inc.—too late, unfortunately, for many organizations to easily extricate themselves from their initial opposition.

I developed the idea of establishing a disability rights organization that supports the right to die when I was an attorney working for the international law firm of McDermott, Will, and Emery. I had been contacted by Barbara Coombs-Lee, executive director of Oregon Compassion in Dying. Apparently, she had read an article that I published in 1992 in the *Western Journal of Medicine*.[4] Amazed as I always am whenever anyone tells me that he or she has read my work, I listened intently to her request that I serve as the lead attorney on an amicus curiae ("friend of the court") brief on behalf of people with disabilities who support the right to assisted dying in the *Vacco v. Quill* and *Glucksberg v. Washington* cases then before the U.S. Supreme Court. An amicus brief is basically a document that represents the arguments and interests of certain constituencies that are not actual parties in a case; its purpose is to inform the court of additional interests that may be affected by the court's decision. The opportunity to present an amicus brief to the U.S. Supreme Court is a difficult offer to refuse, and I had no inclination to turn it down. I immediately requested permission from the firm's partners to accept this case on a pro bono basis. My request was granted.

As it turned out, the most difficult aspect of this assignment was not developing the brief, which, though challenging, was not terribly difficult, but locating clients to represent on it. This was not because people with disabilities opposed my position in the brief. Quite the contrary, when I asked people with disabilities whether they believe that people with terminal illnesses should have the right to assistance from their physicians in ending their lives, the vast majority answered in the affirmative. However, having only individuals represented on the brief would create the perception that only a few people with disabilities supported my position. Ideally, I would have liked to have at least several disability organizations or disability rights organizations represented. Unfortunately, I soon learned that all of these organizations had already solidified their positions in opposition to legalized assisted dying, convinced by Not Dead Yet that in so doing they represented the view of virtually all people with disabilities.

My colleagues at the law firm and I resolved this issue by recruiting several organizations that represent people with AIDS. Because the AIDS community has witnessed this suffering of their friends and family members during the painful and debilitating final stage of the illness, they tend to strongly support the right. Although I truly appreciated their support, which made an enormous difference, this resolution was not ideal for me. I would have liked to represent a broad array of organizations representing, in turn, a broad array of disabilities. Yet we must play the hand we are dealt, and I believe we developed a strong brief on behalf of several AIDS organizations and five prominent individuals with disabilities.

I also thought that this issue was not going to disappear over time; sometime in the future I wanted to establish a disability rights organization that would specifically support the right to die, including the right to assisted dying. There was simply no time to do this when I was drafting the briefs for *Quill* and *Glucksberg*. The opportunity did not arise until five years later, after I left the law firm and joined the faculty of Florida International University. When I did establish AUTONOMY, Inc., I did not do it alone. Barbara Coombs-Lee provided some start-up resources from her organization, as did Estelle Rogers, who was the executive director of the Death with Dignity National Center. (Among the most important of those resources were the services of Jane Ruvelson, who developed a website for AUTONOMY, Inc.)

To ensure the success of the new organization, I needed to recruit highly respected people with disabilities to serve on its board of directors. I could not have assembled a more impressive board. The first recruit, who would become the vice president of the organization and who would give the organization its name, was Hugh Gregory Gallagher, regarded as one of the founders of the modern disability rights movement. He is also considered one of the foremost experts on the Nazi euthanasia program, in which Nazis authorized and implemented the killing of people with disabilities. This expertise has been invaluable in refuting contentions by Not Dead Yet that a right to assisted dying is the first step toward the Nazi situation.

The other board members for AUTONOMY, Inc. include the following remarkable individuals: David Gray, a professor of neurology and occupational therapy at Washington School of Medicine in St. Louis and the former director of the National Institute on Disability and Rehabilitation Research; Lauro Halstead, a clinical professor of medicine at Georgetown University and one of the most respected rehabilitation physicians in the world; Michael Stein, a noted law professor at the College of William and Mary School of Law; and Susan Webb, a leading disability rights advocate who has served on the U.S. Access Board as well as on the board of the National Council on Independent Living. All of these individuals have significant disabilities, and all are prominent members of the national disability community. I myself am a person with high-level quadriplegia resulting from a spinal cord injury suffered in 1973, and I serve as president and chairman of AUTONOMY, Inc.

The Current Status of Physician-Assisted Suicide

Despite my best efforts and those of many other attorneys supporting the right to assisted dying, the U.S. Supreme Court decided in *Quill* and *Glucksberg* that there is no federal constitutional right to assisted suicide in this country.[5] This decision means that states are not required by the Constitution to allow terminally ill individuals to hasten their deaths with the assistance of their physicians. However, the decision also did not prohibit states from allowing the practice, and states may determine whether and under what conditions it will be allowed. In retrospect, this resolution of the broad constitutional issue is not at all surprising; the current Supreme Court is relatively conservative and adverse to the recognition of new constitutional rights. Even at the time, we recognized that it was not likely that the Court would rule in our favor, but these decisions were necessary for the debate to continue at the state level.

Very soon after the U.S. Supreme Court decided these cases, I was involved in this issue at the state level in a case that had gone up to the Florida Supreme Court.[6] The case raised issues similar to those put before the U.S. Supreme Court a few months earlier, but the Florida court was considering whether the state constitution required recognition of a right to assisted dying in Florida, which happens to be my state of residence. The interesting twist in this case was that the Florida constitution, unlike the U.S. Constitution, describes an explicit right to privacy, which protects citizens from undue state interference in their lives. For this reason, and because the Florida Supreme Court had previously recognized that this right to privacy guarantees the right to die for individuals who require medical interventions (ventilators, feeding tubes, and the like) in order to live, we were more optimistic that the court would rule in our favor. We modified our previous brief to focus on Florida law and submitted it to the Florida Supreme Court. At the oral argument, I sat next to Charles Hall, a man with AIDS who was requesting the right to physician assistance in dying. Unfortunately, the Florida Supreme Court denied him this right, and he died several months later precisely the way he had hoped he would not have to—in a morphine-induced stupor.

The resolution of these constitutional issues has shifted the assisted-dying debate to the states. States, including the state of Florida, may enact a right to assisted dying in state legislation or through citizen initiatives at the voting booth, such as the Oregon Death with Dignity Act, which was passed in a citizens' referendum.[7] The Oregon law encountered numerous obstacles on its path to enactment and implementation. Despite several efforts to nullify the law, in the three years it has been fully implemented there has not been a single negative incident.[8] Other states, such as California, Hawaii, and Vermont, have been seriously considering legislation or referendums permitting physician-assisted suicide. Thus far, no such measures have been enacted into law.

The most recent episode in the ongoing soap opera of the assisted-dying debate is that Attorney General Ashcroft, representing his key constituency of right-to-life advocates, reinterpreted the Controlled Substances Act to authorize the prosecution of physicians who prescribe pharmaceuticals with the intent of assisting patients to end their lives. Right-to-die advocates, including AUTONOMY, Inc., successfully challenged the attorney general's directive imposing this policy in federal district court in Oregon. The Department of Justice appealed that decision, however, and we filed another amicus brief with the Ninth Circuit Court of Appeals. In May of 2004, this appeal was rejected, but an appeal to the U.S. Supreme Court is anticipated.

Views of People with Disabilities on Physician-Assisted Dying

Like any politically, ethnically, and religiously diverse community, there is a wide range of opinions among members of the disability community on this issue. Contrary to claims made by Not Dead Yet, there is some evidence that a majority of people with disabilities support a right to assisted suicide for terminally ill individuals.

A recent in-depth study of forty-five individuals with disabilities in Berkeley, California—a stronghold of organizations that oppose a right to assisted suicide —suggests that the community of people with disabilities is deeply divided over whether terminally ill individuals should have a right to end their lives with the assistance of their physicians.[9] The key finding of the study is that "tremendous breadth and diversity of opinion exists with respect to attitudes toward death with dignity legislation."[10] Specifically, 27 percent of the disabled people interviewed supported assisted suicide legislation, 24 percent opposed such legislation, and 49 percent were ambivalent on this issue. However, "virtually all of the 45 respondents expressed a desire for autonomy in life's choices, and all but one respondent (based on religious beliefs) also expressed a desire to choose whether or not to end their lives if faced with a terminal disease or other significant life-changing situations."[11] A member of the study's community advisory committee of six people with disabilities summarized the study results as follows: "There seems to be one public position on behalf of people with disabilities about death with dignity legislation put forward by disability community spokespersons and groups, but when you go deeper into the community there are many different opinions. An individual's opinion seems to depend on their own character [and] personal experience [of self or a loved one] with near-death or death, among many other things."[12]

The Arguments of People with Disabilities

In examining the disability debate over physician-assisted dying, there is a tendency to conceptualize the debate as having two sides. This is consistent with the way American politics is conceptualized generally in terms of Democrats versus Republicans, liberals versus conservatives, the rich versus the poor, and other political bifurcations. In this country, we look at politics much like we watch a football game, rooting for one side or the other even if we are not enthusiastic about either of the teams. We do much the same with disability policy and end-of-life issues, including the debate over assisted dying.

Opposition to Assisted Dying

Disability rights advocates who oppose the right argue that our society has devalued people with disabilities, relegating many of them to institutions in which they cannot achieve their potential. In a society that continues to discriminate against people with disabilities, and in a health care system designed to cut costs no matter what the consequences, they argue, people with terminal illnesses and other disabilities will be coerced into choosing to end their lives.

They further contend that the right to assisted suicide itself is based on traditional prejudices and misconceptions about people with disabilities; that it is premised on a notion that people with disabilities necessarily have a diminished quality of life. They conclude that basing the right to assisted suicide or the availability of related services (such as suicide prevention services) on such misconceptions violates the Americans with Disabilities Act of 1990 and denies them equal protection under the law as mandated by the Fourteenth Amendment to the Constitution.[13]

The right to physician-assisted suicide, opponents argue, cannot be limited to competent individuals in the terminal stage of an illness, and it will inevitably be expanded to cover competent individuals with nonterminal disabilities and incompetent individuals. It cannot be limited to voluntary decisions to self-administer lethal drugs prescribed by a physician but will be expanded to euthanizing people with disabilities against their will. They point to the Netherlands, and even Nazi Germany, as examples demonstrating that the right cannot be contained and will ultimately harm people with disabilities generally. They are particularly opposed to the proposed role of physicians as gatekeepers to assisted suicide, based on a fundamental distrust of the medical profession.[14]

Finally, they contend that disabled people are an oppressed minority and will be coerced into ending their lives against their will. One of the foremost opponents of physician-assisted dying, Paul Longmore, states, "I think that we live in a society that is deeply prejudiced against us, and that we are an oppressed minority. . . . It is one thing to make fundamental choices; it's another thing to have the society that's oppressing us set up mechanisms to facilitate our suicides. Any society that would guarantee assistance in committing suicide by an oppressed person is simply indicating just how oppressive and hypocritical it is."[15]

Support for a Right to Assisted Dying

People with disabilities who support the right, including myself, focus primarily on the autonomy and self-determination of the individual with a disability.[16] We argue that the disability rights–independent living movement is based fundamentally on autonomy, and people with disabilities should be allowed to make all decisions that affect their lives—including the decision to end their lives, with or without assistance. We believe that the disability rights movement in this country stands for the right to self-determination of people with disabilities—our fundamental right to control all aspects of our lives.[17]

The disability rights movement has been successful in securing a broad array of rights on behalf of people with disabilities, based in large part on recognition of these individuals' autonomy. Among these are the rights of people with disabilities to live in their communities (rather than in impersonal institutions), to be free of involuntary sterilization, to raise children, to obtain a public education, to use public transportation, and to have access to places of public accommodation.[18] We believe that competent individuals with disabilities, even those in oppressive circumstances such as exist in many institutions, are capable of autonomy.

We do not believe that the right to assisted suicide is premised on a diminished quality of life for people with disabilities. It is based on respect for the autonomy of terminally ill individuals during their final days. Moreover, it does not deprive people with disabilities of anything, and therefore does not violate the Americans with Disabilities Act or the Equal Protection Clause of the Constitution. It does not deny people with disabilities suicide prevention services, protection against murder, or protection from other abuses. We further contend that, though we must always be vigilant in preventing abuses, the right will not necessarily be expanded to individuals or situations for which it was not intended. Studies of the experience in the Netherlands indicate that the "slippery slope" opponents predict has not occurred in that country.[19]

Analogies to Nazi Germany are particularly misplaced. Nazi Germany conducted an involuntary euthanasia program in which an all-powerful state granted authority to physicians to kill people with disabilities.[20] In our constitutional democracy, we are debating whether dying individuals may choose for themselves whether to end their own lives with the assistance of their physicians. Although there may be some superficial resemblance because both involve physician intervention resulting in death, they are, in fact, diametric opposites. In one case, the state has all the power; in the other, the individual has all the power.

Those who oppose a right to assisted suicide predict that a substantial number of people with disabilities would be killed against their will if assisted suicide were legalized. However, there is no evidence that this has happened to people on life-support systems, who have had the right to die at least since the *Cruzan* decision in 1990.[21] We believe that abuses of assisted suicide, to the extent they are now occurring behind closed doors, are less likely to continue once assisted suicide is legalized and appropriately regulated.[22]

With respect to the oppression argument, disabled people who support the right do not necessarily disagree that disabled people have been subject to a history of oppression but may believe one or more of the following:

· People with disabilities, as a group, are no longer oppressed at this time in our history.

· Even if people with disabilities are an oppressed minority, an individual is not necessarily oppressed simply because he or she has a disability.

· Even if the individual is considered oppressed, this does not necessarily mean the individual is so devoid of autonomy that he or she should not be allowed to control decisions that affect life and death.[23]

The Link between Personal Assistance Services and Physician-Assisted Suicide

The concept of personal assistance services has been deployed on both sides of the legalization debate.[24] One of the primary arguments against a right to assisted suicide that is frequently raised by opponents with disabilities is that until society provides people with disabilities all the resources they need to live independent, dignified lives, we should not even be thinking about providing assistance in ending life. Although this argument generally is not presented in formal philosophical terms, one way to interpret it is that people with disabilities cannot provide "informed consent" to assisted suicide unless and until they have, and are aware of, reasonable options available to live independently. Another more radical interpretation is that people with disabilities, both individually and as a group, are so oppressed by the lack of options offered by society that any decision to end their lives must be presumed to have been coerced.

The example that is virtually always presented to support this set of arguments relates to access to personal assistance services. Opponents of the right to assisted dying discuss situations in which people who were institutionalized or otherwise did not have adequate access to personal assistance services chose to end their lives. Several key cases are frequently presented as evidence against legalization of assisted suicide: the cases of Larry McAfee, Elizabeth Bouvia, and David Rivlin.

Following a motorcycle accident, Larry McAfee was a quadriplegic dependent on a respirator. After being transferred from one nursing home to another, he finally decided that "every day when I wake up there is nothing to look forward to," and he requested permission from a court to have his respirator turned off.[25]

The judge eventually granted his request. Fortunately, McAfee never exercised his right to die. In time, he was able to secure the public resources to live in his community with the aid of personal assistants.

Those with disabilities who oppose a right to physician-assisted suicide cite the McAfee case as evidence of how our society oppresses people with disabilities and as proof that assisted suicide and other manifestations of the right to die should not be permitted in this country. First, they claim that McAfee was so oppressed by a system that did not allow him to live in a noninstitutional setting that any decision to end his life could not be considered truly voluntary. Second, they claim that decisions by the court and medical professionals supporting McAfee's decision to end his life demonstrate strong prejudices against people with disabilities, particularly a belief that they necessarily have a diminished quality of life. These opponents further contend that, while McAfee's request would have been answered with suicide prevention efforts if made by a nondisabled person, McAfee, because of his disabilities, was given support to end his life.[26]

Those of us with disabilities who support a right to physician-assisted suicide agree that our society does not adequately meet the needs of people with disabilities and that much more needs to be done in this regard. We also agree that anyone subject to the nightmare that McAfee endured would probably want to end his or her life. We agree, in particular, that access to personal assistance services must be dramatically improved and that Georgia, his state of residence, certainly should have offered this option to McAfee at an early stage. However, we reject the notion that until life circumstances for people with disabilities are much better, there should be no right to assisted suicide. In fact, if one's life circumstances are sufficiently bad, for whatever reason, suicide may be the only means of escaping what the individual regards as an ongoing nightmare. From the perspective of right-to-die advocates, the McAfee case was actually a right-to-die success story, in that only after McAfee was granted the right to die did he receive the attention, resources, and administrative flexibility he needed to live in his community. In a very real sense, his decision to live was the direct result of having the option to die.

The cases of Elizabeth Bouvia and David Rivlin, on the other hand, were not success stories. They also involved a failure of the system to meet the personal assistance and independent living needs of people with disabilities. Each sought and was granted the right to have life-sustaining interventions withdrawn. Bouvia, who was granted the right to have her feeding tube removed, never exercised the right and continued to live in a small room at a state hospital at a charge of $800 per day.[27] She would have been much better off if the state had simply given her half that money to hire personal assistants in the community. Rivlin did exercise the right to end his life, having his ventilator removed. Although both these cases involved true tragedies, neither tragedy can be attributed to the right to die. Rivlin presumably would have found some way to end his life without the right or would have lived the remainder of his life in institutions.

People with disabilities who oppose the right to die argue that McAfee, Bouvia, and Rivlin were oppressed individuals and that for such individuals any decision to die is coerced. The general "oppressed minority" version of the personal assistance argument against assisted suicide is particularly offensive to people with disabilities who support the right. The contention that all people with disabilities are so oppressed, simply by virtue of their disability status, as to be presumed incapable of making end-of-life decisions reflects the same paternalism that the independent living movement was established to abolish.[28] Whether the disabled population is an oppressed minority is a political and philosophical question upon which people with disabilities are divided.[29]

The question of personal assistance plays into the aid-in-dying debate in another way as well. Those who support a right to physician-assisted suicide argue that some people, particularly those with substantial disabilities, are not able to take their own lives without substantial risk of failing in their efforts and thereby worsening their conditions. For example, a failed attempt could result in severe brain injury or coma. Supporters of the right contend that, rather than forcing these individuals into desperate acts of suicide, typically with inadequate knowledge of how to achieve death successfully, competent assistance should be available to them. The availability of such assistance could provide the individual with an opportunity to reconsider the decision to end his or her life or at least to postpone acting on the decision.

Those with disabilities who oppose the right contend that virtually anyone can end his or her life without assistance. It has been reported that one of the leading opponents actually contended that "[Larry] McAfee could run his electric wheelchair into a lake and drown or crash it down a flight of stairs."[30] It is not clear whether this was a serious suggestion; the most likely consequence of crashing down a flight of stairs would be multiple severe bone fractures and possibly a severe head injury. Although death is clearly a possible outcome of this strategy, it is by no means certain. Driving a wheelchair into a body of water is more likely to result in death, although this outcome would depend largely on how soon the attempted drowning were discovered. Another likely outcome would be a near drowning, resulting in severe brain damage from oxygen deprivation.

There are, of course, more dependable strategies to end one's life, such as shooting, hanging, or drugging oneself. None of these is guaranteed to achieve the desired goal. Moreover, some people with major disabilities, such as quadriplegia or diseases that severely weaken muscles, simply do not have the functional capacity to implement these strategies. Others have dysphagia and cannot swallow pills. Although it is easy to say that anyone can end his or her life independently, the reality is often more complicated, particularly for people with substantial disabilities.

Finally, one suicide strategy appears to be applicable to virtually anyone: voluntary refusal of food and fluids, often referred to as "terminal dehydration."[31] The refusal to eat or drink for an extended period of time will bring about death in a dependable manner without undue risks.[32] This approach has the ethical advantage of being directed and initiated entirely by the consumer and is therefore less subject to criticisms concerning external coercion by others, such as physicians or family members. However, in practice, this approach cannot be implemented independently. Palliative care to address discomfort, such as dry mouth and throat, is typically required. Some sedation is often necessary, and terminal sedation may be indicated if the individual becomes severely agitated.

The arguable problem with this strategy is its time frame. The period of time necessary to achieve death through starvation and dehydration varies from one individual to another and may range from about a week to several weeks, depending in part on the individual's physical condition.[33] For some, dying slowly over a period of one to two weeks may be personally acceptable. For others, the prospect of withering away slowly is appalling and unacceptable. Even more profound than the effect on the individual is the likely effect on family members, friends, assistants, and others who must observe the slow dying process. Because this strategy cannot be implemented comfortably without assistance, the availability of hospice workers to provide comfort care and thereby to spare the family emotional trauma is important.

One commentator, recognizing that both terminal dehydration and physician-assisted suicide have advantages and shortcomings, observes,

> The time required for death by terminal dehydration is likely to make this method seem less humane than physician-assisted suicide. Indeed, it may seem repugnant that a competent, informed patient who resolutely seeks voluntary death must stop eating and drinking and wait for an undeter-

mined period for death to arrive. The vigil of family members awaiting their loved one's death may be burdensome and stressful. Moreover, minimal drinking in response to thirst or the urging of concerned relatives may further prolong the process of dying. Those who die by terminal dehydration typically lapse into unconsciousness before death, which may seem intolerable to some patients and their family members.[34]

The bottom line is that while the strategy of starvation and dehydration is available to virtually anyone, it is not necessarily acceptable to everyone. Those opposed to a right to assisted suicide who argue that assistance by others is unnecessary because anyone can starve himself must answer those who contend that they do not wish to die in that manner. Opponents typically respond that an "easy death" is not a legitimate goal of public policy and that the risks associated with authorizing assistance outweigh the individual's desires. They claim that many people who attempt suicide do not really wish to succeed, which explains the high failure rate of suicide.

Those of us who support the right to assisted suicide argue that it is not humane to force individuals into desperate acts of suicide alone and that with assistance, people are more likely to think through whether they really want to die. It also offers additional opportunities for someone to intervene and convince the individual not to take his or her life. Finally, it allows individuals to postpone their suicides with the knowledge that they can always obtain assistance at a later time if they are not able to implement a suicide strategy alone.

Practical Matters

This abstract, philosophical debate raises some practical, real-world issues. If it is true that some people simply cannot end their own lives in a certain and reasonable manner, First, should we honor requests for assistance by those who require it? Second, if we decide that we should honor the request, who should provide the assistance? And third, if someone is permitted to provide assistance, what type of assistance should be allowed?

Should We Honor Requests?

Obviously, those who differ on whether a right to assisted suicide should be legally recognized will differ on whether we should honor the requests of people with disabilities who cannot end their lives without assistance. Those who support the right to assisted suicide are divided over whether the right should be available to people with nonterminal conditions. The reasons for the division are diverse. Some who would not extend the right believe it should be available only to people with terminal illnesses (that is, those with life expectancies of less than six months). Some probably are concerned that the risk of abuse associated with extending the right is not justified by the benefit to a relatively small number of people. Some simply take the politically pragmatic view that it is easier to pass assisted-suicide legislation for people with terminal illnesses than for people with nonterminal conditions.

Some of those who believe that the right should be extended to people with nonterminal conditions do so for what I would call the wrong reasons. These include some members of the Hemlock Society who have based their position on precisely the types of misconceptions about people with disabilities and their quality of life that the opponents criticize.[35] Others, including myself, are much more ambivalent about extending the right to individuals with nonterminal conditions and conclude in support of the right on the basis of compassion for people who simply are not able to adjust to their disabilities. We conclude that the alternative to forbidding assistance is often desperate acts of suicide by people who do not have the capacity to carry out suicide plans effectively. As discussed earlier, the availability of assistance raises the issue above the surface and creates opportunities for suicide prevention that might not otherwise exist. The Netherlands allows physicians to aid in the death of patients with nonterminal conditions without prosecution, and there is relatively little controversy over this issue in that country.

For all these reasons, people who oppose a right to assisted suicide are particularly opposed to extending the right beyond the terminally ill population.

Who Should Be Allowed to Assist?

If our society ultimately decides that people with nonterminal conditions have a right to assisted suicide, it must be decided who may assist them in ending their lives. Some people with disabilities who oppose the right contend that for a variety of reasons physicians and other health care professionals cannot be trusted to serve in this capacity, claiming that they have substantial biases, misconceptions, and negative attitudes toward people with disabilities.[36] Some even claim that their physicians would be eager to end their lives, if given the opportunity.

Those of us who support the right tend to be more reluctant to accept that our physicians and health care professionals cannot be trusted to assist us with life and death issues and are particularly reluctant to accept the contention that these health care professionals are eager to end our lives. We believe that health professionals who address disability issues can be trained to address death and dying, just as health care professionals at hospices are.

However, if it is determined that health care professionals are not qualified to address these issues, owing to bias or for any other reason, this does not mean that nobody is qualified to assist. Assistance by physicians or other trained health care professionals is probably preferable simply because they are more likely to have the technical knowledge to provide assistance in achieving a certain death. Yet with the right information, any competent and willing adult can provide such assistance, if the law permits. The basic philosophy of personal assistance services is that people with disabilities should be able to receive help from their personal assistants with respect to any task the individual requests and the personal assistant is willing to perform. Although applying this philosophy in the current context may appear morbid, the general principle should still apply.

What Type of Assistance Should Be Allowed?

Several options are available for assistance to those who wish to end their lives. These range from self-administration of a lethal agent to administration of the lethal agent by the assistant. The options available may be limited by the individual's functional limitations. Opponents tend to support the conceptual distinction between self-administration, labeled "assisted suicide," and administration by others, labeled "euthanasia," though they oppose a right to either. Those of us who support the right tend to be divided over whether this distinction is justified. Some believe it offers one additional safeguard that the act is voluntary. Others, including myself, believe that though voluntariness is the key issue, the distinction between self-administration and administration by others is a difference without real meaning. We believe that assistance should be permitted in the manner in which the individual needs it and that people who are not capable of self-administration should not be deprived of any right simply by virtue of their disabilities or arbitrary distinctions.

A New Role for the Disability Debate

Despite the substantial head start of Not Dead Yet and other disability organizations that oppose the right to assisted dying, it appears that there is now recognition that the disability community is divided on this issue. AUTONOMY, Inc. has been effective in communicating the best data available on the opinions of the disability community, indicating that a substantial majority of people with disabilities support the right and that, at the very least, there is a clear division among people with disabilities on this key issue. Both Not Dead Yet and AUTONOMY, Inc. have made strong legal and policy arguments for their particular positions. It is unlikely that either side will dominate the other in this ongoing debate. Consequently, although the disability issues will remain key, they are no longer likely to be dispositive in deciding whether assisted dying should be permitted in our society.

Notes

Editors' note: Andrew died shortly after completing this chapter. It has been minimally edited from the original, with the approval of his brother, Mitchell. The views expressed are Andrew's and do not necessarily represent the positions of Florida International University or any other organization with which he was affiliated.

1. A.I. Batavia, "Disability and Physician-Assisted Suicide," *New England Journal of Medicine* 336 (1997): 1671–73.

2. T.J. Marzen, "National Right to Life Committee and Oregon RTL File Brief in Support of Ashcroft Decision on Assisted Suicide" (2001), www.nrlc.org/news/2001/NRL12/marz.html (accessed March 11, 2003). The Ninth Circuit Court ruled against the Ashcroft measure in May of 2004.

3. Public Opinion Online, Question 004 NEW06090. New York: Louis Harris and Associates, 1995.

4. A.I. Batavia, "A Disability Rights–Independent Living Perspective on Euthanasia," *Western Journal of Medicine* 154 (1991): 616–17.

5. *Washington v. Glucksberg,* 521 U.S. 702 (1997); *Vacco v. Quill,* 521 U.S. 793 (1997).

6. *Krischer v. McIver,* 697 So.2d 97 (1997).

7. Oregon Death with Dignity Act, *Oregon Revised Statutes,* secs. 127.800–127.995 (1995).

8. A.E. Chin, K. Hedberg, G.K. Higginson, and D.W. Fleming, "Legalized Physician-Assisted Suicide in Oregon—The First Year's Experience," *New England Journal of Medicine* 340 (1999): 577–83.

9. P. Fadem, M. Minkler, M. Perry, K. Blum, L.F.J. Moore, J. Rogers, and L. Williams, "Attitudes of People with Disabilities toward Death with Dignity/Physician-Assisted Suicide Legislation: Broadening the Dialogue," *Journal of Health, Politics and Law* 28 (Dec. 2003): 977–1001.

10. Ibid., 984.

11. Ibid., 994.

12. Ibid., 986.

13. See, for example, D. Coleman, "Not Dead Yet," in *The Case against Assisted Suicide: For the Right to End-of-Life Care*, edited by K. Foley and H. Hendin (Baltimore: Johns Hopkins University Press, 2002), 213–37.

14. C.J. Gill, "Health Professionals, Disability and Assisted Suicide: An Examination of Relevant Empirical Evidence and Response to Batavia," *Psychology, Public Policy and Law* 6 (2000): 526–45.

15. B. Corbet, "Assisted Suicide: Death Do Us Part," *New Mobility* 8, no. 43 (1997): 48–51, 50.

16. A.I. Batavia, "The Relevance of Physician Data on the Right to Physician-Assisted Suicide: Can Studies Resolve the Law?" *Psychology, Public Policy and Law* 6 (2000): 546–58.

17. S.S. Pflueger, *Independent Living* (Berkeley, Calif.: Berkeley Planning Associates, 1977); National Council on Disability, *Toward Independence* (Washington, D.C.: National Council on Disability, 1986); *On the Threshold of Independence* (Washington, D.C.: National Council on Disability, 1988); G. DeJong, "Independent Living: From Social Movement to Analytic Paradigm," *Archives of Physical Medicine and Rehabilitation* 60 (1979): 435–46.

18. M. Nagler, *Perspectives on Disability*, 2d ed. (Palo Alto, Calif.: Health Markets Research, 1993); J. West, *The Americans with Disabilities Act: From Policy to Practice* (New York: Milbank Memorial Fund, 1991).

19. P.J. van der Maas, G. van der Wal, I. Haverkate, C.L. de Graff, J.G. Kester, B.D. Onwuteaka-Philipsen, A. van der Heide, J.M. Bosma, D.L. Willens, "Euthanasia, Physician-Assisted Suicide, and Other Medical Practices Involving the End of Life in the Netherlands, 1990–1995," *New England Journal of Medicine* 335 (1996): 1699–1705; G. van der Wal, P.J. van der Maas, J.M. Bosma, B.D. Onwuteaka-Philipsen, D.L. Willens, I. Haverkale, B.J. Kostense, "Evaluation of the Notification Procedure for Physician-Assisted Death in the Netherlands," *New England Journal of Medicine* 335 (1996): 1706–11; M. Angell, "Euthanasia in the Netherlands—Good News? Or Bad?" editorial, *New England Journal of Medicine* 335 (1996): 1675–78, 1676.

20. H.G. Gallagher, *By Trust Betrayed: Patients, Physicians and the License to Kill in the Third Reich* (Arlington, Va.: Vandamere, 1995).

21. *Cruzan v. Director, Missouri Department of Health*, 476 U.S. 261 (1990).

22. L. Shavelson, *A Chosen Death: The Dying Confront Assisted Suicide* (New York: Simon and Schuster, 1995).

23. A.I. Batavia, "The New Paternalism: Characterizing People with Disabilities as an Oppressed Minority," *Journal of Disability Policy Studies* 12 (2001): 107–13.

24. It is important to note that these disability arguments concerning personal assistance services are not the only disability arguments for and against a right to physician-assisted suicide. For example, there is disagreement among members of the disabled population over whether the right is based on a presumption of diminished quality of life for people with disabilities and whether regulatory safeguards against abuse would be effective in protecting those disabled people who are vulnerable.

25. J.P. Shapiro, *No Pity: People with Disabilities Forging a New Civil Rights Movement* (New York: Random House, 1993), 258–59.

26. See, for example, Coleman, "Not Dead Yet," and references therein.

27. Shapiro, *No Pity.*

28. Batavia, "New Paternalism."

29. A.I. Batavia, "Are People with Disabilities an Oppressed Minority, and Why Does This Matter?" *Journal of Disability Policy Studies* 12, no. 2 (2001): 66–67.

30. Shapiro, *No Pity,* 270.

31. J.L. Bernat, B. Gert, and R.P. Mogielnicki, "Patient Refusal of Hydration and Nutrition: An Alternative to Physician-Assisted Suicide or Voluntary Active Euthanasia," *Archives of Internal Medicine* 153 (1993): 2723–27.

32. T.E. Quill and I.R. Byock, "Responding to Intractable Terminal Suffering: The Role of Terminal Sedation and Voluntary Refusal of Food and Fluids," *Annals of Internal Medicine* 132 (2000): 408–14.

33. T.E. Quill, B. Lo, and D.W. Brock, "Palliative Options of Last Resort: A Comparison of Voluntarily Stopping Eating and Drinking, Terminal Sedation, Physician-Assisted Suicide, and Voluntary Active Euthanasia," *Journal of the American Medical Association* 278 (1997): 2099–104, 2099.

34. F.G. Miller and D.E. Meier, "Voluntary Death: A Comparison of Terminal Dehydration and Physician-Assisted Suicide," *Annals of Internal Medicine* 128 (1998): 559–62, 561.

35. D. Humphry, *Final Exit* (Eugene, Ore.: Hemlock Society, 1991), 58–63.

36. Gill, "Health Professionals, Disability and Assisted Suicide"; Batavia, "Relevance of Physician Data on the Right to Physician-Assisted Suicide."

5

When Suffering Patients Seek Death

Eric J. Cassell, M.D., M.A.C.P.

If I am so badly off, death is my harbor.
And this is the harbor of all men, even death,
and this is their refuge.

Epictetus IV.X.22–29

Marcy Thompson* was sixty-two when she became so severely impaired by advancing cancer of the ovary that she chose to die. She was determinedly single and had led a life of books, with which her apartment was filled. With her only family, a sister and nieces, she was distant by preference. Although generally alone, she had been and remained in a long love relationship. Her cancer was discovered after it had spread, and she refused chemotherapy (having researched the topic thoroughly). She stopped working as an editor a few months before her decision because of weakness and fatigue, but she continued to read and write commentary, attended only by a home health aide. Pain, although present, was adequately controlled. She found existence intolerable when she could hardly walk, could no longer read or write critically, and was not, in her estimate, a partner to the man she loved, so she decided to die.

She read about how to end her life and with the aid of her loving friend came into possession of barbiturates sufficient to do so. She informed her doctor of many years, with whose advice she was impatient (she had, after all, read the literature), and her accountant-lawyer about her plan. The latter agreed to come to her apartment the day after she took her medication and then report her death and notify the police and the doctor. Unfortunately, when he discovered the body he became alarmed at the thought that she might still be alive and instead called 911. She was taken to a local hospital where, though thought

---

*Her name is fictitious but the case is true.

to be dead (with a flat EEG), she was placed on life support. She returned to consciousness. The extent of her disease was acknowledged in the record. Pneumonia was treated, despite her refusal of all treatment, and she was kept on suicide watch. She was transferred to the inpatient unit of a hospice.

The psychiatrist at the hospice wrote that she had the capacity to make reasoned decisions and that she was not clinically depressed. However, he recommended that she not be discharged until she had promised not to attempt again to end her life. She returned home sicker than before and worried that soon she would lose control of her situation completely. For a brief period it was legal in New York state to provide aid in dying, and during that time she ended her life with assistance.

Patients who are terminally ill look forward to death not because they want to die but because their suffering has made living intolerable. This chapter addresses the premise that the very sick may request assistance in dying because their suffering is not relieved. The word *suffering* occurs again and again in discussions about whether assistance in death should be legalized. Few commentators stop to say what they mean by the word. Frequently, suffering and symptoms are equated and then confused in a common failure to understand suffering. For example, when "physical" suffering arising from pain is offered as an example, and the fact that pain can be relieved offered as a solution.[1] Suffering isn't physical (or emotional or existential); it is suffering. Suffering is distinct from what initiates it.

The relief of pain is always to be sought, but that may not in itself relieve the suffering; pain and the suffering it causes are different. Suffering isn't something that people get, like (say) bronchitis or appendicitis. It is an afflicted state of being, a specific distress that happens to a particular person on whom has been inflicted unendurable pain or other symptoms, losses, enduring fear, hardship, injury, disaster, grief, sorrow, or care and who has been changed as a result of the burden. When the state of suffering occurs because of sickness, it is the province of medicine and physicians. Why it is so important—why suffering can bring forth in some the desire to die and in others, out of compassion, the desire to assist them in dying—is crucial to understand, as is its relation to sickness. First, however, a word about the dyadic setting in which it occurs.

The Doctor and the Relationship with the Patient

At the heart of the controversy is a specific relationship, that between physician and patient. It is this relationship that defines each of the roles: Patients are patients because they are in the care of physicians, and physicians are physicians because they care for patients. In an individualistic and mechanistic (and even cynical) age, it may be difficult to acknowledge the power of the connection between them that is brought on by sickness. In that context, it was not rare in the past for physicians to assist in the death of patients who were overmastered by their suffering, and current surveys confirm the continuance of the practice. I know this to be true from personal experience and a lifetime spent among doctors. This happens, I believe, when a physician is personally weighed down by the distress suffered by a patient whom he or she knows well. There is evidence that the physicians caring for suffering persons mirror in themselves aspects of the patients' suffering. A death that means a young child is left behind will awaken old memories if the doctor lost a loved one at an early age. The grief of survivors and of dying persons themselves will trigger past deaths and awaken feelings of grief in the physician. It is an aspect of the care of such patients that physicians learn to deal with—not by suppressing the feelings, which is a poor defense, but by acknowledging their presence.

The decision to assist in a patient's death is distressing. Physicians who care for the very sick know about death. They know that nothing can make it any less what it is. Nothing diminishes its profound importance in and to life, the sadness, pain, grief, and loss that may precede and almost inevitably follow death. All these consequences do not occur because a body has died but because a person has died and because survivors are also persons. Physicians, too, are persons. They know, as the persons they are, that the decision to assist a patient in dying is situated in the landscape of death—in the midst of extreme personal distress in patients and those who love them.

It is difficult for nonphysicians to know how indelibly stamped into the doctor's whole being is the injunction not to harm a patient. Physicians actively worry throughout their working lives about hurting patients. They do not need to be reminded that when they assist in death they have done something many consider wrong. For these and for social reasons, the decision to make this a part of a physician's responsibility to his or her patient is not lightly taken, I believe. For some physicians, it is simply an impossible idea because of religious or other beliefs. For those who hold to a purely technical view of caring for patients, assisting in death represents an enlarged emotional and professional commitment that is not easily arrived at. Physicians who have no specific training in palliative care, or who have not previously involved themselves with their patients who are dying, have to work their way toward increased participation in their patients' terminal illness. Generally, they will be taking back the responsibility for day-to-day care from oncologists or other specialists, in itself not a simple matter. They may need to get over their fear of intractable illness or pain and then resolve their fear of opioid analgesics. These are steps that take time and are poorly rewarded except in personal terms. When they finally find themselves able to help a suffering patient die and to resolve the conflicting emotions, I believe, they find it complexly rewarding.

Suffering

The arguments for and against physician-assisted death often have at their core the fact that persons suffer in some terminal illnesses and suffer also in instances of certain diseases that end in severe impairment. All agree that suffering should call forth our most compassionate response; relief of suffering is, after all, the warrant of medicine in probably all cultures. No one denies that suffering is often inadequately addressed, that ignorance of what suffering really is and how to relieve it is widespread, and that hospice and palliative care programs came into existence as a response, in large part, to the failed relief of suffering so common in hospitals and medical centers.

The arguments against assisted death frequently claim that virtually all suffering can be relieved, that in the presence of good hospice care suffering is much less common, that pain, which is a frequent source of suffering, can almost always be controlled, and that when physicians are adequately trained in palliative care there is the possibility of much more effective relief of suffering. Such statements, usually made by opponents of assisted death, seem to argue *in support* of physician-assisted death in instances of intractable suffering by saying that there are only a few cases in which physician-assisted death might be warranted or by pointing out that when adequate palliative care has become widespread, suffering will be lessened. But what about now, when it is widely acknowledged that there is *not* adequate care of the terminally ill? What should be done for the patients whose pain or suffering is not included in the "virtually all," the "almost always," or the "much less common"?

Suggesting that because unrelievable pain or intractable suffering rarely occurs it should be ignored follows a logic that has never motivated the practice of medicine: that because a source of suffering is uncommon it should not be attended to. On the same logic, we would not pursue rare tumors or other strange diseases; we would not expend resources on unusual cases or cases with a small chance of good outcome. Indeed, in medicine's history the opposite has been true—the exception tests the rule (theory). On this logic, communities wouldn't waste large amounts of money and other resources to rescue one young child who has fallen down a well or try to save trapped miners for whom hope of rescue is, at best, small. In fact, we would train physicians only for the diagnosis and treatment of common diseases. On the contrary, from its roots in classical Greece the profession of medicine has responded to sickness in individuals, no matter how unusual, even when communities have failed that test of humanity. The idea of (nonreligious) community involvement in the care of the sick is relatively modern; in the past it fell to individual doctors. Furthermore, there is general agreement that the principles and practices of palliative care, which include the relief of suffering, are not known widely enough in the United States.

Those experienced in palliative care acknowledge that not all pain can be relieved. In the care of suffering patients, even the best physicians sometimes (and not rarely) find their abilities insufficient; the suffering of some patients seems beyond reach. Whatever may be the origin of suffering (for example, pain or the depredations of disease), the loss of a person's intactness—the hallmark of suffering—is related to the specific nature of that person.[2] Whatever may be the origin of suffering, once suffering has started, it is the suffering that is the main problem, not the pain or other symptoms, as awful as they may be.[3] The suffering of some patients *cannot* be relieved because its sources within the patient are inaccessible.

If unrelieved or intractable suffering is a reason to permit or endorse physician-assisted death, then changes in the law should be enacted with appropriate safeguards. If, however, other reasons are at the root of the argument against physician-assisted death, they should be made explicitly clear and be the basis of further discussion. In that instance, it should also be clearly stated that some patients (and their communities) must simply accept unrelieved pain and intractable suffering. The belief that suffering can be relieved in all or "virtually all" cases displays an ignorance of what suffering is and how it comes about.

I chose, as the case with which to open this discussion, a patient whose suffering was precipitated by metastatic cancer of the ovary but was related not to pain but to the increasing inability to live her carefully constructed life as the person she had made herself into over the years. Some might object that her suffering wasn't medical, it was psychological, or maybe existential, or even social, and therefore not the doctors' job. Such divisions into kinds of suffering reveal an ignorance of the nature of suffering. Suffering is always personal. It involves the person, and persons are of a piece. What afflicts one part afflicts the whole, and what afflicts the whole afflicts each part. The belief that had Marcy

Thompson's cancer been treated into remission, she wouldn't be suffering only suggests that the impairments that made her life intolerable came from the cachexia, debility, and weakness of advanced cancer. In another person the same impairments might not have been a source of suffering because they would not have had the same impact on that person's integrity as they did on Marcy's.

The Components of Suffering

One of the difficulties in understanding symptoms and the suffering that may follow from them is the persistence of the idea that a symptom as experienced—for example, pain or dyspnea (shortness of breath)—is the disease speaking, the unmediated result of the pathophysiology (the physiological chain of events leading to the abnormal state) of the disease.[4] For pain, this means the persistence of the model of acute pain and the idea that pain is always secondary to tissue damage, exemplified by what everyone experiences as a result of a splinter, a burn, or a twisted ankle. In acute pain there is usually a direct relation to tissue damage, and where there is tissue damage pain often follows. However, fractures, acute localized inflammation, and rapidly expanding lesions (such as abscesses or fast-growing tumors)—all of which involve tissue damage—are experienced by only a fraction of patients in whom suffering develops or who request assistance in dying.

Nowadays, pain is relatively easy to control, particularly in a hospital or hospice. This fact leads to the incorrect belief that all pain can be controlled if people only know how or have adequate training. While much pain is often controllable (at least in good part) in most patients, it is not unusual for physicians to move the pain that is not easily relieved into other categories by emphasizing, for example, the psychological aspects of the patient's problem. This is, in fact, the final obstacle to understanding: seeing suffering as either physical or psychological—as though if some feature of pain or a patient in pain cannot be explained physiologically, it must be psychological in origin.[5]

Physiology

There has been a recent explosion in knowledge about the physiology of pain. Thirty years ago, a search of the medical literature for information about the physiology of pain would bring up a hundred or so articles. A similar search currently would retrieve thousands of sources. The physiological mechanisms revealed are so interesting that it is difficult to avoid returning again and again to this research to explain this or that manifestation in an individual patient, or as a basis for the choice of treatment for a patient's pain, or believing that further research will lead to a solution of the problems of pain and suffering.[6] Further research into a particular physiological mechanism will not solve the problem of suffering because it does not address the whole person. On the other hand, as the phenomenon called pain appears to double and then re-double in complexity as a result of new discoveries about its physiology, a relatively simple conclusion becomes possible. What has been revealed by newer research (something already apparent in a simpler fashion years ago) is that there is not a direct correspondence between the stimulus that elicits pain and the pain itself. In fact, it is evident that there exist many pathways by which the person's experience of pain can be enhanced, diminished, and changed in character or with respect to where in the body it is experienced.[7]

Given the many different physiological ways to alter the nature of the pain as felt, what determines the person's actual experience? It cannot be simply the pain stimulus itself—whether there is evident tissue damage or not (because that does not match the complexity of pain physiology). It cannot be what is happening in the person's body alone, although physical phenomena such as fever or other discomforts may change the person's experience of the original pain. It must be something about the nature of the person who has the pain.

Emotions

It is commonly believed that if a physical basis for pain cannot be demonstrated —no lesion sufficient to explain the pain can be found, or the pain does not conform to expectations—the pain must be emotional (psychogenic) in origin. Psychogenic pain—in this view—is imaginary pain; the patient feels pain that does not exist, that is not *real* pain. There are, I suppose, rare cases in which patients report pain but nothing else in their behavior or activities supports their claim. Their activities are unchanged, their use of pain relieving medications is not increased, they do not utilize medical services, and their interactions with family and others appear to be unaffected. In other words, all the behavioral changes that usually occur when people are in pain are absent. These are not patients in palliative care programs, patients with serious disease whether or not lesions to cause the reported pain can be demonstrated, or persons whose suffering is of such intensity that they wish assistance in ending their life. Similarly, problems of malingering or using pain as part of drug-seeking behavior are uncommon and should not distract from the central problems that get in the way of understanding pain and suffering.

Fear, panic, or even anger, on the other hand, may aggravate pain, as suffering itself commonly does, and make it difficult to control.[8] Increasing opioid or analgesic dose for pain that is unrelieved because of concurrent emotional distress, anguish, or suffering can lead to persistence of the pain, opioid toxicity, escalating drug costs, increased family distress, greater demands on caregivers, and diminished patient quality of life.[9] This is not rare—even among patients with terminal illness receiving palliative care services—and often accounts for inadequate pain relief and increased suffering despite doses of opioid analgesics that are sometimes astonishingly high.

If neither understanding the physiology of pain nor probing the psychological aspects of illness brings us closer to an understanding of suffering, what will help us understand? What will give us insight into why it is that suffering is personal and why it is the person and not just the body that is involved in suffering? Why is all suffering individual? Why can the same illness or symptoms cause suffering in one person but not in another? Why is it that suffering may involve any aspect of a person from his or her past, family history, relationships with others, work, habits, relationship with the body and others? Why are a few suffering people legitimately intent on ending their lives while others who are also suffering hold on grimly or even gratefully? I think when we see the place of meaning, much of the mystery will be dispelled.

Meaning

Meaning is one of those words that we use all the time; it implies many different things and has been the main concern of philosophers of language for a generation or more. Although meaning is not usually considered as part of medicine, anyone who wants to understand suffering cannot avoid it.

The assignment of meaning to experience (persons, objects, events, relationships, and circumstances) and to words and utterances are activities of thought —mentality. All meanings include bodily aspects (note the inherent physicality of many words such as *push, heavy, tripped, itchy*), sensory perceptions (in all their dimensions), and feelings, with their inherent bodily dimension and physiological concomitants. The activity of mentality in assigning meaning is necessarily accompanied by the bodily dimensions of those meanings. Think of the nausea some people experience as they approach the chemotherapy suite or the sudden feelings of fear as one hears bad news. The bad news doesn't cause the feeling; the feeling of fear is part of the meaning of the bad news. On the other hand, what happens in the body—what is perceived in the skin, muscles, joints, intestines, heartbeat, and through the activity of the nervous system, for example—are bodily experiences. As experiences they are assigned meaning like any other experience. Bodily experiences thus elicit the ideas or concepts that generate meaning. Meaning—ideas, or concepts—generates bodily effects. Meaning is a medium through which thought flows into body and body flows into thought.[10]

The meanings of things—words, objects, events, and relationships—are not simply their dictionary definitions. The repository of meaning also includes what a thing signifies: the frown on the doctor's face signifies bad news, chest pain signifies angina. Meanings also include an element of importance that carries the value—the attitude of the person toward the thing. Importance is always personal; a diagnosis of cancer means I will experience pain and suffering, a negative biopsy means I'm free. The content of meaning is dynamic, not fixed or static. It includes where things come from and what they become. Apples come from trees and can become applesauce. Fall on your wrist on the ice, and you will think not only of the fracture but also of the impairment that is sure to follow. Meanings contain predictions, and predictions lead to the foretaste of experience. Think of how your foot feels when the next step going down is not in its expected place. Walking down a stationary escalator, the failed expectation of sensation as the step risers get smaller produces its own bodily sensation.

In the light of all this, let us look again at illness and symptoms. First, symptoms are bodily sensations. Bodily sensations are not simple straightforward things. Sit down; feel the seat of the chair against your buttocks and thighs— the sensation is immediate. Just as immediate is the assignment of meaning, "This is not my chair." Separating sensation from meaning is difficult. Try it and you will see how complex is even such a simple set of sensations as sitting in a chair. Sitting down produces not just one sensation but multiple fragments of the original sensation. Pain or shortness of breath are also complex, as their meanings are produced in persons and may change or evolve over the duration of the symptom. With the meanings come attributions of cause, or ideas of what to do, and thoughts of seriousness or not, and predictions, leading to changes in the person and the person's behaviors varying from a shift in position to calling for an ambulance.

In other words, symptoms are not simple brute facts of nature; they are actively influenced by the person in whom they occur because they are affected by that person's meaning. They are, in a word, personalized. Meanings are learned in the moment and over a lifetime. Although people may share some meanings, of words, for example, meanings may be highly individual—which is why two people may experience the same thing but react to it differently and also one reason that suffering is *always individual.* Experience confirms or modifies meaning. Meanings and their resultant predictions are not only a result of sensation but modify the ongoing sensation (from moments to months), as well, so that it is reinforced and amplified and other sensations are recruited, or it is diminished. The whole process of the assignment of meaning may occur below awareness (and, most of the time, probably does). Therefore, meanings and their impact may not be conscious or verbalized, or may even not include words.

When people suffer because of pain, two things are apparent; the meaning of the symptom (for example, pain) and the future. Neither the severity of pain alone nor the duration of pain alone explains suffering. Some suffer from even a "mild" pain if they attribute to it a bad meaning—for example, a recurrence of the cancer. What people think will happen is also a determinant—for example, the thought, "If the pain continues, I won't be able to take it." When, at the time they are saying it, they are taking it. Those facts demonstrate that suffering is not something that happens to bodies; *only persons suffer* (because while bodies may exhibit pain, only persons have meanings and ideas of the future). That much has been understood for many years. Why is it in terminal illness (or other serious sickness or events) persons come to the hallmark of suffering, the belief that their *integrity* or *intactness* as persons is so under assault that it has been lost or is threatened?

The Progression from Illness to Suffering

It should now be clear that symptoms—pain, shortness of breath, weakness, inability to walk or work, smelling bad, loss of interest, diarrhea, and so on— are not just facts of nature or events visited on a person by disease. Although these symptoms accompany disease and worsen as the disease progresses, they give rise to meanings and are subsequently personalized as the person assigns meaning to events and changes behaviors and attitudes in response to those meanings. Pain is never just pain; it is *this person's* pain. The same occurs with other symptoms. As the illness deepens, pain, other symptoms and losses of function, and social and emotional losses continue or worsen. The embrace of illness tightens, fed by external events such as the experience with physicians, medical care, and its institutions. The reactions of family, friends, and the surrounding world contribute. There is a continued interpretation of information and accumulation of knowledge (which may or may not be accurate or valid) —nowadays fed by multiple sources, including the Internet. Alternatively, there is no information from the outside, but there is continued rumination and reflection. Meanings become increasingly dire, their predictive aspects change, and *threat* is introduced. The person with amyotrophic lateral sclerosis may have been acclimated to the increasingly severe losses of function. The impairments were conquered by adaptation, perhaps, or with optimism and the help of others. Then something happens, perhaps a minor further loss of function or the failure of an adaptation, and suddenly the person becomes aware of the terror the future holds. The meaning has changed, and suffering begins. Persons see themselves as no longer being the persons they were, as "coming apart," as losing their integrity in comparison with their past, as no longer being intact persons. In one of the few empirical studies of suffering, Daneault and colleagues have shown three consistent characteristics of terminally ill suffering patients that are coherent with this description. These suffering patients feel under assault, as though they were subjected to violence; they feel themselves to be deprived or overwhelmed; and they are in a constant state of apprehension.[11]

Specific aspects of the person are threatened; for example, relationships with family or friends are seen as disappearing.[12] The connections to loved ones may seem to be increasingly attenuated, setting in motion grief and bereavement. Roles—as mother, doctor, executive, or whatever—cannot be maintained, perhaps destroying self-respect. Work and the meaning of work are threatened, injuring self-image. The belief that control of the world is possible disappears. Hopes, dreams, and aspirations for the future are seen as fading beyond redemption, stranding the person in the unsatisfactory present. Unconscious conflicts and repressed trauma may be reactivated by the bombardment of illness and the feeling that everything happening is an attack; the person abused in childhood begins to see the pain and illness as a repetition of the abuse. The relative contribution of these things is different in every individual—perhaps only one thing for this person may set suffering in motion, while for another it will be different or multiple losses.

Central purpose, the sense of being oneself in a world of others, begins to disappear, as purpose narrows and focuses on the threat itself, the disease, the pain, and related phenomenon, so that purpose no longer extends even beyond the sickbed. Internal conflicts appear or worsen—for example, between the needs of the whole person and the needs of his or her body. Loneliness deepens as the suffering person withdraws from others; the caregiving environment is seen as not helping. Through the impact of changing meanings on the body, these events act on the nociceptive process (the physiologic machinery of pain), and the pain (and perhaps other symptoms) becomes increasingly intractable and unresponsive to increasing doses of analgesics. With increasing side effects of opioids and psychotropic drugs, the person's withdrawal advances—aggravated by delirium and confusion.

It is vital to understand that to the suffering person the pain and other physical manifestations of sickness have become of lesser importance as a source of impairment than the suffering itself. Unless the suffering is addressed, the pain often remains intractable. Unless the suffering is addressed, even if the pain is controlled, the suffering may continue. Unrelieved suffering is not rare. If the illness goes away, the suffering will stop (but not be forgotten). Focusing on cure where that is not realistic may only produce more suffering. A focus on suffering specifically for what it is should be one of the marks of good end-of-life care. At the present time that is not true, as can be demonstrated by a walk through the floors of contemporary hospitals. Suffering *can* be treated successfully, even when the symptoms of disease continue. In good hospice and palliative care environments, that is just what happens; it is wonderful to see. A moment's reflection on the nature and evolution of suffering will show, on the other hand, that it is probably impossible to lift all suffering from every patient—Marcy Thompson, for example. Suffering is too individual, and some losses are too intransigent, for sympathy to offer any real comfort or even for sympathetic engagement to be possible.

Some terminally ill patients are not suffering, they are depressed. Such depression can be effectively treated. That someone is going to die of his or her disease is not a sufficient reason for depression. Although suffering and depression have some features in common, and depression itself may be the source of suffering, the two are distinct. (Certainly, one useful distinction is that the terminally ill person whose "depression" does not respond to antidepressants is probably suffering.)

Why is it that only a minority of suffering patients with terminal illness choose to ask for aid in dying? For one thing, not all suffering is the same; some is worse than others. Only the patients know how awful their own suffering is. Some may have beliefs, religious or otherwise, that override their desire to end their suffering. Some are afraid of the reactions of their families and their friends. Some do not want to disappoint or are not willing to risk the disapproval of their doctors or other caregivers. Others are embarrassed to ask for assistance or are afraid of stigma. I think that most hold dear what life they have and do not want to relinquish a drop of it. Experience thus far suggests that most people, sick or otherwise, will not choose to die. Certainly, that is one of the lessons of the rather benign Oregon experience. Some, few as they may be, find their suffering unendurable, and their cry for help should be met, as it has over the centuries, though in a spotty fashion and in a way that serves only a few and has been unfair to most. One of the lessons of Oregon has been that offering aid in dying has improved palliative care and concern with end-of-life treatment. Assisting a patient in dying is not an easy way out. Doctors' driving motivation is to help their patients, to relieve their suffering and make them better—and if cure is not possible, at least to make them feel better. Legal assistance in dying pushes physicians in that direction. Perhaps it will push governments into providing more training and palliative care opportunities.

When terminally ill patients request assistance in dying because of their suffering, and their request meets commonly endorsed safeguards, their request should be honored. Those who disagree on the basis of their own beliefs, religious or otherwise, should feel no compulsion to give aid in dying. I do not believe that palliative care or hospice programs should publicly support assisted death, because to do so might frighten some of their patients. This does not relieve individual physicians of the responsibility to help their suffering patients, even if that help includes assistance in dying when their suffering is unendurable and beyond relief.

Notes

1. F. Cohn and J. Lynn, "Vulnerable People: Practical Rejoinders to Claims in Favor of Assisted Suicide," in *The Case against Assisted Suicide: For the Right to End-of-Life Care,* edited by K. Foley and H. Hendin (Baltimore: Johns Hopkins University Press, 2002), 230–60.

2. E.J. Cassell, "The Nature of Suffering and the Goals of Medicine," *New England Journal of Medicine* 306 (1982): 639–45.

3. E.J. Cassell, *The Nature of Suffering and the Goals of Medicine* (New York: Oxford University Press, 2003 [second edition]), xxx.

4. P.D. Wall, *Pain: The Science of Suffering* (New York: Columbia University Press, 2000), viii.

5. Cassell, *Nature of Suffering and the Goals of Medicine.*

6. R. Twycross, "Palliative Care in the Past Decade and Today," *European Journal of Pain* 3 (1999): 23–29.

7. G.J. Amundson, J.L. Kuperos, and G.R. Norton, "Do Patients with Chronic Pain Selectively Attend to Pain-Related Information? Preliminary Evidence for the Mediating

Role of Fear," *Pain* 72 (1997): 27–32; P.D. Wall and R. Melzack, *Textbook of Pain* (Edinburgh: Churchill Livingstone, 1999).

8. R.V.J. Severeijns, M.A. van den Hout, and W.E. Weber, "Pain Catastrophizing Predicts Pain Intensity, Disability, and Psychological Disability Independent of the Level of Physical Impairment," *Clinical Journal of Pain* 17 (2001): 165–72.

9. B. Mount, personal communication, McGill University, Montreal, Canada, 2000.

10. M. Johnson, *The Body in the Mind* (Chicago: University of Chicago Press, 1997).

11. S. Daneault, V. Lussier, S. Mongeau, P. Paille, E. Hudon, D. Dion, and L. Yelle, "The Nature of Suffering and Its Relief in the Terminally Ill: A Qualitative Study," *Journal of Palliative Care* 20 (2004): 7–11.

12. M. Arman, A. Rhensfedt, L. Lindholm, and E. Hamrin, "The Face of Suffering among Women with Breast Cancer—Being in a Field of Forces," *Cancer Nursing* 25 (2002): 96–103.

PART TWO

Clinical, Philosophical, and Religious Issues about the Ending of Life

6

Why Do People Seek
Physician-Assisted Death?

Robert A. Pearlman, M.D., M.P.H.,
and Helene Starks, M.P.H., Ph.D.

Despite the illegality of physician-assisted death in the United States (except in the state of Oregon), many primary care providers and oncologists have been asked to provide aid in dying.[1] Popular explanations for physician-assisted death include inadequate treatment for pain or other symptoms, depression, hopelessness,[2] and socioeconomic stressors, such as concerns about the burden of increasing dependency on other members of the family and the economic hardship associated with the costs of health care.[3]

What motivates people to pursue physician-assisted death has proved to be both a controversial and a foundational issue in debates regarding the legality of and appropriate clinical response to requests for aid in dying. To date, insights regarding the motivations for assisted death have come largely from three sources: provider impressions, patients who transiently consider physician-assisted death or other means to end their lives under certain conditions, and forced-choice reporting (that is, responding to a checklist of reasons) from patients in Oregon who have pursued physician-assisted death. However, there has been limited direct reporting from patients about the motivation and process that lead them to pursue assisted death.

To address the current gaps in the understanding of physician-assisted death, we conducted a longitudinal, qualitative study of patients who seriously pursued assisted death and their family members.[4] The patients in our study lived an average of ten months between their first request for aid in dying and the time of death. Patients used this time to acquire the means to end their lives. For many, however, simply having medications did not result in their immediate use. These patients engaged in an ongoing evaluation of the value of living versus dying and repeatedly assessed the benefits and burdens of their current experience. Moreover, among the individuals in our study, the pursuit of physician-assisted death was not motivated by any single factor, nor was depression reported as a reason. Rather, the decision to hasten death culminated from an interaction of illness-related experiences, threats to the person's sense of self, and fears about the future.

The reports from these patients and their family members identified opportunities for improving palliative care that might have reduced patients' perceived need to choose aid in dying. However, these accounts also illustrate why a small number of patients will continue to view assisted death as a desirable choice. Some will decide that hospice and palliative care are not for them or that some of the choices offered by palliative care, such as the trade-off between pain management and cognitive function, are not acceptable ones. In addition, some issues, such as the desire to control the dying process and the suffering associated with a loss of sense of self, are not easily addressed even by the most capable health care providers.

"I Can't Do This Anymore"

When Anna was sixty-two years old she was diagnosed with metastatic ovarian cancer. Throughout her life, Anna was organized, energetic, and athletic. She was actively involved in community activities; she was a professional and an involved grandparent. About her illness she said, "I'm trying not to change my life and let cancer steal any more of it than it has to." She also expressed long-standing beliefs about having control over her life and death: "It should be up to me to decide . . . when I've had enough suffering. . . . If I'm at the point where all I can do is lie on a bed all day long, then to me that's probably not living anymore."

Over four years, Anna underwent multiple surgeries and rounds of chemotherapy and radiation. Many of her treatments were quite uncomfortable. She reported that she had been "deathly ill after every [chemotherapy] treatment, just not even able to read or barely even watch television. I would wake up in the morning with dry heaves and being incontinent and rolling out of bed so I wouldn't get the bed messed up. It was really wretched."

Anna talked to her family and sought medications for assisted death in the event she decided to hasten her death. Once she got them, she reported, "I felt I had more energy to fight the cancer and just to live in the present time. It just took a big weight off my shoulders somehow, knowing at least that that was one thing that maybe I didn't have to worry about." It was another three years before Anna used the medication to end her life.

During her illness Anna also experienced painful complications, including bowel obstruction and spinal cord compression. Despite enduring significant amounts of pain, Anna never cited this as the motivation for a hastened death. Her primary concern was that she would die in a hospital, "away from my home with familiar people and familiar surroundings and some privacy and some control."

After exhausting her anticancer treatment options, Anna became very weak, sleeping much of the day, and was unable to perform many of her routine functions. She started bleeding uncontrollably from her bowel as a late side effect of total abdominal radiation and was told that the only treatment was constant transfusions. She told her husband, "Honey, this is it. I can't do this anymore." Over the next thirty-six hours, Anna gathered her family together to say good-bye. She ingested the medication to hasten her death, with twelve loved ones in attendance, and died within two hours.

Factors Motivating Physician-Assisted Death

In our interviews with thirty-five families, we asked questions about the history of the patient's illness, the patient's stated reasons for seeking aid in dying, and other factors influencing the pursuit of physician-assisted death, as well as the manner of death. Our analysis identified nine common factors. No single factor on its own ever accounted for a serious interest in a hastened death. Rather, interest usually arose out of an interactive process involving multiple factors in three broad categories: illness-related experiences (symptoms, functional losses, effects of pain medication, and the like), threats to the person's sense of self (as revealed by his or her desire for control over the circumstances of dying and long-standing beliefs in favor of hastened death), and fears about the future. Table 6.1 presents our assessment of the frequency and importance of these factors in the patients' deliberations.

Illness-Related Experiences

Weakness, tiredness, and discomfort made up one set of motivating concerns for patients who sought aid in dying. Excellent end-of-life care can often ame-

Table 6.1. Motivations for Seeking a Hastened Death

Motivating Factor	Total Patients[a] (N = 35)
Illness-related experiences	
Feeling weak, tired, and uncomfortable	24 (69%)
Loss of function	23 (66%)
Pain or unacceptable side effects of pain medication	14 (40%)
Threats to sense of self	
Loss of sense of self	22 (63%)
Desire for control	21 (60%)
Long-standing beliefs in favor of hastened death	5 (14%)
Fears about the future	
Fears about future quality of life and dying	21 (60%)
Negative past experiences with dying	17 (49%)
Fear of being a burden on others	3 (9%)

Source: Data from R.A. Pearlman, C. Hsu, H. Starks, A.L. Back, J.R. Gordon, A.J. Bharucha, B.A. Koenig, and M.P. Battin, "Motivating Factors for the Pursuit of Physician-Assisted Suicide: Patient and Family Voices," unpublished manuscript.

Note: Motivating factors were rated independently by two investigators as to their role in influencing the pursuit of a hastened death. Four response categories were recorded: "not mentioned," "present but not judged to be influential," "influential," and "very influential." The table records response ratings inferred to be "influential" or "very influential" based on the reading of the transcripts.

[a]Total patients included prospective and retrospective cases. Prospective cases included patients and family members recruited while the patient was alive. Retrospective cases included only surviving family members recruited after the patient's death.

liorate these concerns. However, the functional losses caused by advanced illness are often less amenable to successful intervention, especially when the patient is dying. Approximately two-thirds of the patients in our study described the relation between symptoms brought on by illness and treatment and the resultant loss of function as considerations in their pursuit of assisted death. For example, a woman with ovarian cancer spoke of the effects of chemotherapy: "Of course, with me, with the chemo and things, [there's] just the terrible weakness and the nausea and just not feeling like you can do anything. . . . If it'd been like two weeks after and I was going out to do things—[but] you were still shaky, and you couldn't quite predict how you were going to feel, or you were afraid to make commitments because you weren't sure you were going to be able to carry them out." Physical symptoms often led to a lack of function. For example, one woman described her response to steroids for her chronic lung disease:

> My thighs are so weak I can't get up from the floor, and I don't have energy.
> . . . My arms are withering away. It's ridiculous. And also I take stuff with
> [prednisone] that gives me stomach problems, and I have bowel problems
> —there is no part of me that is functioning routinely. I'm very, very tired,
> and I cough a lot. My cough is worse when I talk a lot, and early in the
> morning it's horrible. I cough all this yucky stuff up and can't talk a lot.
> And I'm so weak, for example, that although I can drive a car, I find it just
> too much to lift my own oxygen tank up and in and out of the car. . . . So
> I'm not living; I'm existing.

Pain and the side effects of treatment for pain were another set of motivating issues for more than a third of the patients in our study. As others have argued, pain can be better managed with excellent end-of-life care.[5] However, the side effects of treatment, especially effects on cognition, will continue to be challenging. For some patients, these side effects are totally unacceptable, and feeling that they must choose between being pain free and being mentally competent creates the desire for another alternative—a hastened death. One woman described her mother's situation as follows:

> She was in a lot of pain. . . . What she feared more than the pain was the ef-
> fect that the pain drugs would have on her. . . . She didn't want to lose her
> rational mind. She didn't want to lose any of her personality or capacity. . . .
> Certainly, [she had a] fear of the pain increasing and causing her to have to
> take more medication . . . enough that she didn't really know what she was
> doing all the time or that she might start drooling or saying stupid things or
> coming across as drunk.

In another case, a man had metastases to his spine causing severe pain that was difficult to control, despite large doses of morphine. Hospice nurses had attempted to control his pain but ended up sedating him completely for twenty-four hours, which he found absolutely unacceptable. His wife told us,

> Pain was an extraordinary factor. He would go out and split kindling . . .
> and I kept saying, "I'm going to have more kindling than Carter has pills."
> And he says, "It gives me something to do, and if I have something to do, I
> don't have to think about how badly it hurts." Pain was an extreme factor
> . . . . and he was not a sissy, not at all. . . . [But] the morphine pump didn't
> do it. He was still taking Roxicet. . . . This had been going on for months,

and so by that time his body had built up a tremendous tolerance. . . . They could knock him out; he could be a vegetable; but that was not what he wanted. . . . If he couldn't function and at least think somewhat clearly, life wasn't worth it. And he did not want to leave me. He did everything possible to set me up, because he knew he was going to die. . . . There was no way you could stop that. And he did everything imaginable to make my life as easy as it could be. But it got to a point where the pain was just intolerable.

Threats to Sense of Self

The literature suggests, indirectly, that depression and hopelessness may motivate some patients to seek a hastened death.[6] However, acute depression was not judged to be an influential factor for any of our participants. The more common motivating issues of a psychological nature pertained to loss of control and sense of self (both experienced by nearly two-thirds of our patients). Most experts in end-of-life care acknowledge that redirecting the loss of sense of self in a dying patient is a daunting challenge and one that is rarely achieved. This form of suffering is profound and is related to losses in relational, social, and community involvement.[7] These losses affect not only what one can do but how one perceives oneself. One woman described her mother's response to progressive losses owing to an autoimmune disorder:

My mother was at age seventy-two before she got sick. She was still very energetic and vibrant, youthful and active and looked ten years younger than she was. And then when she got sick, she started losing her hair, and she became disfigured with this skin condition. . . . She would, literally, have spells when her muscles would be so bad that she would feel paralyzed, and she was in incredible fear of becoming paralyzed and becoming completely incapacitated and immobile. . . . [She wanted to have] control over her own dignity and her own independent life. The things that were meaningful to her in her life were her art, her ability to do her art, and her friends and spending time with her friends and cooking and eating. . . . She was . . . convinced that when she couldn't do any of those things anymore, her life would be meaningless, and she wouldn't want to live anymore.

In another example, a man described his mother's final sense of loss when she could no longer visit with her extensive network of family and friends:

She lost her appetite, her pleasure for food. She lost her strength to go outside and even having . . . people come over. She'd try. She hated to say no, they couldn't visit. . . . She wanted to, but a visit was a painful process. She just didn't have the strength or the concentration . . . to even visit with people anymore. . . . So basically, even having company is a strain, a pain to you, almost more than it's a pleasure to enjoy the people. And that was about the last thing she had left, was just sitting around and enjoying people, and . . . even that went away. Like she said, you get so sick of being sick and tired.

For most patients, sense of self is inextricably connected to ability to function. Moreover, the loss of sense of self creates appreciable anxiety. For example, one woman had metastases to the bone and was at risk for a spinal compression that would lead to paraplegia and incontinence. This functional loss represented more to her than just another accommodation to her illness. Her daughter explained the patient's view about her future:

> She saw this declining physical curve, and that at some point along that she was going to lose significant ability to be the person that she was. And she had already lost a lot—she couldn't go for the long hike anymore, . . . she couldn't go for the long walks, and now she wasn't supposed to work full time, and she was completely exhausted all the time, because she was working and taking care of her big house and all. So she had already seen some things go, and that was acceptable, but she knew at some point she'd be somewhere down on the curve [where] she had given up so many things that it wasn't okay. . . . Rather than wait to get there and have to figure out where that point was, she wanted to just die before it got any worse. And then when her spine started to go, of course, the big threat was losing control of her bowels, [which] was clearly not acceptable.

Fears about the Future

Fears about the future, including fears about the experience of dying, also motivate patients who seek to hasten death. Many of the patients projected that the course of their illness would result in a fate worse than death and preferred to end their lives before they reached this condition. Their judgments about this poor quality of life were often based on their own prognosis, accumulated losses, and fears of becoming a burden on others. For about half of our patients, their fears were also influenced by having witnessed loved ones go through terrible deaths involving pain, what they viewed as pointless use of medical technologies, and images of tubes coming out of every orifice. With better palliative and end-of-life care, fears like these should abate as people see others having better dying experiences. Nonetheless, even the best palliative care cannot prevent all functional losses and loss of sense of self, and thus for some, these fears will remain and motivate them to seek aid in dying.

Implications for End-of-Life Care

Several important implications for clinicians emerge from these case reports. First, that multiple interacting factors prompt patients to seek assisted death challenges health care providers, including those in palliative care, to understand patients' illness and dying experiences holistically. Our patients reported intricate and subtle interactions between physical and functional decline and existential concerns that could not be easily separated or compartmentalized. Our data confirm the familiar recommendation that providers repeatedly assess the patient's concerns about losses and dying in order to understand patients' concerns and tailor end-of-life care to the patient's evolving personal experience.

Second, these narrative accounts also demonstrate the importance to patients of their sense of self and of control over the manner of death. Clinicians need to be sensitive to these deeply personal psychological and existential issues and differentiate them from clinical depression. Although it is important to determine whether depression is driving a request for assisted death, it is equally important to examine other psychological processes.

Finally, the factors that motivate an interest in assisted death are similar to those that prompt people to complete advance directives and forgo life-sustaining treatment: the desire to control the timing and circumstance of one's death.[8] Many people view assisted death as another option that should be available at the end of life. The topics identified in Table 6.1 can serve as a guide in talking to patients about the far-reaching effects of illness, including the quality of the dying experience. Clinicians should explore patients' fears and how they see themselves in light of current and future physical decline and functional losses. Clinicians frequently shut down discussion about aid in dying and, in so doing, thwart opportunities for understanding patients' responses to their dying experience. Instead, clinicians must explore the motivations for these patients' interest in this option and identify ways to ameliorate their suffering.[9] For some patients, however, the amelioration of suffering will come only with death, and these patients may be unwilling to endure a prolonged dying process.

Our study suggests that some dying patients will continue to desire a hastened death in spite of excellent palliative end-of-life care. Some suffering cannot be relieved and will continue or worsen. The question that must be asked is, Are we as a society sufficiently compassionate to allow the choice of a hastened death to terminally ill, competent patients who are receiving state-of-the-art end-of-life care but are still suffering?

Appendix

We interviewed two cohorts of participants: patients who were seriously pursuing physician-assisted suicide and members of their families, and surviving family members of deceased individuals who had seriously pursued or received aid in dying. With the approval of the Human Subjects Division of the University of Washington, we recruited participants through intermediaries, including advocacy organizations that counsel people interested in physician-assisted suicide, hospices, and grief counselors.

Several concerns arise in carrying out research in this context, particularly around participants' decision-making capacity, the sensitive nature of the information collected, and the professional obligations of clinician-researchers. We screened prospective participants to ensure that they were not severely psychiatrically impaired and could competently consent to participate in the study. We also put in place procedures to refer individuals back to the intermediary through which they had been recruited if, during the course of our interview, concerns arose about their capacity.

Physician-assisted suicide is illegal in Washington state, and the possibility that data we collected could be used to incriminate family members, health care providers, and others who assisted a patient with a hastened death was a concern. We took several measures to protect participants' privacy and confidentiality: We asked participants to give oral assent to participate, rather than have them sign a written consent document, and we did not retain any written records containing identifying information. We also edited any identifying content out of interview transcripts and erased all audiotapes of interviews.

Finally, we addressed the question of whether there was a potential role conflict for us as clinicians-researchers: Did we have a professional or legal obligation to warn or intervene to prevent a harm—in this case, the hastened death? The ongoing professional and public debate about the philosophical and ethical questions posed by assisted suicide indicates that there is no settled consensus. In our judgment, after ensuring that participants had capacity, we did not believe that our roles as clinician-researchers carried any duty to warn or to intervene in a patient's decision making.

Notes

1. D.J. Doukas, D. Waterhouse, D.W. Gorenflo, and J. Seid, "Attitudes and Behaviors on Physician-Assisted Death: A Study of Michigan Oncologists," *Journal of Clinical Oncology* 13 (1995): 1055–61; D.E. Meier, C.A. Emmons, S. Wallenstein, T.E. Quill, R.S. Morrison, and C.K. Cassel, "A National Survey of Physician-Assisted Suicide and Euthanasia in the United States," *New England Journal of Medicine* 338 (1998): 1193–1201; E.J. Emanuel, D.L. Fairclough, B.R. Clarridge, D. Blum, E. Breera, W.C. Penley, L.E. Schnipper, and R.J. Mayer, "Attitudes and Practices of U.S. Oncologists Regarding Euthanasia and Physician-Assisted Suicide," *Annals of Internal Medicine* 133 (2000): 527–32.

2. E.J. Emanuel, D.L. Fairclough, E.R. Daniels, and B.R. Clarridge, "Euthanasia and Physician-Assisted Suicide: Attitudes and Experiences of Oncology Patients, Oncologists, and the Public," *Lancet* 347 (1996): 1805–10; K.M. Foley, "Competent Care for the Dying Instead of Physician-Assisted Suicide," *New England Journal of Medicine* 336 (1997): 54–58; T.E. Quill, D.E. Meier, S.D. Block, and J.A. Billings, "The Debate over Physician-Assisted Suicide: Empirical Data and Convergent Views," *Annals of Internal Medicine* 128 (1998): 552–58; H.M. Chochinov, K.G. Wilson, M. Enns, and S. Lander, "Depression, Hopelessness, and Suicidal Ideation in the Terminally Ill," *Psychosomatics* 39 (1998): 366–70; L. Ganzini, W.S. Johnston, B.H. McFarland, S.W. Tolle, and M.A. Lee, "Attitudes of Patients with Amyotrophic Lateral Sclerosis and Their Care Givers toward Assisted Suicide," *New England Journal of Medicine* 339 (1998): 967–73; W. Breitbart, B. Rosenfeld, H. Pessin, M. Kaim, J. Funesti-Esch, M. Galietta, C.J. Nelson, and R. Brescia, "Depression, Hopelessness, and Desire for Hastened Death in Terminally Ill Patients with Cancer," *Journal of the American Medical Association* 284 (2000): 2907–11.

3. Emanuel, Fairclough, Clarridge, et al., "Attitudes and Practices of U.S. Oncologists Regarding Euthanasia and Physician-Assisted Suicide"; M.E. Suarez-Almazor, M. Belzile, and E. Bruera, "Euthanasia and Physician-Assisted Suicide: A Comparative Survey of Physicians, Terminally Ill Cancer Patients, and the General Population," *Journal of Clinical Oncology* 15 (1997): 418–27.

4. R.A. Pearlman, C. Hsu, H. Starks, A.L. Back, J.R. Gordon, A.J. Bharucha, B.A. Koenig, and M.P. Battin, "Motivating Factors for the Pursuit of Physician-Assisted Suicide: Patient and Family Voices," unpublished manuscript.

5. M.J. Field and C.K. Cassel, eds., *Approaching Death: Improving Care at the End of Life* (Washington, D.C.: National Academy Press, 1997); R.S. Morrison, A.L. Siu, R.M. Leipzig, C.K. Cassel, and D.E. Meier, "The Hard Task of Improving the Quality of Care at the End of Life," *Archives of Internal Medicine* 160 (2000): 743–47; D.E. Meier, "United States: Overview of Cancer Pain and Palliative Care," *Journal of Pain and Symptom Management* 24 (2002): 265–69.

6. Emanuel, Fairclough, Daniels, et al., "Euthanasia and Physician-Assisted Suicide"; Quill et al., The Debate over Physician-Assisted Suicide: Empirical Data and Convergent Views"; Chochinov et al., "Depression, Hopelessness, and Suicidal Ideation in the Terminally Ill"; Ganzini et al., "Attitudes of Patients with Amyotrophic Lateral Sclerosis and Their Care Givers toward Assisted Suicide"; Breitbart et al., "Depression, Hope-

lessness, and Desire for Hastened Death in Terminally Ill Patients with Cancer"; S.D. Block and J.A. Billings, "Patient Requests to Hasten Death: Evaluation and Management in Terminal Care," *Archives of Internal Medicine* 154 (1994): 2039–47; E.J. Emanuel, D.L. Fairclough, and L.L. Emanuel, "Attitudes and Desires Related to Euthanasia and Physician-Assisted Suicide among Terminally Ill Patients and Their Caregivers," *Journal of the American Medical Association* 284 (2000): 2460–68.

7. J.V. Lavery, J. Boyle, B.M. Dickens, H. Maclean, and P.A. Singer, "Origins of the Desire for Euthanasia and Assisted Suicide in People with HIV-1 or AIDS: A Qualitative Study," *Lancet* 358 (2001): 362–67.

8. R.A. Pearlman, K.C. Cain, D.L. Patrick, H.E. Starks, M. Applebaum-Maezel, N.S. Jecker, and R.F. Uhlmann, "Insights Pertaining to Patient Assessments of States Worse Than Death," *Journal of Clinical Ethics* 4 (1993): 33–41.

9. A.L. Back, H. Starks, C. Hsu, J.R. Gordon, A. Bharucha, and R.A. Pearlman, "Clinician-Patient Interactions about Requests for Physician-Assisted Suicide: A Patient and Family View," *Archives of Internal Medicine* 162 (2002): 1257–65.

7

Doctor-Patient Communication about Physician-Assisted Suicide

Anthony L. Back, M.D.

For physicians and other clinicians who care for patients with life-threatening illness, the ability to respond to a patient's request for physician-assisted suicide is an important clinical skill. Although Oregon is the only state to have legalized assisted suicide, patients and physicians discuss it nationwide.[1] In a national survey involving 988 terminally ill patients, 60 percent of patients supported physician-assisted suicide in a hypothetical situation, and 10 percent reported they had seriously considered assisted suicide for themselves.[2] In physician surveys, 18–24 percent of primary care physicians and 46–57 percent of oncologists state that they have received a request for aid in dying.[3]

How should a clinician respond to a patient request for assisted suicide? Experts agree on some initial steps: the clinician should ask why the patient is interested in assisted suicide, explore the meanings underlying the request, assess whether palliative care is adequate (especially in addressing depression), and revise the care plan to respond to the patient's concerns. These steps enable clinicians to respond to patient requests regardless of whether the request will persist and regardless of the clinicians' personal beliefs.[4] Beyond this initial response, however, there is controversy about whether the clinician should disclose his or her own moral beliefs about assisted suicide, offer sedation for refractory symptoms or intolerable suffering, or provide a prescription for lethal medication in a state where physician-assisted suicide is illegal.[5]

Expert recommendations for responding to requests for assisted suicide presume that clinicians possess communication skills and palliative care expertise,[6] but little empirical research has been conducted to identify exactly what skills and expertise are required. To date, surveys of physicians indicate that the expertise most relevant to the issue of assisted suicide is the clinician's ability to address nonphysical concerns about dying, such as loss of control and loss of dignity.[7] One qualitative study suggests that the most difficult task for physicians is addressing their patients' existential suffering.[8]

To explore the question of doctor-patient communication around physician-assisted suicide, my colleagues and I conducted an intensive qualitative interview study of patients who seriously had pursued assisted suicide and members of their families.[9] Our primary objectives were to describe the patient's reasons for pursuing assisted suicide, the narrative of events leading to death, and the patient's and family's interactions with physicians and other clinicians. Chapter 6 in this volume addresses patients' motivations for requesting aid in dying. This chapter reports our findings about interactions with clinicians. We asked our subjects to describe their conversations with their physicians and other medical clinicians about assisted suicide. From these data, we identified qualities of clinician-patient interactions that patients and family members valued. In describing these qualities, we hope to provide guidance for clinicians faced with these difficult conversations, regardless of their individual willingness to provide such assistance or its legal status.

Broaching the Topic

Physicians' openness to discussion about assisted suicide was a major theme. Patients and family members highly valued clinicians who were willing to discuss assisted suicide, but many found their own clinicians unwilling to do so. When they encountered a clinician who was willing to discuss assisted suicide, they were able to disclose many of their concerns about dying. They recognized their good fortune because they knew the topic was controversial. As one family member put it, what she wanted was "another sane adult" who could "talk in terms . . . that remove the taboo from the process," giving "a real, clear picture of possible approaches without advocating [physician-assisted suicide]." A counterexample underscores the importance to patients of clinician's openness to discussing assisted suicide: "The conversations were a struggle with [our physician] because we couldn't talk about hastening the death. So there was . . . a part of us that we could not talk about, which made our questions limited. . . . We didn't have access to information that would have allowed our conversations to be more full and more fully informed."

Patients and family members attributed clinicians' reluctance to discuss assisted suicide to a variety of reasons. Some clinicians were unwilling to consider aid in dying because the practice was illegal. These clinicians behaved as if discussions of assisted suicide in and of themselves were illegal and dangerous. One patient observed that "all [my physicians] talk about is the legality of it"; another concluded that clinicians "have to hide their feelings about [assisted suicide], so as not to jeopardize their careers."

In other cases, patients and family members reported that the topic of assisted suicide provoked a strong emotional response from clinicians that made further conversation awkward. One family member described a neurologist as "adamant that [physician-assisted suicide] was a terrible thing and the wrong thing to do. . . . [The conversation] was kind of awful." A patient said that her oncologist became "really uncomfortable" talking about assisted suicide or "anything" about dying, so she would change the subject for his sake. She said, "I learned that he's a baseball fan and much more comfortable if I change the topic to baseball. . . . It's awful when you have to try to make them feel comfortable, but that's the way it is." Other patients reported that clinicians seemed to want to maintain a biomedical focus. One family member of a different patient said, "They won't talk to you about [assisted suicide] even as a possibility. It's like, 'I know that happens, but—what about let's do the chemotherapy.'"

Others said that physicians indicated they would discuss assisted suicide only indirectly. A family member reported that her mother's physician "did lower himself to tell me, if it was Valium, how much she would need" but that "his reaction at the end" was to say that "we never had this conversation." "He was protective [of himself]," she recalled, "not at all sympathetic or comforting."

Patients also faced internal barriers to communicating about assisted suicide. They were fearful of how their providers might react if they raised the topic. One patient, hoping to discuss assisted suicide with one of her physicians, found it was "really a scary thing to try to guess" which doctor to approach. "I . . . went in with fear and trembling. . . . It's a real crap shoot." Patients were also reluctant to admit to vulnerability caused by disease. As one patient put it, "Even though I talk a lot, I do keep a lot of this inner stuff very hidden. . . . They think I'm an incredibly feisty, tough lady . . . and I don't want that image changed."

Exploring Patient Concerns

As chapter 6 indicates, most patients who seriously pursue physician-assisted suicide have more than one concern, and many have lifelong beliefs about the importance of maintaining control over their own lives. Clinician openness to discussing assisted suicide was fundamental to the exploration of patient concerns. Patients felt that a clinician willing to talk about assisted suicide might also be willing to discuss other worries, fears, and vulnerabilities about illness and dying. As one patient said, "Everything was laid out on the table. Oh, you bet, yeah. Because he can't help you—nobody can help you—if they don't know what's going on in your life."

In a different case, a family member described how her father's relationship with the caseworker from an advocacy organization provided a different dimension of care from that by his oncologist. The family member said, "It provided a place where he could talk about his illness. He didn't talk about hastening his death [because he was prepared and did not think it was time]. He's just describing to them what's going on with him and so on. But it's good to have a place like that." Thus patients may use discussion of assisted suicide as a gateway to talking about dying: "It's not that [my friend, the patient] doesn't want to [talk about dying]; that's the sad thing. She's sitting here holding all of this stuff in, and to me the most important events in your life are your transitions, your birth and your death . . . the beginning and the end of this physical existence. But you can't talk to your doctor about it without them getting all weird, [thinking] that you're suicidal or something." During her own interview, this patient wept as she described her frustration trying to talk to one of her doctors. She said, "You're trying to get a doctor to sit down and listen to you . . . but they never, ever get the overall picture." Her clinicians' unwillingness to discuss assisted suicide resulted in missed opportunities to connect with this patient's deepest concerns, which included her quality of life, her prognosis, and her suffering.

Talking about Palliative Care and the Dying Process

One important type of clinician expertise is the ability to describe the natural history of illness and palliative care options in the last days of life. In their survey of Oregon patients, Maria Silveira and her colleagues found a substantial degree of misunderstanding about withholding life-sustaining treatment and hastening death.[10] In our study, patients and families were sensitive to the ways in which clinicians talked—or avoided talking—about these issues. A woman with metastatic ovarian cancer found that she could not get information from her oncologist about how she would die, so she went to a medical library and read a textbook on gynecologic cancer. What she learned was that the dying process from ovarian cancer was "long, protracted, not very happy. . . . [There are] organ failures or blockages or blood poisoning or pneumonia, and it takes a whole combination of things to finally just be fatal." Although she confronted her oncologist with this information, she left without reassurance that she could avoid a long, agonizing death. "I would say, what happens if I stop treatment? How awful is this going to be?" but she never got a direct answer. She sought out another physician, who told her, "You don't have long . . . and it's going to be rough . . . [and] I can't help you." She concluded that physician-assisted suicide was probably the least worst way for her to die. Another patient was told by his physician that in "all the AIDS cases in the city, [his] was the worst thrush they'd ever seen." His partner reported that

> our doctor [said], . . . "you do not want to die of thrush," and then kind of described how it would happen. . . . Basically, he said the thrush would grow and shut off your esophagus, so that you'd not be able to swallow. . . . [My partner] would drool constantly and end up starving to death, because he wouldn't be able to pass any food down. The doctor said, "You don't want to die like that." And that's when [my partner] decided to do a hastened death."

The patient and his partner interpreted the physician's statements, which did not include a medical response to fears of drooling and starving to death, as a tacit endorsement of physician-assisted suicide as the best option in their circumstances. The patient had already been considering assisted suicide, but this conversation marked a turning point in his interest.

Another valued type of palliative care expertise is the ability to define reasonable expectations about dying and then deliver the care needed to fulfill those expectations. One woman with lung cancer was suspicious of doctors and hospitals and believed that "cancer is big business." She declined anticancer therapies but was willing to explore palliative care options. Her physician referred her to hospice, and her experience with them made her rethink her commitment to physician-assisted suicide:

> Before Thanksgiving, I went over to the hospice [an inpatient unit] for respite care. It's a wonderful place. It's absolutely wonderful. Unlike a hospital, you don't see any uniforms; you are not No. 14 or No. 12; you are a person. The only thing that resembles a hospital is the bed and the tray table. Outside of that, there is absolutely nothing that resembles a hospital. There is no noise of anyone being in pain. It's wonderful; it really is. [My] main concern is to be pain free, and they do take care of that.

She ultimately died of progressive cancer, at home with hospice care.

Another case of a patient with advanced AIDS exemplifies what can happen when clinicians over-promise a "pain-free" death:

> The physician encouraged [stopping total parenteral nutrition] as a nice way to go and said that that would be probably a three-week process, maybe four at the most, but probably three. "That's a very pleasant way to die. It's pain-free." . . . We went in and out of the emergency room three times over pain in the last two weeks of his life . . . and he had great, agonizing, lower abdominal pain through it all. So I felt real cheated about that. It wasn't this quiet, pain-free existence. . . . If you're going to make a guarantee that a person is really not going to be in pain, you need to make sure that they're not. And if you don't think that you can make sure, you shouldn't promise.

When dying proved to be neither quiet nor pain free, the patient and his partner began to plan a physician-assisted suicide.

A third type of expertise is individualizing pain control to meet patient goals. In one case, the absence of this expertise led to a death by self-inflicted gunshot. The patient had painful bony metastases to his spine and was "on 800 milligrams of morphine a day—besides all the Roxicet he could manage to keep down." His oncologist referred him to hospice for better pain management. However, the patient and his wife found that their hospice providers had an agenda about pain control that did not allow for the fact that his top priority was to maintain a sense of control over his situation:

> They put him on a morphine pump. It took him a couple of days to adjust it, and they were extremely caring. They hovered. They just about drove him up the wall. [They said,] "We're going to kill your pain." Well, they killed his pain. He was unconscious for almost twenty-four hours. Flat on his back. He had not been able to lay on his back. He was totally out of it. He got up the next day and he said, "I feel like Ray Milland's *Lost Weekend*." [That movie was about] an alcoholic who just went through all sorts of, just, DTs and, you know, it just—really hell on wheels. And that's exactly how my husband felt. He said, "I can't think; I can't do this."

The next morning, the patient fired the hospice and discontinued the pain regimen. "Once the hospice people had knocked him for one loop, he wasn't going to let it happen again," explained his wife. The following day, the patient warned his wife not to follow him outside, where he positioned himself out of sight and shot himself in the head. The hospice nurse wrote in her bereavement card, "At least he got one good night's sleep"—to which his wife responded, "I almost went through the ceiling."

Discussing Beliefs about Physician-Assisted Suicide

Most patients in our study were reluctant to describe details of what they remembered their physicians saying about assisted suicide because of concerns about confidentiality; however, it is apparent from our transcripts that a subset of physicians explicitly disclosed their beliefs about aid in dying. These data indicate that patients are generally respectful of physicians' moral beliefs about assisted suicide and that mismatch between physician and patient beliefs does not necessarily end the doctor-patient relationship:

> My internist simply will not do [physician-assisted suicide], not just because of fear of the law [but] because his approach is he will not end life. . . . I adore my internist, who, when he had more time, used to make house visits to see [my husband when he was dying] and pep him up. Wonderful. So I love this guy; I really do, even though I disagree with him on this issue. I love him, and I respect him as a doctor.

Other patients described clinicians who avoided discussing assisted suicide openly or explicitly, even though they were willing to provide medications for it. In these cases, the clinicians fulfilled requests for assisted suicide with little evaluation: "My husband, with the advice of a doctor friend that lives in [another state], went to his cardiologist . . . and he told the doctor that he needed Seconal. . . . This doctor has known my husband for a long time, and all he said was, 'I trust you have a good reason,' and gave it to him, a prescription for it." In this case, a family member obtained a prescription for assisted suicide from a physician who had never met the patient. This is an extreme example but not unique. Two other patients in our study obtained prescriptions without any medical evaluation. In one of these cases, a family member found that after a visit with the patient's oncologist, the necessary prescriptions had been tucked into her purse without her knowledge.

Negotiating Responsibilities and Boundaries

The Oregon Death with Dignity Act explicitly describes some physician responsibilities when caring for patients who decide to proceed with assisted suicide. When physician-assisted suicide is performed illegally, as in most of the cases in our study, the agreements between doctors and patients about responsibility are usually tacit. Every patient and family member in this study recognized that asking for physician-assisted suicide was a special request that went beyond the usual boundaries of a clinician-patient relationship. Patients were sensitive to subtle ways in which physicians defined their commitment to the doctor-patient relationship:

> The lung guy is very young. He's cute as hell. I like him, but I don't have any emotional involvement with him at all. . . . I wouldn't think of [asking him for assisted suicide]. It would overstep the boundaries of our relationship completely, and he wouldn't do it. . . . It's just not appropriate. I don't have that kind of relationship with him. He's a technician that came in at the last minute, and he does his thing. It [would be] as if I asked a plumber.

When physicians were willing to assist in some way, the patients and family members in our study were relieved and reassured. Even when physicians were willing to assist illegally, the patient, family, and physician sometimes colluded to avoid explicit discussion of medication use. "I'm sure that the doctor realizes what [this prescription for secobarbital] is for," said one family member. "If you say to the doctor 'I need this pill,' and you tell him the next month that you need another thirty-day supply, that's how you stockpile your supply." This sort of collusion keeps the request for physician-assisted suicide in the background but not out of sight. As one family member recalled, "I think [the hospice nurse] knew what we were planning, because she said as she was leaving, 'Now I hope by the time I get to the end of the road, I get a call from you.' . . . And I think she was saying, 'Do whatever you're going to do now.'"

Perhaps because discussion about physician-assisted suicide is often absent or not explicit, many patients and families got little support or instruction beyond the prescription provided by physicians. One example of indirect instruction was given by a physician who said, as he was writing out a prescription for morphine and diazepam, "I'm going to give you a prescription for a hundred each of these; more than fifty would kill you." Other patients and families, however, received information and support from community organizations about assisted suicide.

Yet even clinicians who declined to participate could still maintain an important relationship with a patient and family member if they were able to set clear boundaries about their role. One physician told a family that he had great sympathy for the patient, would provide medical records and medication for pain and symptoms, but was not able to provide a prescription for a lethal dose of barbiturates. The family felt this physician was supportive and had acted appropriately, within his "comfort zone," to help the patient; they called the physician soon after the death to reassure him that things had gone smoothly.

One case illustrates the importance of clinicians' self-awareness of emotional needs and vulnerabilities in maintaining a therapeutic relationship. The physician in this case, as a family member put it, "lacked boundaries." The physician had a reputation for extraordinary dedication and sensitivity and developed an intense relationship with the patient, including daily phone calls, home visits, and long discussions about assisted suicide. A family member said, "I didn't think it was healthy, but [the patient] needed it." After a two-year relationship, the physician was willing to prescribe the medication needed for assisted suicide and be responsible for a backup plan if the medication failed. She was present on the night the patient attempted suicide by using the medication. When the patient's ingestion of medications failed, the physician implemented the backup plan—placing a plastic bag over the patient's head. Following the patient's death, the family member reported that "[the physician] would go over to the hospital to see a patient, and she'd call me at ten o'clock [at night] and say she wanted to come over [to our house] and sit in the room where he died and 'hang out.' And I'd say no, and [the physician] would come over anyway." After a couple of these incidents, the family member wrote the physician requesting that they have no further contact because he felt burdened by these requests; he felt that the physician "really misbehaved, big time."

Technical Competence in Hastening Death

A final type of expertise involves clinicians' knowledge about the lethal potential of medications. When clinicians had this knowledge and were willing to provide a prescription for purposes of assisted suicide, patients and families in our study were reassured that if they ultimately decided to implement the assisted suicide, they would be successful. As one family member said,

> The psychiatrist that [my husband] saw said that he didn't understand why my husband needed to be in hell anymore, or myself, and that he was seeing that a lot had been tried, and he thought that [my husband] should be able to end his life if he wanted. So he began prescribing the correct pills. . . .
> When he had [the prescription], I remember there was just a huge relief on both of our parts and deep gratefulness to that person.

In other cases, patients or family members received instructions from clinicians to increase doses of morphine and diazepam to hasten death. One family member recalled that a hospice nurse, with explicit instructions from the physician, taught him how to unlock a patient-controlled intravenous analgesia device and administer a lethal dose of morphine. "They told us that within three to four hours his heart would stop and it would be over. . . . Very specific. And we were never told any alternative. We were never told it might not work. . . . And of course, it didn't work." After twelve hours, the patient woke up, and his partner spent days frantically searching for information and support. The family member called the physician and hospice nurse for help, but "when I asked what went wrong, they had no idea." The patient finally came up with the idea of dissolving secobarbital tablets in saline and injecting the solution intravenously. In another case, a physician who did anticipate medication failure instructed a family member to use meat tenderizer purchased at a grocery store to prepare a lethal intravenous injection.

The Moment of Death

The importance of the physician's capacity to be present with complex emotions is also evident at the bedside of patients who are actively dying as a result of assisted suicide. One physician who volunteered to be present at an assisted suicide was unable to conceal awkward feelings. The family member recalled that he "didn't do anything. He just kind of showed up and sort of said, 'Oh, gosh, look, he's still alive; what a surprise.'" In contrast, physicians who could contribute to an appropriate bedside environment were prized. One family member described a physician who carefully reconfirmed a patient's wishes at the bedside in a way that left open the possibility of changing her mind without loss of face. "He was so gentle. . . . If I had it to do it over again, I can't think of a doctor I would rather have involved. He handled it in such a dignified and kind way."

Some patients ritualized their deaths in ways that provided closure for themselves and their families, and in most instances their physicians were unaware of these rituals. One patient assembled four generations of her family, sat with them in a circle, and led a carefully planned good-bye ritual that included readings, singing favorite songs, listening to specific pieces of music, and finally eating yogurt—the patient's portion laced with lethal medication. This patient left behind photo albums, with thousands of pictures of family life, that she had organized in preparation for her death and a personal letter to each family member, to be opened after her death. Although this did not result from doctor-patient communication, it exemplifies an opportunity for life closure that doctors may wish to raise with patients in discussions about dying.

Preparing Family Members for the Aftermath

In our study, family members were involved to varying degrees in planning and implementing a patient's assisted death and in after-death logistics. Family members were most involved when the attempt failed or when a planned euthanasia was implemented. Although most family members supported their loved one's choice about hastening death, they often experienced ambivalence. They appreciated the deep emotional intimacy engendered by discussion about dying and physician-assisted suicide yet often had to deal with difficult and unexpected events when the patient's plans were implemented. Finally, the need to maintain secrecy had an enduring impact on family members. Strikingly, none of the family members in our data set recalled physicians' preparing them for what could follow their loved one's hastened death, and several suggested that having some preparatory knowledge of what to expect would have been helpful. Family members, in retrospect, wished they'd had information about dealing with their grief and possibly guilt, the difficulty of maintaining secrecy, and the need for backup plans in case of medication failure. This suggests another communication opportunity for physicians who care for patients who decide to pursue physician-assisted suicide.

Improving Doctor-Patient Communication about Aid in Dying

The literature on communication about physician-assisted suicide has focused on how physicians should respond to these requests.[11] Existing recommendations stress the importance of clarifying the request, exploring the reasons underlying it, emphasizing that the patient will not be abandoned, and providing excellent palliative care. Taken in the context of other studies, the data presented here indicate some additional important lessons in doctor-patient communication about physician-assisted suicide. First, aid in dying may be a patient concern that is often blocked by physicians. Our finding that clinicians displayed varying degrees of openness to discussion about assisted suicide, and about broader discussions of dying, as well, leads us to wonder whether published surveys of physicians actually underestimate the degree to which patients wish to talk about assisted suicide. When physicians say that their patients never ask about it, that may be because the physicians themselves block the discussion. Peter Maguire has described how clinicians block and avoid cancer patients' concerns about dying.[12] Our data suggest that some physicians behave similarly with regard to assisted suicide.

For some patients, talking about physician-assisted suicide may be a starting point for discussions about death and dying. In a medical culture that views death as a failure, dying patients may feel that they have failed.[13] Assisted suicide provides a different kind of end-of-life story for patients, one that emphasizes individual values and personal choice;[14] data about experience under Oregon's Death with Dignity Act underscore the importance of autonomy for patients who choose physician-assisted suicide.[15] Our data indicate that assisted suicide can serve as the starting point for discussions that go beyond the right to die to explore concerns about dying. Recognizing this can enable clinicians to probe beyond the issue of assisted suicide. In addition to asking, "Why are you considering assisted suicide?" physicians should ask, "What is happening now that leads you to think about assisted suicide?" and "What has your family said about your desire to consider assisted suicide?"

The timing of when in the course of illness the patient first raises the topic of physician-assisted suicide may provide some indication as to how quickly he or she will implement a plan for assisted death. Kohlwes and his colleagues interviewed twenty physicians who had experience with requests for assisted suicide.[16] These physicians distinguished between early and late requests. When requests occurred early in the disease process, physicians felt that the primary reasons for the discussion of assisted suicide were related to patients' fears of the dying process. Physicians felt these early requests were generally exploratory rather than serious. One physician noted,

> In my experience, the people that ask it [early] usually aren't serious about it. . . . It's usually not someone who's imminently planning to end their life; they just want to talk about it and find out what my thoughts are, so we'll discuss what might happen to them when they are really ill or dying and how to control symptoms. . . . But I can't think of somebody who's asked early on who's really been in the planning stages to do it.

This is quite consistent with our finding that assisted suicide can be a starting point for talking about dying.

Kohlwes also identifies the question, "Why do you want to die now?" as a way of exploring the issues underlying the request for assisted suicide. As one of his physician respondents noted, the question, "Why now?"

> leads to all kinds of things. It leads you to, "I don't like the pain regimen that you've come up with." "I don't like the drugs I'm taking." "I'm

depressed." It leads you to, "My family is getting tired of taking care of me," or "I don't want to be a burden to my family," or "I can't afford the care"; or it leads you to "I'm overwhelmingly guilty about being gay," or having cancer, or whatever. It leads you to any number of places. Then you have some opportunities to talk about it or even to do something about it.

In dealing with a request for aid in dying, a therapeutic relationship between patient and doctor may be as important as a prescription for physician-assisted suicide. The combination of openness to discussions about assisted suicide and expertise in dealing with the dying process are what make a continued clinician-patient relationship possible when a patient pursues a hastened death. Our data suggest that even for this highly selected group, a therapeutic relationship may be even more important to patients interested in assisted suicide and their family members than a lethal prescription. When the patients in our study approached their clinicians about assisted suicide, they were usually looking for more than just a prescription. They were looking for someone with whom they could build a therapeutic alliance—a person who could act as a sounding board or guide them through the dying process. Although several existing guidelines for responding to requests for assisted suicide address the request as a single event, our data emphasize the importance of the process of responding to a request over time in the context of a clinician-patient relationship. As part of building an authentic relationship, it may also be important for physicians to choose a time to disclose their own beliefs about assisted suicide. Disclosure should be made at a time when patients would be least likely to interpret it as rejection of their concern or abandonment.

Clinicians responding to requests for assisted suicide should be mindful of their own boundaries. Our data show that clinician underinvolvement and overinvolvement can both be problematic in dealing with patients requesting aid in dying. These behaviors may reflect the clinician's personal emotions. Based on clinical experience and a careful reading of psychological and psychiatric literature, Block and Billings and Miles have outlined how the personal emotions of clinicians might influence their behavior in dealing with a patient considering assisted suicide.[17] For clinicians, these issues of personal emotion, which may include self-awareness, boundaries, and transference or countertransference, require attention because they can facilitate or complicate the clinical relationship.[18] Our findings reinforce other work noting how important it is for clinicians to monitor their own feelings and establish boundaries in their relationships with patients.[19]

Finally, clinicians should be mindful of the impact of assisted suicide on family members and should include them in discussions about it with the patient as they unfold. After an assisted suicide, family members should be screened for signs of complicated grief. They may need special counseling because commonly available bereavement groups may not be appropriate forums in which to discuss the events surrounding a hastened death. Physician-assisted suicide may place family members at risk for disenfranchised grief.

The conversations about assisted suicide that doctors and their patients engage in often touch the core of what it means to be a physician and what it means to die. In the midst of the controversy surrounding physician aid in dying, these discussions can provide a rich meeting point for both physicians and patients.

Notes

1. A.E. Chin, K. Hedberg, G.K. Higginson, and D.W. Fleming, "Legalized Physician-Assisted Suicide in Oregon—The First Year's Experience," *New England Journal of Medicine* 340 (1999): 577–83; D.E. Meier, C.A. Emmons, S. Wallenstein, T.E. Quill, R.S. Morrison, and C.K. Cassel, "A National Survey of Physician-Assisted Suicide and Euthanasia in the United States," *New England Journal of Medicine* 338 (1998): 1193–201.

2. E.J. Emanuel, D.L. Fairclough, and L.L. Emanuel, "Attitudes and Desires Related to Euthanasia and Physician-Assisted Suicide among Terminally Ill Patients and Their Caregivers," *Journal of the American Medical Association* 284 (2000): 2460–68.

3. Emanuel et al., "Attitudes and Desires Related to Euthanasia and Physician-Assisted Suicide among Terminally Ill Patients and Their Caregivers"; A.L. Back, J.I. Wallace, H.E. Starks, and R.A. Pearlman, "Physician-Assisted Suicide and Euthanasia in Washington State: Patient Requests and Physician Responses," *Journal of the American Medical Association* 275 (1996): 919–25; E.J. Emanuel, D.L. Fairclough, E.R. Daniels, and B.R. Clarridge, "Euthanasia and Physician-Assisted Suicide: Attitudes and Experiences of Oncology Patients, Oncologists, and the Public," *Lancet* 347 (1996): 1805–10.

4. K.M. Foley, "Competent Care for the Dying Instead of Physician-Assisted Suicide," *New England Journal of Medicine* 336 (1997): 54–58; L.L. Emanuel, "Facing Requests for Physician-Assisted Suicide: Toward a Practical and Principled Clinical Skill Set," *Journal of the American Medical Association* 280 (1998): 643–47; T.E. Quill, C.K. Cassel, and D.E. Meier, "Care of the Hopelessly Ill: Proposed Clinical Criteria for Physician-Assisted Suicide," *New England Journal of Medicine* 327 (1992): 1380–84; S.D. Block and J.A. Billings, "Patient Requests to Hasten Death: Evaluation and Management in Terminal Care," *Archives of Internal Medicine* 154 (1994): 2039–47; S.D. Block and J.A. Billings, "Patient Requests for Euthanasia and Assisted Suicide in Terminal Illness: The Role of the Psychiatrist," *Psychosomatics* 36 (1995): 445–57; L.L. Emanuel, C.F. von Gunten,

F.D. Ferris, and R.K. Portenoy, *Education for Physicians in End-of-Life Care (EPEC) Trainer's Guide* (Chicago: American Medical Association, 1999).

5. T.E. Quill and I.R. Byock, "Responding to Intractable Terminal Suffering: The Role of Terminal Sedation and Voluntary Refusal of Food and Fluids," *Annals of Internal Medicine* 132 (2000): 408–14; D. Orentlicher, "The Supreme Court and Physician-Assisted Suicide: Rejecting Assisted Suicide but Embracing Euthanasia," *New England Journal of Medicine* 337 (1997): 1236–39; D.P. Sulmasy, W.A. Ury, J.C. Ahronheim, M. Seigler, L. Kass, J. Lantos, R.A. Burt, K. Foley, R. Payne, C. Gomez, T.J. Krizek, E.D. Pellegrino, and R.K. Portnoy, "Publication of Papers on Assisted Suicide and Terminal Sedation," *Annals of Internal Medicine* 133 (2000): 564–66; T.E. Quill, "Death and Dignity: A Case of Individualized Decision Making," *New England Journal of Medicine* 324 (1991): 691–94.

6. Emanuel, "Facing Requests for Physician-Assisted Suicide"; Quill, Cassel, and Meier, "Care of the Hopelessly Ill"; Block and Billings, "Patient Requests to Hasten Death"; Emanuel et al., *Education for Physicians in End-of-Life Care Trainer's Guide*.

7. Back et al., "Physician-Assisted Suicide and Euthanasia in Washington State"; G. van der Wal, J.T. van Eijk, H.J. Leenen, and C. Spreeuwenberg, "Euthanasia and Assisted Suicide II: Do Dutch Family Doctors Act Prudently?" *Family Practice* 9 (1992): 135–40.

8. R.J. Kohlwes, T.D. Koepsell, L.A. Rhodes, and R.A. Pearlman, "Physicians' Responses to Patients' Requests for Assisted Suicide," *Archives of Internal Medicine* 161 (2000): 657–63.

9. A.L. Back, H. Starks, C. Hsu, J.R. Gordon, A. Bharucha, and R.A. Pearlman, "Clinician-Patient Interactions about Requests for Physician-Assisted Suicide: A Patient and Family View," *Archives of Internal Medicine* 162 (2002): 1257–65.

10. M.J. Silveira, A. DiPiero, M.S. Gerrity, and C. Feudtner, "Patients' Knowledge of Options at the End of Life: Ignorance in the Face of Death," *Journal of the American Medical Association* 284 (2000): 2483–88.

11. Foley, "Competent Care for the Dying Instead of Physician-Assisted Suicide"; Emanuel, "Facing Requests for Physician-Assisted Suicide"; Quill, Cassel, and Meier, "Care of the Hopelessly Ill"; Block and Billings, "Patient Requests to Hasten Death"; Block and Billings, "Patient Requests for Euthanasia and Assisted Suicide in Terminal Illness"; Emanuel et al., *Education for Physicians in End-of-Life Care Trainer's Guide*.

12. P. Maguire, "Improving Communication with Cancer Patients," *European Journal of Cancer* 35 (1999): 1415–22.

13. M.J. Field and C.K. Cassel, eds., *Approaching Death: Improving Care at the End of Life* (Washington, D.C.: National Academy Press, 1997).

14. D. Humphry, *Final Exit* (Eugene, Ore.: Hemlock Society, 1991).

15. Chin et al., "Legalized Physician-Assisted Suicide in Oregon."

16. Kohlwes et al., "Physicians' Responses to Patients' Requests for Assisted Suicide."

17. Block and Billings, "Patient Requests to Hasten Death"; S.H. Miles, "Physicians and Their Patients' Suicides," *Journal of the American Medical Association* 271 (1994): 1786–88.

18. D.H. Novack, A.L. Suchman, W. Clark, R.M. Epstein, E. Najberg, and C. Kaplan, "Calibrating the Physician: Personal Awareness and Effective Patient Care," *Journal of the American Medical Association* 278 (1997): 502–9; N.J. Farber, D.H. Novack, and M.K. O'Brien, "Love, Boundaries, and the Patient-Physician Relationship," *Archives of Internal Medicine* 157 (1997): 2291–94; M. Balint, *The Doctor, His Patient, and the Illness* (New York: International Universities Press, 1957).

19. "The Inner Life of Physicians and Care of the Seriously Ill," *Journal of the American Medical Society* 286 (2001): 3007–14.

8

When Hastened Death Is
Neither Killing Nor Letting Die

Tom L. Beauchamp, Ph.D.

There are two fundamental moral issues about physician-assisted hastening of death: Are physicians morally justified in complying with requests by patients who ask for assistance? Is there an adequate moral basis to justify the legalization of physician-assisted hastening of death at the patient's request? Legal developments in the United States have encouraged us to frame virtually all moral questions as ones of legalization. As important as legalization is, however, the question whether physicians are morally justified in complying with requests for aid in dying presents a more fundamental moral issue. Accordingly, my concern here is with the moral justification of *individual acts* of hastening death.

The thesis that physician-assisted hastening of death is morally prohibited has commonly been grounded in the premises that there is a defensible and relevant distinction between letting die and killing and that physicians may let patients die but cannot kill them. I do not reject the distinction between killing and letting die; indeed, I offer an analysis that makes sense of it. Nonetheless, I argue that this distinction is fatally flawed as a means of treating the major problems of physician-assisted death that face medicine and society today. Physician-assisted hastening of death need not involve either killing or letting die; and even if an act is one of killing or letting die, it must be shown whether the act is justified or unjustified. The categories of "killing" and "letting die" therefore need to be redirected to the key moral issue that should drive discussions of physician-assisted death, which is the liberty to choose and the justification (if any) for limiting that liberty.[1]

The Conceptual Foundation of the
Distinction between Killing and Letting Die

In examining the conceptual foundation of the distinction between killing and letting die, the first question is whether physicians *kill* patients by *causing* their deaths either through interventions or through intentional noninterventions. In medical tradition, the term *killing* has understandably carried meanings of wrongfulness and blameworthiness. However, in contexts external to traditional medical morality, *killing* does not imply wrongful behavior; it refers only to causal action that brings about another's death. In settings both within and outside medicine, *letting die* refers to intentionally not intervening so that disease, system failure, injury, or circumstance causes death.

In ordinary discourse, medicine, and law these conceptions are conspicuously vague. Some cases of letting die count also as acts of killing, thereby undermining the hypothesis that these terms distinguish two different sets of cases. For example, health professionals kill patients—that is, cause patients to die—when they intentionally let them die in circumstances in which a duty exists to keep the patients alive, such as a patient with pneumonia who could easily be cured and wants to be cured but is "allowed to die" by a physician who chooses not to "intervene." In much of the literature of medical ethics, it is unclear how to distinguish killing from letting die so as to avoid even this elementary problem of cases that satisfy the conditions of both categories.

A widely accepted account of letting die holds that intentionally forgoing a medical technology qualifies as letting die, rather than killing, only if an underlying disease or injury is intentionally allowed to cause death when death might be delayed by employing that technology.[2] According to this view, if a medical technology is intentionally withdrawn or withheld, a natural death occurs when natural conditions do what they would have done had the technology never been initiated (that is, when existing conditions take their natural, undeterred course). By contrast, killing occurs if an act of a person or persons, rather than natural conditions, causes an ensuing death.

This account misses its mark unless other conditions are added to it, but additional conditions threaten to undermine the very point of the account. One condition that must be added is that any withholding or withdrawing of a medical technology must be *justified;* an unjustified withholding or withdrawing that releases natural conditions is a killing. This brings a moral consideration of justified action into the heart of the conceptual analysis of letting die. To see why this condition of justified withholding or withdrawing must be added, consider the case of a physician who either mistakenly (through negligence) or maleficently (through ill intent) removes a life-sustaining medical technology from a patient who wants to continue living. This action lacks justification; indeed, it is unjustified. We could not reasonably say, "The physician did not cause the patient's death; he only allowed the patient to die of an underlying condition." In this case, the physician did cause the death, and the physician therefore cannot be said to have let the patient die.

Now change the patient's wishes. Suppose that the patient autonomously refused the technology that sustains life. In this circumstance, it would not be correct to say that the physician caused the death. Whether the physician did or did not *cause* death is determined in these circumstances by whether the act was *validly authorized*. If the act is validly authorized, it is a letting die; if it is not validly authorized, it is a killing. The reason for forgoing a medical technology is therefore the key condition in conceptually distinguishing killing and letting die in cases of withholding or withdrawing life-sustaining interventions. A physician lets a patient die if he or she has valid authorization for withholding or withdrawing treatment. Fundamentally "letting die" is validly authorized nonintervention in circumstances in which patients die (when and in the precise manner they do) as a result. By contrast, a comparable action or inaction is a *killing* when

- the physician had a duty to treat,
- the physician withheld or withdrew a life-sustaining technology without authorization, and
- the patient subsequently died for lack of that technology.

The critical point is that a physician is the relevant cause of death and thereby kills a patient if he or she has no valid authorization for withholding or withdrawing treatment, but the physician lets the patient die if he or she does have valid authorization for withholding or withdrawing treatment. Of course, physicians also may kill in so-called active ways. I confront this problem in due course.

Letting Die Based on Medical Futility

Thus far I have argued that the following conditions are (conceptually) sufficient conditions of letting die in medicine:

1. the patient validly refused a medical technology that is essential to the patient's continued existence,

2. the physician withheld or withdrew the refused life-sustaining technology, and
3. the patient subsequently died for lack of the technology.

To say that these conditions are conceptually sufficient for letting die is not to say that they are either necessary conditions or the only set of sufficient conditions. Withdrawing or withholding a medically futile technology can be the main reason why we categorize an action as one of letting die. Accordingly, the following conditions form a second set of (conceptually) sufficient conditions of letting die in medicine:

1′. a medical authority appropriately judged that a medical technology is futile to achieve the goals for which it was initiated (though it has to this point kept the patient alive),
2′. the physician withheld or withdrew the futile technology, and
3′. the patient subsequently died for lack of the technology.

A common, but incorrect, thesis is that letting die occurs in medicine *only if* "ceasing *useless* medical technologies" eventuates in the patient's death.[3] This account rightly connects letting die to futility (as in [1′]–[3′]) but wrongly assumes that in the circumstance of letting die, technologies *must* be futile. As demonstrated in the previous section, medical futility is not a necessary condition of letting die. A patient's valid refusal of a medical technology makes a circumstance one of letting die even if the technology is not futile.

In the case of (1′)–(3′), the physician's *intention* may also need to be of one type rather than another to qualify as letting die, but I will not here pursue this question about proper intention. What does need an additional comment is the language in (1′) of "a medical authority appropriately judged." As the previous analysis suggests, in the medical context letting die is conceptually tied to *acceptable* acts, where acceptability derives either from a well-substantiated judgment of the futility of a technology or from a valid refusal of the technology. In the case of a valid refusal, there exists no problem about responsibility for the death because the refusal itself justifies the physician's conduct; the refusal nullifies what would otherwise be an injury or maltreatment and makes the case one of letting die. A judgment of futility does not as transparently provide justification, but a well-substantiated judgment of futility clearly can be the basis of a justified act of withholding or withdrawing a technology.

The language of letting die is used in medical contexts to express a moral judgment. A letting die is a justified act; it is not morally neutral or unjustified.

Despite this general feature of medical discourse, it is an open question, so far as I can see, whether physicians kill or let die when they nonnegligently make a *mistaken* judgment about a patient's condition (after which the patient refuses treatment) or about the futility of a treatment. Assessment of such hard cases is likely to turn on special features of the cases. For present purposes, suffice it to say that a conscientious and knowledgeable physician who makes a reasoned and justifiable determination of futility in light of all the information that could be gained in the circumstances lets the patient die and does not kill the patient, even if the judgment of futility turns out to have been mistaken.

Do Physicians Kill Patients When They Assist in Hastening Death?

A necessary condition of killing a patient is that the actions or inactions of the physician cause the patient's death. However, the criteria of causing death in the medical setting need clarification. The conscientious and informed physician who either makes a justifiable determination of futility or follows a patient's valid refusal does not cause the patient's death even if, in the circumstances, the technology withdrawn or withheld is causally necessary for the patient's continued existence. The physician's act of withholding or withdrawing is a necessary (or "but for") condition of the patient's death as the death occurred, but the physician is not the *cause* in the pertinent sense here, which is that of being causally responsible. A physician is not responsible for the consequences of withholding or withdrawing a technology the patient has refused, even if the physician is a contributing cause of those consequences. By contrast, the previously mentioned physician who maleficently removed a medical technology from a patient who wanted to continue living *is* the cause of death, is causally responsible for the outcome, and indeed killed the patient.

Why is the first physician not the cause, whereas the second is the cause? "The cause" judgments (or singular causal judgments) are relative to the prevailing criteria in a given context of investigation. In the circumstance of physician-caused death, judgments of causation (and, derivatively, of killing) turn on whether a physician intervened in an unwarranted manner in a course of events that could reasonably have been expected to take place. When the physician has specific warrant for action or inaction (for example, when the physician has a valid authorization from a patient) and the patient's death is a consequence of acting or not acting, the physician is not the cause of death. Rather, the cause is disease, injury, system failure, or perhaps the decision of another party who authorized the physician's conduct.

To illustrate some of these abstract points and make them more transparent, consider the following thought experiment: Two patients occupy a semiprivate hospital room, both having the same illness and both respirator dependent. One has refused the respirator; the other wishes to remain on the respirator. A physician intentionally flips a master switch that turns off both respirators; the physician is aware that both respirators will shut down. The two patients die in the same way at the same time of the same physical causes and by the same physical action of the physician. (Thus all variables are held constant except that one patient authorized the physician's action and the other did not.) Although the two patients die of the same physical causes, they do not die of the same causes of interest to law, medicine, and morality, because the proximate cause—that is, the cause responsible for the outcome—is not the same in the two otherwise identically situated patients. Consistent with the analysis provided previously, this thought experiment shows that a valid authorization transforms what would be a maleficent act of killing into a nonmaleficent act of letting die.

From both a legal and a moral point of view, one reason why physicians do not injure, maltreat, or kill patients when they withhold or withdraw medical technology is that a physician is morally and legally obligated to respect a valid refusal. Since a valid refusal of treatment binds the physician, it would be absurd to hold that these legal and moral duties require physicians to cause the deaths of their patients and thereby to kill them.

Quite apart from killing by means of withholding or withdrawing a treatment, killing can and occasionally does occur through a physician-initiated "active" means to death. Here is a conceptually clear example: Paul Mills was a patient in the Queen Elizabeth II Health Sciences Center in Halifax, Nova Scotia. Mills had undergone ten unsuccessful operations for throat cancer. He was dying, and a life-support system had been withdrawn at the request of his family. It was thought that he would die a natural death within a few hours. However, the heavy sedation he had been given was not having its intended effect. Mills was suffering from infection and experiencing "tremendous discomfort" and "excruciating pain," according to hospital officials. On November 10, 1996, Nancy Morrison, Mills's physician, administered to Mills a dose of potassium chloride. Mills died shortly thereafter. His family was unaware of the injection. On May 6, 1997, Dr. Morrison was indicted for first-degree murder; these charges were thrown out on February 27, 1998, for lack of legal evidence sufficient to sustain the charge of first-degree murder.[4]

Dr. Morrison did not, and would not, describe her act as "killing," let alone as "murder." She viewed it as a compassionate act of assistance in dying. It may indeed have been an act of this description. However, Dr. Morrison had no specific authorization for her act, and she was the cause of Mills's death in the way and at the time that his death occurred; she was causally responsible for the death, and she killed Mills. Whether she killed him *justifiably* is another matter, and one now to be considered.

Is Killing by Physicians Morally Permissible?

I have proposed that in cases of killing a patient the physician is causally responsible (a proximate cause), and in cases of letting die the physician is not causally responsible (not the proximate cause). This proposal so far conforms to legal and medical traditions. Now, however, I depart from those traditions.

It does not follow from the fact that a physician kills a patient that the physician acts unjustifiably. Outside of traditional thinking about medical morality, it is clear that to correctly apply the label "killing" or the label "letting die" to a set of events cannot determine whether one type of action is better or worse than the other or whether either is acceptable or unacceptable.[5] Rightness and wrongness in killing depend exclusively on the merit of the justification underlying an act of killing, not on the type of action it is.

Outside of medical tradition there are several generally accepted justifications for killing, including killing in self-defense, killing to rescue a person endangered by another person's immoral acts, and killing by misadventure (accidental, nonnegligent killing while engaged in a lawful act). These excusing conditions establish that we cannot prejudge an action as wrong merely because it is a killing.[6] I hereafter assume this morally neutral sense of *kill* to see where it can and should take us in contexts of physician-hastened death.

Even though medical tradition has emphatically condemned physician killing, it is conceptually and morally open to physicians (and society) to reverse tradition and come to the conclusion that medicine and the social context have changed and that it is time to permit certain forms of assisted death that involve killing.[7] Medical morality has never been self-justifying, and traditional practices and standards in medicine may, in the face of social change, turn out to be indefensible limits on the liberty to choose. Even if, in medicine, killing is usually wrong and letting die only rarely wrong, this outcome is still contingent on the features of the cases that typically appear in medicine. The general wrongness of killing and the general rightness of letting die are not surprising features of the moral world inasmuch as killings are rarely authorized by appropriate parties, and cases of letting die generally are validly authorized. Be that as it may, the *frequency* with which one kind of act is justified, by contrast to the other kind of act, is not relevant to the moral (or legal) justification of either kind of act.

The justifiability of any particular type or instance of killing is therefore an open question, and we cannot assert without looking at a particular case (or type of case) that killing is morally worse than allowing to die. The way to decide whether killing is wrong in the medical circumstance of a request for hastened death is to determine what makes it wrong in general. Causing a person's death is wrong, when it *is* wrong, not simply because someone is the responsible (or proximate) cause but because an unjustified harm or loss to the deceased has occurred—for example, the person has been deprived of opportunities and goods that life would otherwise have afforded. A person must unjustifiably suffer a setback to personal interests (a harm) that the person would not otherwise have experienced.[8]

It is a complicated question whether patient-authorized killing by physicians involves any form of harm to the patient, but we can here circumvent this question. It is a generally accepted principle even of Hippocratic medicine that physicians may, under various conditions, legitimately harm patients to avoid graver or more burdensome harms. Invasive surgery that requires recuperation is a paradigm case. Because death is sometimes the more inviting of two unwelcome outcomes, physicians may have sound reasons to help their patients by causing the lesser harm.[9] If a patient chooses death as a release from a desperate and harmful circumstance, then killing at that patient's request involves no clear wrong even if it does involve a harm. Shortening life can avoid a state of burdens to a patient that is virtually uncompensated by benefits.[10]

This form of aid to patients might harm society by setting back its interests, and this harm might constitute a sufficient reason not to legalize physician-hastened death. However, this consequence would not change the status of the act as a legitimate form of physician assistance to a patient.

The Place of Autonomous Requests

A *request* by a competent patient for assistance in hastening death does not have the same moral authority and binding force as a competent *refusal* of technology that would sustain life. Patients have a right to refuse and, correlatively, physicians have an obligation to comply with the refusal; but there is no comparable right or obligation in the case of a request. Autonomous refusals by patients compel physician nonintervention, but autonomous requests by patients do not necessarily compel physician intervention. Nonetheless, it does not follow that requests from patients fail to justify acts of physician assistance in hastened death.

Under many circumstances in medicine, a request by patients for aid authorizes assistance by a physician. For example, a request for help in reducing pain warrants interventions to meet the request. Why is a favorable response by a physician to a request for assistance in facilitating death by hastening it different from a favorable response to requests for assistance in facilitating death by easing it? The two acts of physician assistance appear to be morally equivalent as long as there are no other differences in the cases. That is, if the disease is relevantly similar, the request by the patient is relevantly similar, the desperateness of the patient's circumstance is relevantly similar, and so on, then responding to a request to provide the means to hasten death (thought of by some as killing) seems morally equivalent to responding to a request to ease death by withdrawing treatment, sedating to coma, and the like (thought of by many as letting die).

In cases of requested active assistance, requested passive nonintervention, and various borderline cases between the active and the passive (for example, administering fatal medication when the intended goal was only to ease pain or terminally sedate), a patient is seeking the best means to quit a life of unrelieved misery. In each case, persons reach a judgment that lingering in life is, on balance, worse than death. The person who hastens death by ingesting fatal medication, the person who forgoes nutrition and hydration, the person who requests terminal sedation, and the person who forgoes life-sustaining technologies may each be selecting what for him or her is the best means to end unrelievable burdens.

Denial of help to a patient in these bleak circumstances renders life more burdensome from the patient's perspective (or, in the case of not prescribing a fatal medication, takes the decision away from the patient). It is not important that these acts are of a certain type (suicide, say) but only that they are acts of a type that can be justified.

The issue is also not whether valid requests by patients place a *duty* on physicians to hasten death.[11] The question is whether valid requests render it *permissible* for a physician to lend aid in hastening death. A physician with a professional commitment to help a patient die as the patient chooses has made a moral commitment that differs from the commitment made by a physician who draws the line in opposition to all forms of assistance in hastening death. There are intermediate forms of physician commitment, as well. A physician who, in principle, accepts the permissibility of assistance may still refuse to honor a particular request by a patient for assistance on grounds that the patient's condition has not reached a point beyond which standard measures of palliative support are adequate to relieve the patient's suffering or distress. Even a sympathetic physician who is willing to assist a patient at a specific point in the evolution of his or her condition may justifiably refuse a patient's premature request for a hastened death.

Is the Distinction between Killing and Letting Die Relevant to Physician-Assisted Death?

Many assume that the distinction between killing and letting die is relevant to contemporary issues of physician-assisted death. This assumption is suspect. Some forms of physician-assisted hastening of death do not appear to involve either killing or letting die. A physician who prescribes a lethal medication at a patient's request is not the cause (the proximate cause) of the patient's death and so does not kill the patient. Nor does this physician let the patient die. Neither the condition of killing nor that of letting die is satisfied. Since the prescription of fatal medication dominates much of the current discussion about hastened death, the irrelevance to these actions of the distinction between killing and letting die merits more discussion than it has received.

The fundamental ethical issue about physician-assisted hastening of death is whether it is morally acceptable for physicians to help seriously ill, injured, or suffering persons reach their goals in a manner that both the patient and the physician find appropriate. Of course, a decision to hasten death is not justified merely because a patient and a physician *believe* that it is justified. Moral justification of acts of hastening death requires more than patient requests and agreements between patients and their physicians. Acts of hastening death lack justification if a physician has inattentively misdiagnosed the case, if the patient's capacity to make autonomous judgments is significantly impaired, if manipulative family pressures are profoundly influencing either the physician or the patient, and the like.

If no such invalidating condition exists and the physician and the patient both act autonomously, then the choice of a hastened death is justified. One way to express this thesis is that unless a valid liberty-limiting principle warrants intervention to prevent an act of hastened death, there is no moral basis for condemning or punishing the envisioned autonomous acts of patients and their willing physicians. The question of the morality of physician-assisted hastening of death is fundamentally the question of which, if any, liberty-limiting principle justifiably prevents such choices from being effected. Although I have not considered here whether there is any such valid liberty-limiting principle, I would be pleased if I had prepared the way for this question to become the central issue—freeing us from the burden of the unproductive and overvalued distinction between killing and letting die.

Notes

1. The line between killing and letting die is relied on in the codes and guidelines of numerous professional associations; see American Medical Association, Council on Ethical and Judicial Affairs, "Physician-Assisted Suicide," Report 59, December 1993. A version of this report was published as "Physician-Assisted Suicide," *Journal of the American Medical Association* 267 (1992): 2229–33. See also "Physician-Assisted Suicide," *Current Opinions*, H-270.965; "Euthanasia," *Current Opinions*, E-2.21; "Decisions Near the End of Life," *Current Opinions*, H-140.966; "Voluntary Active Euthanasia," *Current Opinions*, H-140.987 (updated June 1996); Canadian Medical Association, *Code of Ethics*, secs. 18–20 (approved October 15, 1996); Canadian Medical Association, Policy Statement, "Euthanasia and Assisted Suicide" (June 19, 1998), which replaces the previous policy entitled "Physician-Assisted Death" (1995); World Medical Association, *Resolution on Euthanasia* (Washington, D.C.: World Medical Association, 2002), reaffirming the *Declaration of Euthanasia* (Madrid: World Medical Association, 1987).

In the formulations of these professional bodies, as in most nations and, effectively, in all traditions of medical ethics, killing is prohibited and letting die permitted under specified conditions. Despite this remarkable convergence of opinion, a cogent and pertinent analysis of the distinction between killing and letting die relevant to medicine remains elusive; see D. Orentlicher, "The Alleged Distinction Between Euthanasia and the Withdrawal of Life-Sustaining Treatment: Conceptually Incoherent and Impossible to Maintain," *University of Illinois Law Review* 3 (1998): 837–59; T.L. Beauchamp, ed., *Intending Death* (Upper Saddle River, N.J.: Prentice Hall, 1996); J. McMahan, "Killing, Letting Die, and Withdrawing Aid," *Ethics* 103 (1993): 250–79; L.O. Gostin, "Drawing a Line Between Killing and Letting Die: The Law, and Law Reform, on Medically Assisted Dying," *Journal of Law, Medicine and Ethics* 21 (1993): 94–101; H.M. Malm, "Killing, Letting Die, and Simple Conflicts," *Philosophy and Public Affairs* 18 (1989): 238–58; B. Steinbock and A. Norcross, eds., *Killing and Letting Die,* 2d ed. (New York: Fordham University Press, 1994).

2. F. Cohn and J. Lynn, "Vulnerable People: Practical Rejoinders to Claims in Favor of Assisted Suicide," in *The Case against Assisted Suicide: For the Right to End-of-Life*

Care, edited by K. Foley and H. Hendin (Baltimore: Johns Hopkins University Press, 2002), 230–60, esp. 246–47; D. Callahan, *The Troubled Dream of Life* (New York: Simon and Schuster, 1993), chap. 2; and various articles in *By No Extraordinary Means,* edited by J. Lynn (Bloomington: Indiana University Press, 1986), 227–66.

3. W. Gaylin, L.R. Kass, E. D. Pellegrino, and M. Siegler, "Doctors Must Not Kill," *Journal of the American Medical Association* 259 (1988): 2139–40 (emphasis added). See also L.R. Kass, "Neither for Love nor Money: Why Doctors Must Not Kill," *Public Interest* 94 (1989): 25–46. It is sometimes added, as a condition, that patients must be dependent upon life-support systems; see R.E. Cranford, "The Physician's Role in Killing and the Intentional Withdrawal of Treatment," in *Intending Death,* edited by T.L. Beauchamp (Upper Saddle River, N.J.: Prentice Hall, 1996), 150–62, 160.

4. The facts about this case have been drawn from several articles that appeared from 1996 to 1999 in Canadian newspapers and medical journals. Some parts of the case rely on reports provided to me by Canadian physicians who investigated the case.

5. In effect, this proposal is made in J.R. Rachels, "Active and Passive Euthanasia," *New England Journal of Medicine* 292 (1975): 78–80; and D.W. Brock, "Voluntary Active Euthanasia," *Hastings Center Report* 22, no. 2 (1992): 10–22.

6. Compare Rachels, "Active and Passive Euthanasia"; J.R. Rachels, "Killing, Letting Die, and the Value of Life," in *Can Ethics Provide Answers? And Other Essays in Moral Philosophy,* by J.R. Rachels (Lanham, Md.: Rowman and Littlefield, 1997), 69–79; R.W. Perrett, "Killing, Letting Die and the Bare Difference Argument," *Bioethics* 10 (1996): 131–39; Brock, "Voluntary Active Euthanasia."

7. Compare H. Brody and F.G. Miller, "The Internal Morality of Medicine: Explication and Application to Managed Care," *Journal of Medicine and Philosophy* 23 (1998): 384–410, 397; G. Seay, "Do Physicians Have an Inviolable Duty Not to Kill?" *Journal of Medicine and Philosophy* 26 (2001): 75–91.

8. Compare A. Buchanan, "Intending Death: The Structure of the Problem and Proposed Solutions," in *Intending Death,* edited by T.L. Beauchamp (Upper Saddle River, N.J.: Prentice Hall, 1996), 34–38; M. Hanser, "Why Are Killing and Letting Die Wrong?" *Philosophy and Public Affairs* 24 (1995): 175–201; and reflections on the roles of intention and the "right not to be killed" in D.W. Brock, "A Critique of Three Objections to Physician-Assisted Suicide," *Ethics* 109 (1999): 519–47, 537.

9. F.M. Kamm, "Physician-Assisted Suicide, Euthanasia, and Intending Death," in M.P. Battin, R. Rhodes, and A. Silvers, eds., *Physician-Assisted Suicide: Expanding the Debate* (New York: Routledge, 1998), 26–49; T. Nagel, "Death," in *Mortal Questions,* by T. Nagel (Cambridge: Cambridge University Press, 1979); and F.M. Kamm, *Morality, Mortality,* vol. 1 (New York: Oxford University Press, 1993), chap. 1.

10. See Kamm, "Physician-Assisted Suicide, Euthanasia, and Intending Death," and some later formulations in her "Physician-Assisted Suicide, the Doctrine of Double Effect, and the Ground of Value," *Ethics* 109 (1999): 586–605, esp. 588ff.

11. Although I am not here raising this question, Kamm has presented an "argument for a duty of a physician"; see Kamm, "Physician-Assisted Suicide, the Doctrine of Double Effect, and the Ground of Value," 589.

9

Physician-Assisted Suicide as a Last-Resort Option at the End of Life

Dan W. Brock, Ph.D.

Palliative care, to relieve suffering rather than to effect cure, is the standard of care when terminally ill patients find that the burdens of continued life-prolonging treatment outweigh the benefits.[1] To better relieve suffering near the end of life, physicians need to improve their skills in palliative care and routinely discuss it with patients earlier in the course of terminal illness. In addition, access to palliative care needs to be improved, particularly for those Americans who lack health insurance. However, even the highest-quality palliative care fails or becomes unacceptable for some patients, some of whom request help hastening death. Between 10 and 50 percent of patients in programs devoted to palliative care still report significant pain one week before death.[2] Furthermore, patients request a hastened death not principally because of unrelieved pain but because of a wide variety of unrelieved physical symptoms in combination with loss of meaning, dignity, and independence.[3]

How should physicians respond when competent, terminally ill patients whose suffering is not relieved by palliative care request help in hastening death?[4] If the patient is receiving life-prolonging interventions, the physician should consider discontinuing them, in accordance with the patient's wishes. Some patients may voluntarily stop eating and drinking. If the patient has unrelieved pain or other symptoms and accepts sedation, the physician may legally administer terminal sedation. However, in all countries but the Netherlands and Belgium, physicians are legally prohibited from participating in physician-assisted suicide in response to such patient requests; in Switzerland, physicians and nonphysicians are permitted to participate in assisted suicide for "altruistic motives."[5] In the United States, physician-assisted suicide is permitted only in Oregon. The U.S. Supreme Court decisions that determined that there is no constitutional right to physician-assisted suicide placed great emphasis on the importance of relieving pain and suffering near the end of life.[6] The Court acknowledged the legal acceptability of providing pain relief even to the point of hastening death, if necessary, and left open the possibility that states might choose to legalize physician-assisted suicide under some circumstances, as Oregon has done.

Voluntarily stopping eating and drinking, terminal sedation, and physician-assisted suicide are all potential interventions of last resort for competent, terminally ill patients who are suffering intolerably, in spite of intensive efforts to palliate, and desire a hastened death. Many opponents of physician-assisted suicide defend the current legal status of these options, arguing that, along with forgoing life-sustaining treatment, voluntarily stopping eating and drinking and terminal sedation constitute adequate and appropriate options for hastening death, obviating the need for legalization of physician-assisted suicide. However, in my view, the differences between these practices and physician-assisted suicide do not justify the continued prohibition of assisted suicide.

Definitions and Clinical Comparisons

Voluntarily Stopping Eating and Drinking

By voluntarily stopping eating and drinking, a patient who is otherwise physically capable of taking nourishment makes an explicit decision to discontinue all oral intake and then is gradually "allowed to die," primarily of dehydration or some intervening complication.[7] Depending on the patient's preexisting condition, the process will usually take one to three weeks; it can take longer if the patient continues to take some fluids. Voluntarily stopping eating and drinking has several advantages. Many patients lose their appetites and stop eating and drinking in the final stages of many illnesses, without any intention of hastening death. Ethically and legally, the right of competent, informed patients to refuse life-prolonging interventions, including artificial hydration and nutrition, is firmly established, and voluntary cessation of "natural" eating and drinking could be considered an extension of that right. Because not eating or drinking requires considerable patient resolve, the voluntary nature of the action and the patient's settled resolve to die should be clear. Voluntarily stopping eating and drinking also protects patient privacy and independence, so much so that it potentially requires no participation by a physician.

The main disadvantages of the practice as a means to hasten death are that it may last for weeks and may initially increase suffering because the patient may experience thirst and hunger. Subtle coercion to proceed with the process, especially once it is already under way, may occur if patients are not regularly offered the opportunity to eat and drink, yet such offers may be viewed as undermining the patient's resolve or expressing disagreement with the patient's choice. Some patients, family members, or health care providers may find the notion of "dehydrating" or "starving" a patient to death to be morally repugnant. For patients whose current suffering is severe and unrelievable, the process would be unacceptable without sedation and analgesia. If physicians are not involved, palliation of symptoms may be inadequate, the decision to forgo eating and drinking may not be informed, and cases of treatable depression may be missed. Patients are likely to lose mental clarity toward the end of this process, which may undermine their sense of personal integrity and dignity or raise questions about whether the action remains voluntary. Although several articles, including a moving personal narrative, have proposed voluntarily stopping eating and drinking as an alternative to other forms of hastened death,[8] there are no data about how frequently such decisions are made or how acceptable they are to patients, families, or health care providers.

Terminal Sedation

The term *terminal sedation* refers to the administration of sedative drugs at the end of life; it is not, strictly speaking, a form of assisted death. With terminal sedation, the suffering patient is sedated to unconsciousness, if need be, usually through ongoing administration of barbiturates or benzodiazepines, and all life-sustaining interventions, including nutrition and hydration, are withheld. Generally, the patient then dies of dehydration, starvation, or some other intervening complication.[9] Although death is inevitable, it usually does not take place for days or even weeks, depending on clinical circumstances. Because patients are deeply sedated during this terminal period, they are believed to be free of suffering.

Since sedation to relieve suffering is a long-standing and uncontroversial aim of medicine, and the subsequent withholding of life-sustaining therapy has wide legal and ethical acceptance, terminal sedation is probably legally permissible under current law.[10] The 1997 U.S. Supreme Court decisions in *Vacco v. Quill* and *Washington v. Glucksberg* gave strong support to terminal sedation, saying that pain in terminally ill patients should be treated even to the point of rendering the patient unconscious or hastening death.[11] Terminal sedation is already openly practiced by some palliative care and hospice groups in cases of unrelieved suffering, with a reported frequency from 0 to 44 percent of cases.[12]

Terminal sedation has other practical advantages. It can be carried out in patients with severe physical limitations. The time delay between initiation of terminal sedation and death permits second-guessing and reassessment by the health care team and the family. Because the health care team must administer medications and monitor effects, physicians can ensure that the patient's decision is informed and voluntary before initiating sedation. In addition, many proponents believe that it is appropriate to use terminal sedation in patients who lack decision-making capacity but appear to be suffering intolerably, provided the patient's suffering is extreme and otherwise unrelievable and the surrogate or family agrees.

Nonetheless, terminal sedation has many of the same risks associated with physician-assisted suicide, as well as some that assisted suicide lacks.[13] Unlike physician-assisted suicide, the final actors are the health care providers, not the patient. Terminal sedation could therefore be carried out without explicit discussions with alert patients who appear to be suffering intolerably, or even against their wishes. Some competent, terminally ill patients reject terminal sedation. They believe that their dignity will be violated if they are unconscious for a prolonged time before they die or that their families will suffer unnecessarily while waiting for them to die. Terminal sedation may not be possible for patients who wish to die in their own homes because it generally requires admission to a health care facility. In some clinical situations, it cannot relieve the patient's symptoms, as occurs when a patient is bleeding uncontrollably from an eroding lesion or a refractory coagulation disorder, cannot swallow secretions because of widespread oropharyngeal cancer, or has refractory diarrhea from AIDS. There is some controversy in the anesthesia literature about whether heavily sedated persons are actually free of suffering or are simply unable to report or remember it.[14] Although such patients are probably not conscious of their condition once sedated, their death is unlikely to be dignified or remembered as peaceful by their families. When patients find their condition intolerable but are not in substantial pain, physicians may deem sedating them to the point of unconsciousness medically inappropriate. Finally, there may be confusion about the physician's ethical responsibility for contributing to the patient's death.[15]

Physician-Assisted Suicide

With physician-assisted suicide, the physician provides the means, usually a prescription of a large dose of barbiturates, by which a patient can end his or her life.[16] Although the physician is morally responsible for this assistance, the patient has to carry out the final act of using the means provided. Physician-assisted suicide has several advantages. Access to a lethal dose of medication may give some patients the freedom and reassurance to continue living, knowing they can escape if and when they feel the need to do so.[17] Because patients have to ingest the drug by their own hand, their action is likely to be voluntary and done with resolve. Once the patient makes a decision in favor of death, physician-assisted suicide does not require a lingering period of days or weeks and so provides what patients and families may view as a more humane and dignified death. Physicians report being more comfortable with assisted suicide than with voluntary active euthanasia,[18] presumably because their participation is indirect.

Opponents of physician-assisted suicide believe that it violates traditional moral and professional prohibitions against intentionally contributing to a patient's death.[19] It also has several practical disadvantages. Self-administration does not guarantee competence or voluntariness. The patient may have impaired judgment at the time of the request or of the act or may be influenced by external pressures. Since there is often a substantial period of time between the provision and use of the means for assisted suicide, and since physicians are often not present when the means are used, there is often no evaluation and assurance of competence or voluntariness at the time of use. Physician-assisted suicide is limited to patients who are physically capable of taking the medication themselves. Because it is not always effective,[20] families may be faced with a patient who is vomiting, aspirating, or cognitively impaired but is not dying. Patients brought to the emergency department after ineffective attempts are likely to receive unwanted life-prolonging treatment. Requiring physicians to be present when patients ingest the medication has practical difficulties and could coerce an ambivalent patient to proceed, yet their absence may leave families to respond to medical complications alone.

Although physician-assisted suicide is illegal in all states but Oregon, no physician has ever been successfully prosecuted for his or her participation.[21] Several studies have documented a secret practice of physician-assisted suicide in the United States. In Washington state, 12 percent of physicians responding to a survey had received genuine requests for assisted suicide within the year studied.[22] Twenty-four percent of requests were acceded to, and more than half of those patients died as a result. A study of Oregon physicians showed similar results.[23] Physician-assisted suicide is usually conducted covertly, without consultation, guidelines, or documentation. Public controversy about legalizing the practice continues in the United States. Although referendums to legalize physician-assisted suicide have been defeated in several states, an Oregon referendum was passed in 1994 that legalized it, subject to certain safeguards.[24] After a series of legal challenges, the Oregon referendum was resubmitted to the electorate in November 1997 and passed by a substantial margin. Several years' experience with assisted suicide in Oregon indicates that the practice largely operates within intended limits.[25] The U.S. Supreme Court ruled that laws in the states of Washington and New York prohibiting physician-assisted suicide were not unconstitutional but simultaneously encouraged public discussion and state experimentation through the legislative and referendum processes.[26]

Voluntarily stopping eating and drinking, terminal sedation, and physician-assisted suicide each have complex sets of advantages and disadvantages. For each practice, particular advantages and disadvantages may be more or less important with a specific patient seeking a hastened death. No one of these practices has a clearly superior balance of advantages over disadvantages in all cases. This implies that physician-assisted suicide should not be prohibited while voluntarily stopping eating and drinking and terminal sedation are permitted.

Ethical Comparisons between the Practices

Many normative ethical analyses use the doctrine of double effect and the distinction between active and passive assistance to distinguish between currently permissible acts that may hasten death (forgoing life-sustaining treatment and high-dose pain medications) and physician-assisted suicide, which is generally impermissible.[27] Using similar arguments, terminal sedation and voluntarily stopping eating and drinking have been argued to be ethically preferable alternatives to assisted suicide.[28] However, there are more problems with the doctrine of double effect and the active-passive distinction than are often acknowledged, and terminal sedation and voluntarily stopping eating and drinking are more complex and less easily distinguished ethically from physician-assisted suicide than proponents seem to realize.

Doctrine of Double Effect

The doctrine of double effect distinguishes between effects that a person intends (both the end sought and the means taken to the end) and consequences of the action that are foreseen but unintended.[29] In evaluating the case at hand, as long as the physician's intentions are good and other conditions are satisfied, it is permissible for him or her to perform actions with foreseeable consequences that would be wrong to directly intend. In this view, intentionally causing death is morally impermissible, even if desired by a competent patient whose suffering could not otherwise be relieved. But if death comes unintentionally as the consequence of an otherwise well-intentioned intervention, even if foreseen with a high probability or even certainty, the physician's action can be morally acceptable. The unintended but foreseen bad effect must also be proportional to the intended good effects.

The doctrine of double effect has been important in generating acceptance of the use of sufficient pain medications to relieve suffering near the end of life.[30] When high-dose opioids are used to treat pain, neither the patient nor the physician intends to accelerate death, but both are willing to accept the risk of unintentionally hastening death in order to relieve the pain. Recent experience suggests, however, that medications sufficient to relieve pain rarely, in fact, result in a hastened death.[31] Double effect has also been used to distinguish terminal sedation from physician-assisted suicide.[32] Relief of suffering is intended in both options, but death is argued to be intended with assisted suicide and merely foreseen with terminal sedation. It is important to distinguish between the patient's and the physician's intentions. The patient's intention in terminal sedation and physician-assisted suicide will typically be to die. The physician's intention in terminal sedation, on the other hand, may be to relieve suffering by sedating the patient and to respect the patient's refusal of nutrition and hydration, foreseeing but not intending the patient's death. In physician-assisted suicide, as well, the physician need not intend the patient's death. He or she may only intend to relieve the patient's anxiety about dying, hoping, expecting, and intending that the patient will not use the means provided. Thus according to the doctrine of double effect, the physician's role in assisted suicide may not always be impermissible. The doctrine does not support a systematic difference between voluntarily stopping eating and drinking or terminal sedation and physician-assisted suicide.

According to the doctrine of double effect, intentionally taking innocent human life is always morally impermissible, whereas doing so foreseeably but unintentionally can be permissible when it produces a proportionate good. As applied to end-of-life medical decision making, this problematically gives more moral weight to the intentions of the physician than to the wishes and circumstances of the patient. An alternative view is that it is morally wrong to take the life of a person who wants to live, whether doing so intentionally or foreseeably. In this view, what can make terminal sedation morally permissible is that the patient gives informed consent to it, not that the physician only foresees but does not intend the patient's inevitable death. More generally, some commentators have argued that the difference between effects intended as a necessary means to a good end versus effects foreseen but unintended as necessary to reach that same end cannot bear the moral importance that the doctrine of double effect gives it.[33] In each case, the effect of death may be unavoidable in the circumstances but judged acceptable to reach the end of relieving the patient's suffering.

The issue of intention is further complicated because the determination of what is intended by the patient or physician is often controversial and unclear and because practices that are universally accepted may involve the intention to hasten death in some cases.[34] Death is not always intended or sought when competent patients forgo life support; sometimes patients simply do not want to continue a particular treatment but hope, nevertheless, that they can live without it. However, some patients find their circumstances so intolerable, even with the best of care, that they refuse further life support with the intent of bringing about their death. There is broad agreement that physicians must respect such refusals, even when the patient's intention is to die.[35] Physicians may sometimes share the patient's intention when they also believe that an earlier death will be best for the patient, and then their removal of life support would be highly problematic when analyzed according to the doctrine of double effect.

The Distinction between Active and Passive Physician Involvement

According to many normative ethical analyses, active measures that hasten death are unacceptable, whereas passive or indirect measures that achieve the same ends would be permitted.[36] The active-passive distinction is typically understood to mirror the distinction between killing and allowing to die. Passive measures that hasten death—that is, allow a patient to die—are typically believed to be justified in circumstances in which active measures—that is, killing —would not be justified. When the patient is allowed to die, the underlying disease, not the physician's action, is said to be the cause of death. However, how the distinctions between active and passive and between killing and allowing to die should be drawn, as well as how they apply to these three practices, remains controversial.[37]

Stopping life-sustaining therapies is typically considered passive assistance in dying, and the patient is said to be allowed to die of the underlying disease, no matter how proximate the physician's action and the patient's death. Physicians, however, sometimes experience their role in stopping life-sustaining interventions as very active.[38] For example, there is nothing psychologically or physically "passive" about taking someone off a mechanical ventilator if that person is incapable of breathing on his own, and some commentators have argued that these are cases of justified killing.[39] Voluntarily stopping eating and drinking is argued to be a variant of stopping life-sustaining therapy, and the patient is said to die of the underlying disease.[40] However, the notion that this is passively "letting nature take its course" is unpersuasive because patients with no underlying disease would also die if they completely stopped eating and drinking. Death is the result of the patient's decision to refuse food and fluids, not a consequence of his underlying disease.

Physician-assisted suicide and terminal sedation are also challenging to evaluate according to the active-passive or kill–allow to die distinctions. Physician-assisted suicide is *active* in that the physician provides the means whereby the patient may take his or her life and thereby contributes to a cause of death that is new and different from the patient's disease. However, the physician's role in assisted suicide is *passive* or indirect in that the patient administers the lethal medication. Neither killing nor allowing to die appears clearly to apply to the physician's role in assisted suicide. In physician-assisted suicide, the patient takes his or her own life, whereas the physician only assists the patient by providing the means for doing so. The psychological and temporal distance between the prescribing and the act may also make physician-assisted suicide seem indirect.[41] These ambiguities may allow the physician to characterize his or her actions as passive or indirect.[42]

Terminal sedation is *passive* in that the administration of sedation does not directly cause the patient's death and the withholding of artificial feedings and fluids is commonly considered passively allowing the patient to die.[43] However, some physicians and nurses may consider it very *active* to sedate to unconsciousness someone who is seeking death and then to withhold life-prolonging interventions, including food and fluids. Furthermore, the notion that terminal sedation is merely "letting nature take its course" is problematic because often the patient dies of dehydration from the withholding of fluids, not from his or her underlying disease.

However these different interventions are properly characterized by the active-passive distinction, some commentators have challenged the moral significance of the difference.[44] If the difference lacks moral importance, then it will not be important whether a particular intervention is active or passive. The application and the moral importance of both the active-passive distinction and the doctrine of double effect are notoriously controversial and should not serve as the primary basis of determining the morality of these practices.

Voluntariness

I suggest that the patient's wishes and competent consent are more ethically important than whether the acts are categorized as active or passive or whether death is intended or unintended by the patient or physician.[45] With competent patients, none of these acts would be morally permissible without the patient's voluntary and informed consent. Any of these actions would violate a competent patient's autonomy and would be both immoral and illegal if the patient did not understand that death was the inevitable consequence of the action or if the decision was coerced or contrary to the patient's wishes. The ethical principle of autonomy focuses on patients' rights to make important decisions about their lives, including what happens to their bodies, and may support genuinely autonomous forms of these acts.[46] There is no systematic difference in these three practices grounded in voluntariness.

Because most of these acts require cooperation from physicians, and, in the case of terminal sedation, the health care team, the autonomy of participating medical professionals also warrants consideration. Because terminal sedation, voluntarily stopping eating and drinking, and physician-assisted suicide are not part of usual medical practice and they all result in a hastened death, health care providers should have the right to determine the nature and extent of their own participation. All physicians should respect patients' decisions to forgo life-sustaining treatment, including artificial hydration and nutrition, and provide standard palliative care, including skillful pain and symptom management. If society permits some or all of these practices (currently, terminal sedation and voluntarily stopping eating and drinking are openly tolerated), physicians who choose not to participate because of personal moral considerations should at a minimum discuss all available alternatives in the spirit of informed consent and respecting patient autonomy. Physicians are free to express their own objections to any of these practices as part of the informing process, to propose alternative approaches, and to transfer care to another physician if the patient continues to request actions to hasten death that they find unacceptable.

Proportionality

Physicians have moral and professional obligations to promote their patients' best interests or well-being and to avoid causing unnecessary harm.[47] The concept of proportionality requires that the risk of causing harm must bear a direct relationship to the danger and immediacy of the patient's clinical situation and the expected benefit of the intervention.[48] The greater the patient's suffering, the greater risk the physician can take of potentially contributing to the patient's death, as long as the patient understands and accepts that risk. For a patient with lung cancer who is anxious and short of breath, the risk of small doses of morphine or anxiolytics is warranted. At a later time, if the patient is near death and gasping for air, more aggressive sedation is warranted, even in doses that may well cause respiratory depression. Although proportionality is an important element of the doctrine of double effect, it can be applied independently of this doctrine. All plausible moral theories accept that, other things being equal, the benefits from our actions should where possible exceed their harms. Sometimes patients' suffering cannot be relieved despite optimal palliative care, and continuing to live offers only torment that will inevitably end in their death; in these circumstances, continued life is no longer a benefit but is now a burden to the patient.[49] Such extreme circumstances sometimes warrant extraordinary medical actions, and the forms of hastening death under consideration in this chapter may satisfy the requirement of proportionality. The requirement of proportionality, which all health care interventions should meet, does not support any principled ethical distinction between these three options.

Conflict of Duties

Unrelievable, intolerable suffering at the end of life may create for physicians an explicit conflict between their ethical and professional duty to relieve suffering and their understanding of their ethical and professional duty not to use at least some means of deliberately hastening death.[50] Currently, physicians who believe they should respond to such suffering by acceding to the patient's request for a hastened death may find themselves caught between their duty to the patient as a caregiver and their duty to obey the law as a citizen.[51] Usually, though not always, solutions can be found in the intensive application of palliative care or within the currently legitimized options of forgoing life supports, voluntarily stopping eating and drinking, or terminal sedation. Situations in

which these may not be adequate include terminally ill patients with un-
controlled bleeding, obstruction from nasopharyngeal cancer, and refractory
AIDS diarrhea or patients who believe that spending their last days iatrogeni-
cally sedated would be meaningless, frightening, or degrading. Clearly, the
physician has a moral obligation not to abandon patients with refractory suffering;[52] hence those physicians who cannot provide some or all of these options
because of moral or legal reservations should search assiduously with the
patient for mutually acceptable solutions or seek to transfer care to another
physician willing to provide them.

Safeguards

In the United States, health care is undergoing radical reform driven more by
market forces than by commitments to quality of care,[53] and 43 million persons are currently uninsured. Capitated reimbursement could provide financial
incentives to encourage terminally ill patients to hasten their deaths. Physicians'
participation in hastening death by any of these methods can be justified only
as a last resort when standard palliative measures are ineffective or unacceptable to the patient.

Safeguards to protect vulnerable patients from the risk of error, abuse, or
coercion must be constructed for any of these practices that are ultimately accepted. These risks, which have been extensively cited in the debates about
physician-assisted suicide,[54] also exist for terminal sedation and voluntarily
stopping eating and drinking and even for forgoing life-sustaining treatment.
Terminal sedation and voluntarily stopping eating and drinking could be carried out without ensuring that optimal palliative care has been provided. This
risk may be particularly great if voluntarily stopping eating and drinking is carried out without physician involvement. In terminal sedation, physicians who
unreflectively believe that death is unintended, or that it is not their explicit
purpose, may fail to acknowledge the inevitable consequences of their action
as their responsibility.

The typical safeguards proposed for regulating physician-assisted suicide are
intended to allow physicians to respond to unrelieved suffering while ensuring
that adequate palliative measures have been attempted and that patient decisions are autonomous.[55] These safeguards need to balance respect for patient
privacy and autonomy with the protection of vulnerable patients by adequately
overseeing and controlling these interventions. Similar professional safeguards
should be considered for terminal sedation and voluntarily stopping eating and

drinking, even if these practices are already sanctioned by the law. The challenge of safeguards is to be flexible enough to be responsive to individual patient circumstances and rigorous enough to protect vulnerable persons.

Safeguards should ensure that the following conditions have been met:

- *Palliative care has proved ineffective or is unacceptable.* Excellent palliative care must be available yet either insufficient to relieve intolerable suffering for a particular patient or unacceptable to that patient.
- *Informed consent has been given.* Patients must be competent and be fully informed about and capable of understanding their condition, the treatment alternatives, and the risks and benefits of these alternatives. Requests for a hastened death must be enduring and free of undue influence and should normally be initiated by the patient so as to avoid subtle coercion. Waiting periods must be flexible, depending on the nearness of inevitable death and the severity of immediate suffering.
- *Diagnosis and prognosis are clear.* Patients must have a clearly diagnosed disease whose prognosis, including the degree of uncertainty about outcomes and how long the patient might live, is understood.
- *An independent second opinion has been sought.* A consultant with expertise in palliative care should review the case. Specialists should also review any questions about the patient's diagnosis or prognosis. If there is uncertainty about treatable depression or about the patient's mental capacity, a psychiatrist should be consulted.
- *Accountability can be established.* Explicit processes for documentation, reporting, and review should be in place to ensure accountability.

The restriction of any of these methods to those who are terminally ill involves a trade-off. Some patients who suffer greatly from incurable but not terminal illness and are unresponsive to palliative measures will be denied access to a hastened death and forced to continue suffering against their will. Other patients whose request for a hastened death is denied will avoid a premature death because their suffering can subsequently be relieved with more intensive palliative care. Some would restrict physician-assisted suicide (and perhaps terminal sedation) to terminally ill patients because of current inequities of access, concerns about errors and abuse, and lack of experience with the process. Because of the inherent waiting period, the great resolve required, and the opportunity for reconsideration, voluntarily stopping eating and drinking might be allowed for those who are incurably ill, but not imminently dying, if they meet all other criteria. Initially restricting assisted suicide to the terminally ill would allow assessment of how realistic the risks and abuses feared by opponents are before extending the practice to patients who are not terminally ill. If any methods are extended to those who are incurably but not terminally ill, safeguards should be more stringent, including substantial waiting periods and mandatory assessment by psychiatrists and specialists, because the risk and consequences of error are increased.

The clinical, ethical, and policy differences and similarities among these three practices need to be debated openly, both publicly and within the medical profession. Some may worry that a discussion of the similarities between voluntarily stopping eating and drinking and terminal sedation, on the one hand, and physician-assisted suicide, on the other, may undermine the desired goal of optimal relief of suffering at the end of life.[56] Others may worry that a critical analysis of the principle of double effect or the active-passive distinction as applied to voluntarily stopping eating and drinking and terminal sedation may undermine efforts to improve pain relief or to ensure that patients' or surrogates' decisions to forgo unwanted life-sustaining therapy are respected.[57] However, hidden, ambiguous practices, inconsistent justifications, and failure to acknowledge the risks of accepted practices may also undermine the quality of terminal care and put patients at unwarranted risk.

Allowing a hastened death only in the context of access to good palliative care puts it in its proper perspective as a small but important facet of comprehensive care for all dying patients.[58] Currently, terminal sedation and voluntarily stopping eating and drinking are probably legal and are widely accepted by hospice and palliative care physicians. However, they may not be readily available because some physicians may continue to have moral objections and legal fears about these options. Physician-assisted suicide is illegal in most states but may be difficult if not impossible to successfully prosecute if it is carried out at the request of an informed patient. In the United States, there is an underground, erratically available practice of assisted suicide.

Explicit public policies about which of these three practices are permissible, and under what circumstances, could have important benefits. Those who fear a bad death would face the end of their lives knowing that their physicians could respond openly if their worst fears were to materialize. For most, reassurance will be all that is needed, because good palliative care is generally effective. Explicit guidelines for the practices that are deemed permissible can also encourage clinicians to explore why a patient requests hastening of death, to search for palliative care alternatives, and to respond to those whose suffering is greatest.[59]

I have argued that an assessment of the advantages and disadvantages of voluntarily stopping eating and drinking, terminal sedation, and physician-assisted suicide shows that no one practice is systematically better than the others and that each may be superior to the others in particular cases. In their ethical assessment, neither the doctrine of double effect nor the active-passive distinction support permitting voluntarily stopping eating and drinking and terminal sedation (as well as forgoing life support) while prohibiting physician-assisted suicide. I have argued that these are not the central issues for their ethical assessment in any case. Instead, the conditions of voluntariness and proportionality are central to ethical assessment of the practices, and they provide no basis for distinguishing voluntarily stopping eating and drinking and terminal sedation from physician-assisted suicide in public and legal policy. Physician-assisted suicide should be added to voluntarily stopping eating and drinking and terminal sedation as a permissible means of hastening death.

Notes

This chapter is based on an earlier paper, Timothy E. Quill, Bernard Lo, and Dan Brock, "Palliative Options of Last Resort: A Comparison of Voluntarily Stopping Eating and Drinking, Terminal Sedation, Physician-Assisted Suicide, and Voluntary Active Euthanasia," *Journal of the American Medical Association* 278 (1997): 2099–3004.

1. K.M. Foley, "Pain, Physician-Assisted Suicide, and Euthanasia," *Pain Forum* 4 (1995): 163–78; American Medical Association, Council on Scientific Affairs, "Good Care of the Dying Patient," *Journal of the American Medical Association* 275 (1996): 474–78; T.E. Quill, *Death and Dignity: Making Choices and Taking Charge* (New York: Norton, 1993); American Board of Internal Medicine, End-of-Life Patient Care Project Committee, *Caring for the Dying: Identification and Promotion of Physician Competency* (Philadephia, American Board of Internal Medicine, 1996).

2. Foley, "Pain, Physician-Assisted Suicide, and Euthanasia"; G.A. Kasting, "The Nonnecessity of Euthanasia," in *Physician-Assisted Death*, edited by J.D. Humber, R.F. Almeder, and G.A. Kasting (Totowa, N.J.: Humana, 1993), 25–43; N. Coyle, J. Adelhardt, K.M. Foley, and R.K. Portenoy, "Character of Terminal Illness in the Advanced Cancer Patient: Pain and Other Symptoms During the Last Four Weeks of Life," *Journal of Pain and Symptom Management* 5 (1990): 83–93; J. Ingham and K. Portenoy, "Symptom Assessment," *Hematology/Oncology Clinics of North America* 10 (1) (1996): 21–39.

3. A.L. Back, J.I. Wallace, H.E. Starks, and R.A. Pearlman, "Physician-Assisted Suicide and Euthanasia in Washington State: Patient Requests and Physician Responses," *Journal of the American Medical Association* 275 (1996): 919–25; P.J. van der Maas, J.J.M. van Delden, and L. Pijnenborg, *Euthanasia and Other Medical Decisions Concerning the End of Life* (Amsterdam: Elsevier, 1992).

4. T.E. Quill, B. Coombs Lee, and S. Nunn, "Palliative Treatments of Last Resort: Choosing the Least Harmful Alternative," *Annals of Internal Medicine* 132 (2000): 488–93.

5. S. Hurst and A. Mauron, "Assisted Suicide and Euthanasia in Switzerland: Allowing a Role for Nonphysicians," *British Medical Journal* 326 (2003): 271–73.

6. *Vacco v. Quill,* 117 S.Ct. 2293 (1997); *Washington v. Glucksberg,* 117 S.Ct. 2258 (1997).

7. J.L. Bernat, B. Gert, and R.P. Mogielnicki, "Patient Refusal of Hydration and Nutrition: An Alternative to Physician-Assisted Suicide or Voluntary Active Euthanasia," *Archives of Internal Medicine* 153 (1993): 2723–27; L.A. Printz, "Terminal Dehydration: A Compassionate Treatment," *Archives of Internal Medicine* 152 (1992): 697–700; D.M. Eddy, "A Conversation with My Mother," *Journal of the American Medical Association* 272 (1994): 179–81; T.E. Quill and I. Byock, "Responding to Intractable Terminal Suffering: The Role of Terminal Sedation and Voluntary Refusal of Food and Fluids," *Annals of Internal Medicine* 132 (2000): 408–14.

8. Bernat, Gert, and Mogielnicki, "Patient Refusal of Hydration and Nutrition"; Printz, "Terminal Dehydration"; Eddy, "A Conversation with My Mother."

9. N.I. Cherney and R.K. Portenoy, "Sedation in the Management of Refractory Symptoms: Guidelines for Evaluation and Treatment," *Journal of Palliative Care* 10 (1994): 31–38; R.D. Troug, D.B. Berde, C. Mitchell, and H.E. Grier, "Barbiturates in the Care of the Terminally Ill," *New England Journal of Medicine* 327 (1991): 1678–81; R.E. Enck, *The Medical Care of Terminally Ill Patients* (Baltimore: Johns Hopkins University Press, 1994); C. Saunders and N. Sykes, *The Management of Terminal Malignant Disease,* 3d ed. (London: Hodder Headline Group, 1993), 1–305; Quill and Byock, "Responding to Intractable Terminal Suffering"; E.H. Loewy, "Terminal Sedation, Self-Starvation, and Orchestrating the End of Life," *Archives of Internal Medicine* (2001): 329–32; J.D. Cowan and D. Walsh, "Terminal Sedation in Palliative Medicine—Definition and Review of the Literature," *Support Cancer Care* 9 (2001): 403–7.

10. T. Morita, S. Tsuneto, and Y. Shima, "Proposed Definitions for Terminal Sedation," *Lancet* 358 (2001): 335–36.

11. G. Craig, "Is Sedation without Hydration or Nourishment in Terminal Care Lawful?" *Medical Legal Journal* 62, no. 4 (1994): 198–201.

12. *Vacco v. Quill; Washington v. Glucksberg;* Foley, "Pain, Physician-Assisted Suicide, and Euthanasia"; Coyle et al., "Character of Terminal Illness in the Advanced Cancer Patient"; Cherney and Portenoy, "Sedation in the Management of Refractory Symptoms"; Troug et al., "Barbiturates in the Care of the Terminally Ill"; Enck, *Medical Care of Terminally Ill Patients;* Saunders and Sykes, *Management of Terminal Malignant Disease;* I.R. Byock, "Consciously Walking the Fine Line: Thoughts on a Hospice Response to Assisted Suicide and Euthanasia," *Journal of Palliative Care* 9 (1993): 25–28; B. Ventafridda, C. Ripamonti, F. DeConno, M. Tamburini, and B.R. Cassileth, "Symptom Prevalence and Control During Cancer Patients' Last Days of Life," *Journal of Palliative Care* 6 (1990): 7–11.

13. H. Brody, "Causing, Intending, and Assisting Death," *Journal of Clinical Ethics* 4 (1993): 112–17; J.A. Billings, "Slow Euthanasia," *Journal of Palliative Care* 12 (1996): 21–30.

14. N. Moerman, B. Bonke, and J. Oosting, "Awareness and Recall During General Anesthesia. Facts and Feelings," *Anesthesiology* 79 (1993): 454–64; J.E. Utting, "Awareness: Clinical Aspects; Consciousness, Awareness, and Pain," in *General Anesthesia*, edited by M. Rosen and J.N. Linn (London: Butterworths, 1987), 171–79, 184–92.

15. Brody, "Causing, Intending, and Assisting Death"; Billings, "Slow Euthanasia."

16. Foley, "Pain, Physician-Assisted Suicide, and Euthanasia"; Quill, *Death and Dignity;* D.W. Brock, "Voluntary Active Euthanasia," *Hastings Center Report* 22, no. 3 (1992): 10–22.

17. T.E. Quill, "Death and Dignity: A Case of Individualized Decision Making," *New England Journal of Medicine* 324 (1991): 691–94; B. Rollin, *Last Wish* (New York: Warner, 1985).

18. J.S. Cohen, S.D. Fihn, E.J. Boyko, A.R. Jonsen, and R.W. Wood, "Attitudes toward Assisted Suicide and Euthanasia among Physicians in Washington State," *New England Journal of Medicine* 331 (1994): 89–94; J.G. Bachman, K.H. Alchser, D.J. Doukas, R.L. Lichtenstein, A.D. Corning, and H. Brody, "Attitudes of Michigan Physicians and the Public toward Legalizing Physician-Assisted Suicide and Voluntary Euthanasia," *New England Journal of Medicine* 334 (1996): 303–9; P.R. Duberstein, Y. Conwell, C. Cox, C.A. Podgorski, R.S. Glazer, and E.D. Caine, "Attitudes toward Self-Determined Death: A Survey of Primary Care Physicians," *Journal of the American Geriatric Society* 43 (1995): 395–400.

19. W. Gaylin, L.R. Kass, E.D. Pellegrino, and M. Siegler, "Doctors Must Not Kill," *New England Journal of Medicine* 259 (1988): 2319–40.

20. T.A. Preston and R. Mero, "Observations Concerning Terminally Ill Patients Who Choose Suicide," *Journal of Pharmaceutical Care in Pain and Symptom Control* 1 (1996): 183–92; P.V. Admiraal, "The Use of Euthanatics" [in Dutch], *Nederlands Tijdschrift Geneeskd* 139 (1995): 265–68.

21. Quill, *Death and Dignity.*

22. Back et al., "Physician-Assisted Suicide and Euthanasia in Washington State."

23. M.A. Lee, H.D. Nelson, V.P. Tilden, L. Ganzini, T.A. Schmidt, and S.W. Tolle, "Legalizing Assisted Suicide: Views of Physicians in Oregon," *New England Journal of Medicine* 334 (1996): 310–15.

24. A. Alpers and B. Lo, "Physician-Assisted Suicide in Oregon: A Bold Experiment," *Journal of the American Medical Association* 274 (1995): 483–87.

25. K. Hedberg, D. Hopkins, and M. Kohn, "Five Years of Legal Physician-Assisted Suicide in Oregon," *New England Journal of Medicine* 348 (2003): 961–64.

26. *Vacco v. Quill; Washington v. Glucksberg; Compassion in Dying v. Washington,* 79 F.3d 790 (9th Cir. 1996); *Quill v. Vacco,* 80 F.3d 716 (2d Cir. 1996).

27. Foley, "Pain, Physician-Assisted Suicide, and Euthanasia"; American Medical Association, "Good Care of the Dying Patient"; American Board of Internal Medicine, *Caring for the Dying;* President's Commission for the Study of Ethical Problems in Medicine and Biomedical and Behavioral Research, *Deciding to Forego Life-Sustaining Treatment: Ethical, Medical and Legal Issues in Treatment Decisions* (Washington: U.S.

Government Printing Office, 1983); Hastings Center, *Guidelines on the Termination of Life-Sustaining Treatment and Care of the Dying* (Bloomington: University of Indiana Press, 1988).

28. Bernat, Gert, and Mogielnicki, "Patient Refusal of Hydration and Nutrition"; Printz, "Terminal Dehydration"; Troug et al., "Barbiturates in the Care of the Terminally Ill"; Byock, "Consciously Walking the Fine Line."

29. Brody, "Causing, Intending, and Assisting Death"; Billings, "Slow Euthanasia"; D.B. Marquis, "Four Versions of the Double Effect," *Journal of Medicine and Philosophy* 16 (1991): 515–44; F. Kamm, "The Doctrine of Double Effect: Reflections on Theoretical and Practical Issues," *Journal of Medicine and Philosophy* 16 (1991): 571–85; T.E. Quill, R. Dresser, and D. Brock, "The Rule of Double Effect: A Critique of Its Role in End-of-Life Decision Making," *New England Journal of Medicine* 337 (1997): 1768–71.

30. Foley, "Pain, Physician-Assisted Suicide, and Euthanasia"; American Medical Association, "Good Care of the Dying Patient"; American Board of Internal Medicine, *Caring for the Dying;* President's Commission for the Study of Ethical Problems, *Deciding to Forego Life-Sustaining Treatment;* Hastings Center, *Guidelines.*

31. N. Sykes and A. Thomas, "Sedatives in the Last Week of Life and the Implications for End of Life Decision Making," *Archives of Internal Medicine* 163 (2003): 342–44.

32. Cherney and Portenoy, "Sedation in the Management of Refractory Symptoms"; Troug et al., "Barbiturates in the Care of the Terminally Ill"; Saunders and Sykes, *Management of Terminal Malignant Disease;* Byock, "Consciously Walking the Fine Line."

33. Brody, "Causing, Intending, and Assisting Death"; Billings, "Slow Euthanasia"; D.B. Marquis, "Four Versions of the Double Effect"; F. Kamm, "The Doctrine of Double Effect: Reflections on Theoretical and Practical Issues"; T.E. Quill, R. Dresser, and D. Brock, "The Rule of Double Effect: A Critique of Its Role in End-of-Life Decision Making."

34. Brody, "Causing, Intending, and Assisting Death"; A. Alpers and B. Lo, "Does It Make Clinical Sense to Equate Terminally Ill Patients Who Require Life-Sustaining Interventions with Those Who Do Not?" *Journal of the American Medical Association* 277 (1997): 1705–8.

35. Foley, "Pain, Physician-Assisted Suicide, and Euthanasia"; American Medical Association, "Good Care of the Dying Patient"; Quill, *Death and Dignity;* American Board of Internal Medicine, *Caring for the Dying;* President's Commission for the Study of Ethical Problems, *Deciding to Forego Life-Sustaining Treatment;* Alpers and Lo, "Does It Make Clinical Sense?"

36. Foley, "Pain, Physician-Assisted Suicide, and Euthanasia"; American Medical Association, "Good Care of the Dying Patient"; American Board of Internal Medicine, *Caring for the Dying;* President's Commission for the Study of Ethical Problems, *Deciding to Forego Life-Sustaining Treatment;* Hastings Center, *Guidelines;* T.L. Beauchamp and J.F. Childress, *Principles of Biomedical Ethics,* 3rd ed. (New York: Oxford University Press, 1994).

37. Brody, "Causing, Intending, and Assisting Death"; Brock, "Voluntary Active Euthanasia."

38. M.J. Edwards and S.W. Tolle, "Disconnecting a Ventilator at the Request of a Patient Who Knows He Will Die: The Doctor's Anguish," *Annals of Internal Medicine* 117 (1992): 254–56.

39. Brock, "Voluntary Active Euthanasia."

40. Bernat, Gert, and Mogielnicki, "Patient Refusal of Hydration and Nutrition"; Printz, "Terminal Dehydration."

41. Cohen et al., "Attitudes toward Assisted Suicide and Euthanasia among Physicians in Washington State"; Bachman et al., "Attitudes of Michigan Physicians and the Public toward Legalizing Physician-Assisted Suicide and Voluntary Euthanasia"; Duberstein et al., "Attitudes toward Self-Determined Death."

42. Brody, "Causing, Intending, and Assisting Death"; T.E. Quill, "The Ambiguity of Clinical Intentions," *New England Journal of Medicine* 329 (1993): 1039–40.

43. Cherney and Portenoy, "Sedation in the Management of Refractory Symptoms"; Troug et al., "Barbiturates in the Care of the Terminally Ill"; Byock, "Consciously Walking the Fine Line."

44. Brock, "Voluntary Active Euthanasia."

45. D. Orentlicher, "The Legalization of Physician-Assisted Suicide," *New England Journal of Medicine* 335 (1996): 663–67; M.A. Drickamer, M.A. Lee, and L. Ganzini, "Practical Issues in Physician-Assisted Suicide," *Annals of Internal Medicine* 126 (1997): 146–51; M. Angell, "The Supreme Court and Physician-Assisted Suicide—The Ultimate Right," editorial, *New England Journal of Medicine* 336 (1997): 50–53.

46. Brock, "Voluntary Active Euthanasia"; Beauchamp and Childress, *Principles of Biomedical Ethics.*

47. Beauchamp and Childress, *Principles of Biomedical Ethics.*

48. Ibid.; M.A.M. de Wachter, "Active Euthanasia in the Netherlands," *Journal of the American Medical Association* 262 (1989): 3316–19.

49. T.E. Quill and R.V. Brody, "'You Promised Me I Wouldn't Die Like This': A Bad Death as a Medical Emergency," *Archives of Internal Medicine* 155 (1995): 1250–54.

50. De Wachter, "Active Euthanasia in the Netherlands"; J.V.M. Welie, "The Medical Exception: Physicians, Euthanasia and the Dutch Criminal Law," *Journal of Medicine and Philosophy* 17 (1992): 419–37.

51. De Wachter, "Active Euthanasia in the Netherlands."

52. T.E. Quill and C.K. Cassel, "Nonabandonment: A Central Obligation for Physicians," *Annals of Internal Medicine* 122 (1995): 368–74.

53. E.J. Emanuel and A.S. Brett, "Managed Competition and the Patient-Physician Relationship," *New England Journal of Medicine* 329 (1993): 879–82; R.S. Morrison and D.E. Meier, "Managed Care at the End of Life," *Trends in Health Care, Law and Ethics* 10 (1995): 91–96.

54. W. Gaylin, L.R. Kass, E.D. Pellegrino, and M. Siegler, "Doctors Must Not Kill," *Journal of the American Medical Association* 259 (1988): 2139–40; J. Teno and J. Lynn, "Voluntary Active Euthanasia: The Individual Case and Public Policy," *Journal of the American Geriatric Society* 39 (1991): 827–30; Y. Kamisar, "Against Assisted Suicide—Even a Very Limited Form," *University of Detroit Mercy Law Review* 72 (1995): 735–69.

55. T.E. Quill, C.K. Cassel, and D.E. Meier, "Care of the Hopelessly Ill: Proposed Clinical Criteria for Physician-Assisted Suicide," *New England Journal of Medicine* 327 (1992): 1380–84; H. Brody, "Assisted Death: A Compassionate Response to a Medical Failure," *New England Journal of Medicine* 327 (1992): 1384–88; F.G. Miller, T.E. Quill, H. Brody, J.C. Fletcher, L.O. Gostin, and D.E. Meier, "Regulating Physician-Assisted Death," *New England Journal of Medicine* 331 (1994): 119–23; C.H. Baron, C. Bergstresser, D.W. Brock, C.F. Cole, N.S. Dorfman, J.A. Johnson, L.E. Schnipper, J. Vorenberg, and S.H. Wanzer, "Statute: A Model State Act to Authorize and Regulate Physician-Assisted Suicide," *Harvard Journal on Legislation* 33 (1996): 1–34.

56. Teno and Lynn, "Voluntary Active Euthanasia"; Kamisar, "Against Assisted Suicide."

57. B. Mount and E.M. Flanders, "Morphine Drips, Terminal Sedation, and Slow Euthanasia: Definitions and Facts, Not Anecdotes," *Journal of Palliative Care* 12 (1996): 31–37.

58. Foley, "Pain, Physician-Assisted Suicide, and Euthanasia"; American Medical Association, "Good Care of the Dying Patient"; Quill, *Death and Dignity;* American Board of Internal Medicine, *Caring for the Dying.*

59. De Wachter, "Active Euthanasia in the Netherlands"; Quill and Cassel, "Non-abandonment"; M.A. Lee and S.W. Tolle, "Oregon's Assisted-Suicide Vote: The Silver Lining," *Annals of Internal Medicine* 124 (1996): 267–69; S.D. Block and J.A. Billings, "Patient Requests to Hasten Death: Evaluation and Management in Terminal Care," *Archives of Internal Medicine* 154 (1994): 2039–47; T.E. Quill, "Doctor, I Want to Die. Will You Help Me?" *Journal of the American Medical Association* 270 (1993): 870–73.

10

Death

A Friend to Be Welcomed,
Not an Enemy to Be Defeated

John Shelby Spong, A.B., M.Div., Honorary D.D., D.H.L.

It is a unique experience for a representative of the Christian church to be invited to contribute to a book on the issue of choice at the end of human life. Typically, this is not an arena in which traditional Christians feel comfortable. Although the church has by and large made peace with what is generally called "passive euthanasia"—that is, the suspension of artificial life-support systems to allow death to take its natural course—organized religion generally draws the line at that boundary. For me, however, that limitation is a sign of an unwillingness to debate the real issues. This reticence is based on certain unspoken moral presuppositions that I believe have simply become inoperative through the remarkable advances in medical knowledge and technology. Far from being the place where the debate ends, in my mind "passive euthanasia" is where the real discussion begins.

Because I will be viewed by some religious leaders as a distinctively minority voice, I find it necessary to state my credentials by starting this chapter with a brief spiritual autobiography. I come at the issues of assisted suicide, active euthanasia, and the freedom to die with dignity from a specifically religious position. Religion is not tangential to my life. Indeed, I identify myself first and foremost as a committed and practicing Christian. I have never lived apart from that identity. I was even born in an Episcopal hospital. I was baptized as an infant, nurtured in a church-school setting, confirmed as a young adolescent, and I was active in my church's teenage and university programs. I wanted to do nothing but be a priest from the time of my earliest memory. I entered that profession, after my theological preparation, at the ripe old age of twenty-four. I served my church as a priest for twenty-one years. My church elected me to be one of its bishops when I was forty-four years old. I served as a bishop for twenty-four years, retiring in 2000 as the senior sitting Episcopal bishop in the United States. Far from being a fringe voice, I am someone who has lived at the heart of the Christian church. I have no context from which to address these end-of-life issues other than that of one who has spent my personal and professional life deep inside the boundaries of organized religion.

Yet I am passionate in my conviction that the time has come when Christians must relinquish their negativity toward those activities that are aimed at assistance in dying, active euthanasia, and physician-assisted suicide. I see all of these initiatives as being within the religious context, which begins with the assertion that life is holy and that this holiness must be served in all we do. It is from the standpoint of what I define as Christian ethics, which are rooted in the sacredness of life, that I bear my witness that assisted suicide can and does operate within that specifically religious framework.

I believe that if and when a person arrives at that point in human existence when death has become a kinder alternative than hopeless pain and when a chronic dependency on narcotics begins to require the loss of personal dignity, then the basic human right to choose how and when to die should be guaranteed by law and respected by our communities of faith. I have spoken publicly in favor of this conviction for years but always assumed that I was a lonely single voice within my church. Then I decided to test that premise; in my role as bishop, I appointed a task force in our diocese to study these issues and to bring their conclusions to our diocese's decision-making body for a vote up or down. That task force was cochaired by a laywoman, who was a professor of nutrition at a small Roman Catholic college in New Jersey, and an Episcopal priest, who before his ordination had been a professor of political science at Louisiana State University.

After a year of study, including open hearings across the state, this task force drafted a report to place before the convention of the Diocese of Newark, which covers all of northern New Jersey. After a three-hour public debate, covered by all the major media from the metropolitan New York area, this convention endorsed, by a two-to-one majority, physician-assisted suicide "as a moral option for Christians."[1] That convention was made up of 600 people, approximately 450 of them elected lay people and 150 ordained clergy from our various and diverse congregations. This was one of the first times that an official body within a mainline Christian church in the United States had taken a positive stand on this question. Empowered by that witness I testified, as the leader of that diocese, before a House of Representatives committee of the

Congress of the United States, stating my support for making this a legal right for all of our citizens. Representative Henry Hyde of Illinois presided over that hearing. The Congress regrettably did not agree with me.

Later, the Supreme Court of the United States, in a unanimous decision, refused even to open this subject for debate by providing us with a minority opinion. So there is work to be done, vast amounts of work. Our task is to educate the public, the lawmakers, and the judges of this nation as to the rightness of this cause. One major factor in that educational process will be to turn the opinion of the religious communities. It is my hope that this chapter might be a factor in that necessary and vital campaign.

I want my readers and my fellow Christians first to seek to understand the sources of the religious negativity that hover around all end-of-life issues. That is the first step that must be taken before progress and change can be accomplished in religious circles. Because I am both a Christian and a supporter of the right to determine how and when I will die, I want to demonstrate that one does not have to abandon a traditional religious commitment in order to embrace what I now regard as a compelling new freedom. Indeed, I present myself to you as a living illustration that a person can join together the principle that we should have some choice in how we die with the Christian conviction that life is ultimately holy. I recognize that this is not an easy assignment in either camp. I will doubtless be forced to defend my participation in this book to the majority of those who live in my faith community. I suspect that the editors and publisher will have to defend their invitation to a bishop to be part of this book to the majority of its readers. So let me begin that process and build that case.

The story of Judeo-Christian faith opens in the book of Genesis with the assertion of life's sacredness. The creation narrative presents us with a portrait of human life as having been made in the divine image. From this assertion, Christians have derived the principle that the power to live or die is not a decision that properly resides in human beings. That power, it is typically said, resides in God alone. Therefore, the traditional Christian concludes, no one can be given the liberty of ending his or her life under any circumstances. That principle permeates contemporary Christian thinking. Yet a look at Christian history reveals that it has been randomly and inconsistently applied.

In the course of our history it can be easily documented that Christians have never left the power to die exclusively in God's hands. Christians have fought religious wars in which people were killed quite deliberately. God did not kill them; Christian human beings did. Many of these victims were people of other religious convictions. Christians have justified these political acts of violence with elaborate arguments about what constitutes a "just war." I do not want to argue on this occasion either the pacifist position or the just-war position. I simply want to note that in this arena Christians have not left the power of life and death in God's hands alone. Rather, they have abrogated this power to themselves. Thus it is hard to maintain that the power to make life and death decisions must be left in God's hands alone.

Christians have also employed the practice of capital punishment in the nations of the Western world for almost all our history. It is only recently, and quite frankly in the more secularized nations of Western Europe, that the debate on the morality of capital punishment has led some nations to ban the practice as cruel and inhumane punishment. However, the records of history show that Christian rulers in ostensibly Christian nations, aided and abetted by the prevailing religious hierarchies of the Christian churches, have shown no reluctance whatsoever in claiming the right to take the power of life and death from God and to place that power squarely into their own very human hands.

Christians have over the years of their history used their power to execute their critics again and again as part of their way of enforcing religious beliefs. Giordano Bruno was burned at the stake in 1600 by the religious authorities of his day because he taught that the earth was not the center of the universe. That was, of course, a point of view contrary to the prevailing Christian synthesis.

The Inquisition used the same tactic at many different fiery stakes to execute thousands of human beings for the sin of heresy or for the "crime," as they thought of it, of being a Jew. The Crusades, officially sponsored by the Vatican, also caused the death of many Jews in Europe because the Jews were the only "infidels" that the Crusaders could locate when their romantic journeys to free the holy land from nonbelievers failed, as most of them did, to reach their appointed destination. The Christian church has also, with enormous ignorance, enforced its prejudice against homosexual persons by burning so many of them at the stake that the little stick that ignited the fire, called a "faggot," became a derisive slang term applied to the homosexual person.

If human beings who call themselves Christians have had no scruples about endorsing war, killing religious enemies, or imposing the sentence of death upon those who violate either the norms of faith or the boundaries of prejudice under a particular set of circumstances in the past, is it still appropriate for Christians to suggest that one cannot elect death for himself or herself under a different set of circumstances in the present? It seems to me that a certain irrational inconsistency is operating here, which needs to be pointed out to any faith community that espouses such claims.

In each of the historical instances I have cited, it will be quickly argued by my religious critics that the people who did these things were motivated, perhaps mistakenly but nonetheless sincerely, by their commitment to the sacredness of life. It was not, they will say, that the principle under which they were acting was wrong but rather that it was applied improperly. In warfare, they will contend, it was the desire to save life that caused Christians to take up arms against a supposed enemy who threatened their own lives. In state-ordered or even church-ordered executions, they will contend, the goal was to protect the lives of the citizens by dispatching permanently those who were guilty of violating what were assumed to be the ultimate boundaries on humanity. This extreme punishment was justified as the only way to guarantee that these victims would never violate life again.

Even in religious persecutions, they will argue, lives were snuffed out because those in authority determined that the continued existence of heresy or heretics would lead people astray and thus violate the ultimate sacredness of life. So as dreadful and wrong as this inquisitional behavior now seems to have been in our eyes as enlightened people of today, my critics will say, it could still be argued that this behavior was nonetheless deemed to have been done in the service of affirming life's sacredness. One must not therefore suggest, they will conclude, that these illustrations can be properly used to pretend that human beings have the right to take their own lives under any set of circumstances.

Suicide, they contend, is always wrong, always a violation of the holiness of life and of the God whom they believe to be the Source of that Life. It is an interesting but unconvincing argument. Its weakness is best seen, however, when these same religious people play what has traditionally been their favorite and final trump card. The Bible condemns suicide in any form, they assert. That, presumably, concludes all debate.

The most amazing thing, however, about people who seek to end an argument by quoting the authority of the Bible is that most of these quoters are woefully ignorant of the content of the Bible itself. I have discovered in my life that no one is a strict biblical literalist, not even Jerry Falwell or Pat Robertson. They are all what I would call "selective literalists." They simply ignore those parts of the biblical text that have become inoperative or inconvenient. They quote only those portions of the text that, they assume, buttress their position. It is a religious power play. It is their attempt to say, "If you disagree with me you are really disagreeing with God." Yet history has not treated this power play very kindly.

The Bible was quoted in the thirteenth century to support the divine right of kings and to oppose the Magna Carta. The Bible lost: there is no king anywhere in the world today who rules by divine right. If a king or queen rules at all, even symbolically, it is by the consent of the people.

The Bible was quoted in the seventeenth century to prove that Galileo was wrong and that the sun really did rotate around the earth. The Bible lost. In 1992 the Vatican finally admitted that Galileo had been right and the church had been wrong. The correction came four hundred years too late, but better late than never. It is because of Galileo that we are today a space-age people.

The Bible was quoted in the eighteenth and nineteenth centuries to justify the institution of slavery. Even the popes have owned slaves. Once again, the Bible lost the battle, and slavery, thank God, has been recognized as a great moral evil. Yet it left behind two bastard stepchildren, segregation and apartheid, and they, in turn, left a culture of racism with which many people are still infected. Senator Trent Lott of Mississippi revealed that poignantly in 2002. Yet Senator Lott's forced resignation as majority leader of the U.S. Senate made it clear that the back of racism has now been broken. Racism is now, quite obviously, a political liability of major proportions, and every politician will go to school on that example. The effects of this long-practiced racism linger on, but the fact remains that the literal Bible was forced to retreat from this fight defeated, chastened, and badly wounded.

In the nineteenth and twentieth centuries, the Bible was again quoted to keep women in positions of second-class citizenship in most of the nations of the Western world. Once more, the Bible lost. Women in the United States won the right to vote by constitutional amendment in 1920. Women first entered the cabinet of the president of the United States in the person of Frances Perkins in 1932. Women entered the Congress, the governors' mansions, and the Supreme Court as the years of the twentieth century rolled on.

Women also invaded the world of medicine, law, science, business, the priesthood, corporate boardrooms, and ultimately the ranks of the chief executive officers of Fortune 500 companies, like Lucent Technology, e-Bay, and Hewlett-Packard, all in that much-maligned but still impressive century of progress. The only battle still engaged by the religious community against the emancipation of women is found in the political struggle to ban abortion. That effort is driven by the attempt to give to the as yet male-controlled government the right to determine what a woman can do legally with her own body. That, too, is a losing fight. Only an administration with an ideology more powerful than its desire to stay in office will continue to press that issue. *Roe v. Wade* is safe even from an attorney general like John Ashcroft. He will, I predict, serve his constituents with rhetoric only, not with action, or with action that cannot succeed, because he and the members of the administration he represents know how to count votes.

The Bible was once again quoted in the twentieth and twenty-first centuries to uphold traditional religious prejudice against homosexual people. That is also a fight that the Bible is losing and will lose as medical and scientific evidence mounts daily, making it abundantly clear that sexual orientation is a given and not chosen. Sexual orientation is part of who people are, not what people do. Sexual orientation is thus more like left- or right-handedness than it is about moral defect. When this definition fully permeates the consciousness of this nation, as it is very close to doing today, then one more ancient prejudice buttressed by biblical quotations will come to an end. The Bible cannot continue to be used in such an ill-informed and dramatically wrong way.

So to have the Bible quoted by the religious community today to bring a final solution to all end-of-life discussions is hardly something to be feared. It is only the last gasp of a dying religious imperialism. It needs only to be countered with informed data.

Suicide is mentioned infrequently in the biblical narrative. Only three of those suicide narratives have risen to the place where they serve as illustrations that are used in the debate on the morality of willful attempts to end one's own life. The first of these is found in the story of King Saul, the predecessor to King David in Jewish history. Saul had been mortally wounded in the battle of Mount Gilboa, when the Jews were fighting against the Philistines. He begged his armor bearer to strike him with his sword to end his suffering and to hasten his inevitable death. When the armor bearer refused, Saul fell on his own sword and ended his life (1 Samuel 31:1–4).

The second involves a man named Ahithophel, one of King David's advisers, who ate daily at the royal table. Ahithophel betrayed King David, who as king was called "the Lord's anointed." When Ahithophel was discovered, the text says, he went out and hanged himself (2 Samuel 17:23).

The third case is Judas Iscariot, whose story was clearly shaped by the account of Ahithophel. He also ate at the Lord's table. He also was said to have betrayed one known as "the Lord's anointed." When Judas was discovered he, like Ahithophel, also went out and hanged himself (Matthew, chaps. 26 and 27).[2]

The biblical writers assumed that for Ahithophel and Judas Iscariot, suicide was an appropriate punishment for their crimes. Although the Bible appears to be generally negative about suicide, it does not condemn King Saul, who hastened his inevitable death to avoid needless suffering, nor does it seem to condemn those who take somebody else's life. That appears to be true even with the commandment, "Thou shalt not kill," as part of the Bible's legal code.

The Bible prescribes the death penalty for such crimes as worshiping false gods; for being disobedient; for talking back to or cursing one's parents; for being a medium, a wizard, or a witch; and for committing adultery. The Bible also prescribes the death penalty for having sex with one's mother-in-law. Few people ever quote this verse about one's mother-in-law (probably because it is hard to imagine anyone being guilty of such an act); it is found in Leviticus 20:14.

My point is a simple one. The Bible actually has little to say about suicide. Furthermore, if the Bible and the Christian tradition are assumed to regard life as too sacred for one to seek release from it under any circumstances, does life not also become too sacred to have it taken away by another? If that conclusion is not drawn, how can one draw the conclusion that suicide is always evil?

As a Christian, I affirm this conviction that life is sacred, that it is the ultimate gift from God. Because I hold this belief, I am committed to living every moment I am given as deeply, richly, and fully as I can. However, the times in which we live, as well as the shape of our developed consciousness in many areas of life, have changed dramatically through the ages. Christians must also take cognizance of that.

Human knowledge has expanded enormously, which means that "new occasions teach new duties," as the poet James Russell Lowell once observed.[3] I today can no longer just quote the biblical wisdom of antiquity as if that is the final answer to anything. I cannot be just a passive observer of life. It is not enough simply to assert that I am a committed Christian. I am also a citizen of the twenty-first century. I must take my place in history seriously.

I am the beneficiary of a vast revolution in scientific and medical thinking. I possess a reservoir of data that was not available to the people who wrote the Bible. This is the gift of the modern world to me. I have watched life expectancy expand remarkably. I live in a world of quadruple heart bypasses, radiation and chemotherapy, laproscopic surgical procedures, organ transplants, prostate specific antigen tests, Pap smears, miracle drugs, and incredible life-support systems. My grandfather died of pneumonia, before the development of penicillin. I have had two diseases that I do not believe my grandparents would have survived.

I live in a privileged part of the world and in a privileged generation. I rejoice in all of these human achievements. Let there be no mistake, however, about what is happening. These stirring achievements represent human beings' taking on the power we once ascribed only to God. We have, by our own knowledge and expertise, put our hands on the decisions regarding life and death. We cannot and must not now refuse to engage these decisions at the end of our own lives. We have pushed back the boundaries of death inexorably. We have enabled this generation to live in a way that previous generations could never have imagined. We have watched human life actually evolve to a point at which it must accept Godlike responsibilities. The time has come to celebrate that, not to hide from it in the language of piety.

I see the religious community today trembling in the face of our own human audacity and seeking to hide from the responsibility inherent in our own human achievements, none of which we would be willing to surrender. Why else would we hesitate before this final boundary called death? Why would we resist so vigorously the reality that now we must take a hand in our death decisions? When medical science expands the boundary and the quality of life, Christians do not complain. Rather, we rejoice because we believe it affirms our conviction that life is holy.

It is one thing, however, to expand life and quite another to postpone death. When medical science shifts from expanding the length and quality of life and begins simply to postpone the reality of death, why are we not capable of saying that the sacredness of life is no longer being served, and therefore Christians must learn to act responsibly in the final moments of life?

What happens to both our courage and our faith? Is a breathing cadaver, with no hope of restoration, an example of the sacredness of life? Is intense and unrelieved suffering somehow a virtue? I do not think so. Do we human beings, including those of us who claim to be Christians, not have the right to say, "That is not the way I choose to die?" I believe we do.

Is death really the enemy of our humanity, as St. Paul once stated? Much Christian thinking has been based on that definition. Well, let it be said by a bishop of the church: *St. Paul was wrong*—here and in several other places. I often wonder how it was that the words of this man ever came to be called "The Word of God." When Paul said, "I hope those who unsettle you would mutilate themselves" (Galatians 5:12), was that the word of God? Paul was a child of his era, responding to his own presuppositions and living with his own prejudices. They are not my presuppositions. I prefer to think of death not as an enemy but as a friend, even a brother, as St. Francis of Assisi once suggested. The time has therefore come, I believe, for Christians to embrace death not as an enemy to be defeated but as an aspect of life's holiness to be embraced.

Death is life's shadow. It walks with us through the course of our days. We embrace death as a friend because we honor life. I honor the God of life whom I serve by living fully. It does not honor God to cling to an existence that has become an empty shell.

I do not honor life when I fail to see that death and finitude are what give our humanity its precious quality. Death is not a punishment for sin, as Paul also once suggested and as classical Christianity has long maintained. Death is an aspect of life, a vital aspect that gives life its deepest flavor, its defining sensitivity.

Death has a way of ringing the bell on all procrastination. It is because life is finite, not infinite, that we do not postpone the quest for meaning indefinitely. It is because of the presence of death with us on our life's journey that we do not fail to take the opportunity to say "I love you," to invest ourselves in primary relationships, to do what needs to be done now, not tomorrow, to build a better world now. Death says you do not have forever to make a difference. Death is what gives conscious life its uniqueness. Remove death from life and life becomes enduring boredom, an endless game of shuffleboard. We make life precious by embracing the reality of death, not by repressing it or denying it. Our present burial customs of applying makeup to the faces of the deceased so that they look natural and using artificial grass to cover the dirt of the grave rise out of our attempt to deny the truth and indeed the fear of our mortality. They do not arise out of our affirmation about the wonder and beauty of life.

I, for one, want to live my life by squeezing every ounce of joy out of every moment I am given. I want to expand my life to its fullest extent. That is the way I choose to affirm the sacredness of life. I want to drink deeply of life's sweetness, to scale its heights and plumb its depths. I want to do all I can do to affirm life and, yes, to postpone death at least until life's quality has been so compromised that it is no longer life as I believe God intended it. At that time I want to embrace death as my friend, my companion who has walked with me from the moment of my birth.

I want to live my days surrounded by those I love, able to see my wife's beautiful smile and feel the touch of her hand. I want to share in the joy and vitality of my children and grandchildren. When those realities are taken away, I want to leave this world, and those I love, with a positive vision. I want them to see in me one who lived and loved deeply and well until living and loving deeply and well was no longer possible. I want them to remember me as a person who was vital to the end, in possession of all that makes me who I am, and as one who died well. My deepest desire is always to choose death with dignity over a life that has become either hopelessly painful and dysfunctional or empty and devoid of all meaning.

That is the only way I know that would allow me to honor the God in whose image I was created. That is the way I want to acknowledge the relationship I have had with God, which has grown from a dependent and immature one into the maturity of recognizing that to be human is to share with God in the ultimate life-and-death decisions. That is how I hope and expect to celebrate life's holiness and to honor life's creator. That does not seem to me to be too much to ask my faith to give me or my government to guarantee for me.

I think this choice should be legal. I will work, therefore, through the political processes to seek to create a world in which advance directives are obeyed and physicians assist those who so choose to die at the appropriate time. I also think the choice to do this should be acclaimed as both moral and ethical—a human right, if you will; and I will work through the ecclesiastical processes of my church and all the forces of organized religion to change consciousness, to embrace new realities, and to enable Christians and other people of faith to say that we are compelled in this direction because we believe that God is real and that life is holy. The God whom I experience as the source of life can surely not be served by those in whom death is simply postponed or not allowed to serve its natural function.

I close with a text, because people seem to believe that a clergyman must have a text for every speech that he or she delivers. In the tenth chapter of John's gospel, these words are attributed to Jesus of Nazareth, who stands at the center of my faith tradition. Articulating his purpose, he says, "I came that they might have life and have it abundantly" (John 10:10). It is that abundant life that is the ultimate gift of God. I walk into the source of that abundant life in the way I live. I want also to walk into the source of that abundant life in the way I die.

I see no contradiction between the faith I cherish and principles of having some choice and control over how we die. I embrace the right to die with dignity as my choice, with the hope that others who do not share my faith perspective will join me, to stand at the side of those today who support physician-assisted suicide at the request of the patient when all other doorways to the fullness of life have been exhausted. I hope they will welcome me as their religious ally even as I welcome them as my partners in the struggle to assert that life is ultimately holy. I am a Christian who has been led by my faith to champion the legal, moral, and ethical right that I believe should be recognized for every individual—to die with dignity and to have the freedom to choose when and how that dignified death might be accomplished.

Notes

The substance of this chapter was delivered as the keynote address at the annual meeting of the Hemlock Society in San Diego, California, on January 11, 2003.

1. This report in its entirety can be found on the Diocese of Newark website at www.dioceseofnewark.org.

2. There is also a reference to the death of Judas in chapter 1:8 of the Book of Acts, which scholars agree was written by Luke, that seems to contradict Matthew's account of Judas's suicide. For readers interested in a fuller treatment of the role of Judas in the Christian story, I refer you to chapter 16 of my book, *Liberating the Gospels: Reading the Bible with Jewish Eyes* (New York and San Francisco: HarperCollins, 1996). That chapter is entitled "Judas Iscariot: A Christian Invention?"

3. This phrase comes from the poem entitled "Once to Every Man and Nation Comes the Moment to Decide" and is quoted from the *The Episcopal Hymnal,* #519 (New York: Church Pension Fund, 1940).

PART THREE

Open Practice in a Legally Tolerant Environment

11

The Oregon Experience

Linda Ganzini, M.D., M.P.H.

With enactment of the Oregon Death with Dignity Act in November 1997, Oregon became the first jurisdiction in the United States to legalize physician-assisted suicide. The Death with Dignity Act, as enacted, allows a treating physician to prescribe a lethal dosage of medication for the purposes of self-administration to a patient who is over eighteen years of age, a resident of Oregon, capable (that is, has decision-making capacity), and diagnosed with a terminal illness (with an estimated life expectancy of less than six months). To minimize the risk that patients will impulsively take lethal medication and to ensure that treatments for depression and physical symptoms are first considered, the law further requires that the patient make one written and two oral requests over a period of fifteen days; that both the prescribing physician and a consulting physician confirm the diagnosis, prognosis, and the patient's capability; that the physician inform the patient of all feasible alternatives, including comfort care, hospice care, and pain control; and that the prescribing or consulting physician refer the patient to a psychiatrist or psychologist for further assessment if he or she believes that the patient's judgment is impaired by a mental disorder, such as depression. The Death with Dignity Act explicitly prohibits death by lethal injection and does not permit physicians to honor a no-longer-competent patient's request for assisted suicide set out in an advance directive.[1]

History of the Death with Dignity Act

The Oregon Death with Dignity Act was originally passed in 1994 by a slim margin of 51 percent to 49 percent through a statewide, voter-initiated referendum (similar propositions in the neighboring states of Washington and California had failed), but implementation was delayed when Judge Michael Hogan of the U.S. District Court issued an injunction prohibiting enactment. In the fall of 1997, the Ninth Circuit Court of Appeals upheld the law, clearing the way for enactment. That same year, the Oregon legislature, uncertain whether Oregonians had been sufficiently thoughtful in casting their ballots, referred the measure back to the voters, who endorsed it a second time by a vote of 60 to 40 percent.

In November 2001 U.S. Attorney General John Ashcroft reinterpreted the Controlled Substances Act as prohibiting physicians from prescribing barbiturates with the intent to hasten death. (To date, all deaths by physician-assisted suicide in Oregon have been from barbiturates.) Judge Robert Jones of the U.S. District Court for Oregon issued a restraining order preventing implementation of the reinterpretation. In September 2002 Ashcroft appealed this decision to the U.S. Court of Appeals for the Ninth Circuit, but in May 2004 this appeal was denied. A further appeal to the U.S. Supreme Court seems likely. If the Department of Justice eventually prevails, the physicians who prescribed barbiturates, the only medically prescribed substances that could reliably cause a safe and peaceful death, would run a substantial risk of losing their Drug Enforcement Agency licenses despite the fact that physician-assisted suicide would remain legally permissible under the state's Death with Dignity Act.[2]

Throughout the three years of uncertainty regarding the law, there was vigorous ongoing debate in Oregon about its merits and risks. The Oregon medical community remained divided, failing to take a strong unified stand against the law. Anticipating that the law might prevail, the Oregon Health and Science University's Center for Ethics and Health Care convened a task force to develop guidance for physicians who might receive requests; its report was published in March 1998.[3] The first lethal prescription under the act was written in spring 1998.[4]

The political debate about the Oregon Death with Dignity Act included a series of speculations about why patients might choose assisted suicide and the attitudes of health care providers about this practice. Experts hypothesized that patients who pursue physician-assisted death have treatable conditions, such as pain and depression, lack social support, and are motivated by financial concerns or a desire not to burden their families.[5] Commentators suggested that requests for assisted suicide would be rare if patients received adequate palliative care.[6] Many worried that women, minorities, and the poor, all of whom may have limited access to health care, including palliative care options, would disproportionately choose legalized physician-assisted suicide,[7] while others suggested that physicians would be less likely to agree to participate in assisted suicide if they had greater knowledge, skills, and levels of comfort in caring for dying patients.[8]

Furthermore, at the time the Death with Dignity Act was passed the delivery of medical care was being radically reorganized in an effort to stem escalating health care costs, and there was concern that managed care would promote physician-assisted suicide as a less expensive alternative to good palliative and hospice care.[9] Finally, it was suggested that legalizing assisted suicide would divert resources and attention from efforts to improve care for dying patients. Commentators argued that resources would be better spent improving access to palliative care than legalizing assisted suicide.[10]

In the absence of reliable data, however, most of what was asserted about both the risks and the advantages of legalizing assisted suicide was largely conjecture. Empirical data from several sources, including reports by the Oregon Department of Human Services (ODHS) and studies of legalized assisted suicide in Oregon, present an opportunity to begin to test these hypotheses.

Data on the Effects of the Death with Dignity Act

In the six years since the Death with Dignity Act was enacted, 171 patients have died by lethal prescription in Oregon, representing approximately one in one thousand deaths in the state.[11] Information about the effect of the law is contained in reports published by the ODHS.[12] The Death with Dignity Act requires each physician who writes a prescription for lethal medication to submit a report to the ODHS at the time the prescription is written, verifying that the physician has complied with the law's safeguards. (Physicians are not required to file reports on patients who are evaluated for assisted suicide but for whom a prescription is not written.) From the time the law took effect through the end of 2002, the ODHS interviewed each prescribing physician as well as nineteen family members of patients who received lethal prescriptions.[13] Table 11.1 summarizes characteristics of patients who have died by lethal prescription under the Death with Dignity Act.

A second source of information is a series of surveys of health care professionals on their views about the law and their experiences with patients who have requested assisted suicide. Findings from these surveys are summarized in table 11.2. Surveys conducted before enactment of the Death with Dignity Act in 1997 focused on attitudes about assisted suicide and concerns about the law

Table 11.1. Demographic Characteristics of 171 Patients Who Died by Medication under the Oregon Death with Dignity Act, 1998–2003

Characteristic	N	Percentage
Sex		
Male	90	53
Female	81	47
Race		
White	166	97
Asian	5	3
Other	0	
Education		
Less than high school	16	9
High school graduate	51	30
Some college	35	21
Baccalaureate or higher	69	40
Disease		
Malignancy	135	79
Amyotrophic lateral sclerosis	13	8
Other	23	13
Hospice enrollment		
Enrolled	145	85
Declined by patient	24	14
Unknown	2	1
Insurance		
Private	102	61
Medicare or Medicaid	64	38
None	2	1
Unknown	3	2
Reported end-of-life concern		
Loss of autonomy	145	87
Diminished ability to engage in enjoyable activities	138	83
Loss of dignity	31	82
Loss of control of body functions	97	58
Burden on family or others	60	36
Fear of inadequate pain control	37	22
Financial concerns	4	2
Median age in years 70		

Source: Data from www.dhs.state.or.us/publichealth/chs/pas.

Table 11.2. Attitudes of Oregon Health Care Professionals toward Physician-Assisted Suicide and the Oregon Death with Dignity Act

Professional Category	Survey Year	N	Response Rate	Attitude toward Legalization of Physician-Assisted Suicide (percentage)			Attitude toward the Oregon Death with Dignity Act (percentage)		
				Support	Neutral	Oppose	Support	Neutral	Oppose
Hospice nurses	2001	306	71				48	16	36
Hospice social workers	2001	91	78				72	5	13
Physicians[a]	1999	2,641	66				51	17	31
	1995	2,761	70	60	10	30			
Emergency-room physicians	1995	248	70	69	7	23			
Psychologists	1996	461	74				78		21
Psychiatrists	1995	321	77				56		44

Sources: L. Ganzini, D.S. Fenn, M.A. Lee, R.T. Heintz, and J.D. Bloom, "Attitudes of Oregon Psychiatrists toward Physician-Assisted Suicide," *American Journal of Psychiatry* 153 (1996): 1469–75; M.A. Lee, H.D. Nelson, V.P. Tilden, L. Ganzini, T.A. Schmidt, and S.W. Tolle, "Legalizing Assisted Suicide: Views of Physicians in Oregon," *New England Journal of Medicine* 334 (1996): 310–15; T.A. Schmidt, A.D. Zechnich, V.P. Tilden, M.A. Lee, L. Ganzini, H.D. Nelson, and S.W. Tolle, "Oregon Emergency Physicians' Experiences with, Attitudes toward, and Concerns about Physician-Assisted Suicide," *Academic Emergency Medicine* 3 (1996): 938–45; D.S. Fenn and L. Ganzini, "Attitudes of Oregon Psychologists toward Physician-Assisted Suicide and the Oregon Death with Dignity Act," *Professional Psychology: Research and Practice* 30 (1999): 235–44; L. Ganzini, T.A. Harvath, A. Jackson, E.R. Goy, L.L. Miller, and M.A. Delorit, "Experiences of Oregon Nurses and Social Workers with Hospice Patients Who Requested Assistance with Suicide," *New England Journal of Medicine* 347 (2002): 582–88; L. Miller, T.A. Harvath, E.R. Goy, A. Jackson, M.A. Delorit, and L. Ganzini. "Attitudes and Experiences of Oregon Hospice Nurses and Social Workers Regarding Assisted Suicide," *Palliative Medicine* 2004 (in press).

[a]Includes internists, surgeons, neurologists, gynecologists, radiation oncologists, family practitioners, and general practitioners.

among primary care physicians, emergency care physicians, psychiatrists, and psychologists.[14] Surveys conducted following enactment include information about actual experiences with requesting patients. For example, in a 1999 survey, 144 physicians (of 2,641 eligible to prescribe under the law who responded to a survey) reported that 206 patients had requested a lethal prescription; these physicians gave detailed descriptions of 143 patients.[15] In another study, among 306 hospice nurses and 91 hospice social workers surveyed in 2001, 45 percent reported having cared for at least one patient who explicitly requested assisted suicide, and 30 percent reported having had a patient who actually received a lethal prescription.[16] In further research, in-depth qualitative interviews with thirty-five physicians who received requests for assisted suicide sought to elicit concerns and experiences that were not asked about in surveys.[17]

Studies of patients are less common. From 1995 to 1997, colleagues and I surveyed one hundred patients with amyotrophic lateral sclerosis (ALS) regarding their desire for assisted suicide and associated factors.[18] In a follow-up project in 2000, researchers located thirty-eight family caregivers of patients who had subsequently died and interviewed them regarding the persistence of the patient's interest in assisted suicide over time.[19] Silveira and colleagues surveyed 728 patients in general internal medicine and family practice clinics regarding their understanding of the law and end-of-life choices in Oregon.[20] I have completed comprehensive psychiatric clinical assessments of seventeen Oregon patients who have requested assisted suicide under the law.

Several important limitations of the Oregon data should be noted. Although response rates were high in all the surveys, this may not overcome a response bias. For example, among physicians surveyed, those who did not support the law were less likely to give complete information about patients who wanted assisted suicide (87 percent versus 71 percent).[21] No studies of patients actually in the process of requesting assisted suicide have been conducted; and except for the interviews conducted by the ODHS[22] and those by Robert Pearlman and Helene Starks reported in chapter 6 of this volume, there have been no studies of families' views and experiences around physician-assisted suicide. More data would help overcome these limitations, but financial support for such studies, whether from federal agencies or private foundations, is difficult to obtain.

Were other states to legalize physician-assisted suicide, they might report different results. Oregon residents have a strong sense of social cohesion that may have mitigated some of the social and clinical concerns about the law; and Oregon's social experiment was preceded by development of a comprehensive palliative care system. (Like many states, however, Oregon has experienced a considerable economic downturn, which may affect the state's commitment to providing almost universal access to hospice.)

Do Health Care Professionals Support Assisted Suicide?

Oregon health care professionals vary in their support of the Death with Dignity Act, with the highest support among psychologists and hospice social workers (see table 11.2).[23] Even among those who are more divided in their support, such as Oregon physicians and hospice nurses, approximately half of respondents support the law.[24] Overall, respondents report that their views on assisted suicide have not changed since the law passed in 1994, though among the small proportion who have changed their minds, twice as many are more supportive rather than more opposed to the law.[25]

Yet although half of Oregon physicians support the law, only one-third are willing to prescribe a lethal medication themselves.[26] Qualitative interviews reveal that most physicians who would decline to do so themselves would assist a patient in finding a physician who was willing to prescribe.[27] Although 36 percent of hospice nurses do not support the law (see table 11.2), only 3 percent of all nurses surveyed would actively oppose a patient's choice on this issue, and 12 percent would transfer a patient who requested a lethal prescription to another provider.[28] In other words, two-thirds of Oregon hospice nurses who oppose the law are nonetheless willing to care for a patient who requests assisted suicide, and only one in twelve would actively oppose a patient's choice to pursue it. Qualitative interviews reveal that practitioners who are morally opposed to assisted suicide experience a conflict between their desire not to abandon the patient and their reluctance to participate in assisted suicide.[29]

Are Patients Who Choose Assisted Suicide Socially Disadvantaged?

As noted earlier, one concern has been that disadvantaged populations would be disproportionately represented among patients who chose assisted suicide. Experience in Oregon suggests this has not been the case. In the United States, socially disadvantaged groups have variably included ethnic minorities, the poor, women, and the elderly. Compared with all Oregon residents who died between January 1998 and December 2002, those who died by physician-assisted suicide were more likely to be college graduates, more likely to be Asian, somewhat younger, more likely to be divorced, and more likely to have cancer or amyotrophic lateral sclerosis.[30] Similarly, in our study of ALS patients, my colleagues and I found those who expressed an interest in requesting assisted suicide generally had higher-than-average levels of education.[31] Moreover, although 2.6 percent of Oregonians are African American, no African American patients have chosen assisted suicide.[32] Only 2 of the 171 patients who died by physician-assisted suicide did not have health insurance (for three patients it was not known whether they had health insurance at the time of death—see table 11.1), and only 2 percent of physicians reported that a patient in their care who died by assisted suicide chose it because of financial concerns.[33] Hospice nurses and social workers concur that financial concerns and poor social support are rarely important reasons for these requests.[34]

Does Fear of Being a Burden Influence Patients' Decisions for Assisted Suicide?

The available data suggest that patients' worries about burdening others with their care are somewhat important reasons for wanting physician-assisted suicide. Table 11.3 reports ODHS data from physicians whose patients died by assisted suicide. Thirty-eight percent of physicians of patients who died by assisted suicide reported that concern about being a burden was important to the request.[35] Physicians reported that among patients who requested assisted suicide, 10 percent who viewed themselves as a burden received lethal prescription compared with 47 percent who did not view themselves as a burden.[36] Yet hospice nurses reported that only 11 percent of family members of patients who received lethal prescriptions were more burdened by caring for their ill relative than other families of hospice patients, whereas 31 percent were less burdened.[37] My assessments of patients who have requested assisted suicide support this finding: their concerns about being a burden to their families appear to reflect patients' own perceptions of the dying process as being without value rather than attitudes communicated to them by others.

Are Patients Who Choose Assisted Suicide Depressed?

As defined in the *Diagnostic and Statistical Manual* (DSM-IV) of the American Psychiatric Association, major depressive disorder is characterized by low mood or inability to experience pleasure nearly every day for more than two weeks and is associated with feelings of worthlessness, thoughts of suicide, and physical

Table 11.3. Reasons for Requesting or Receiving a Lethal Prescription

Reason	Patients Receiving Lethal Prescription[a] (N = 82)		Patients Requesting Lethal Prescription[b] (percentage) (N = 143)
	Median Score	Interquartile Range	
Control and independence issues			
Inability to perform personal care or fear of inability	4.0	3.0–5.0	31
Loss of or fear of losing independence	4.0	4.0–5.0	57
To control circumstances of death	5.0	5.0–5.0	53
Wanted to die at home	5.0	3.0–5.0	28
Existential and meaning issues			
Life tasks complete	3.0	2.0–5.0	18
Loss of or fear of losing dignity	4.0	3.75–5.00	42
Poor quality of life or fear of poor quality of life	4.0	4.0–5.0	55
Ready to die	5.0	4.0–5.0	54
Saw existence as pointless	5.0	3.0–5.0	47
Unable to pursue pleasurable activities	4.0	3.0–5.0	30
Physical symptoms			
Dyspnea or fear of worsening dyspnea	3.0	1.0–5.0	27
Fatigue or fear of worsening fatigue	3.0	2.0–5.0	31
Loss of bowel or bladder function or fear of loss	3.0	1.0–4.5	N/A
Mental confusion or fear of mental confusion	3.0	1.0–4.0	22
Nausea or fear of worsening nausea	2.0	1.0–3.0	8
Pain or fear of worsening pain	4.0	3.0–5.0	43
Psychosocial issues			
Depression or other psychiatric disorder	2.0	1.0–3.0	20
Lack of social support	1.0	1.0–2.0	6
Perceiving self as burden to others or fear of becoming a burden	4.0	3.0–5.0	38
Perceiving self as financial drain to others or fear of becoming a financial drain	2.0	1.0–3.0	11

Sources: Data from L. Ganzini, H.D. Nelson, T.A. Schmidt, D.F. Kraemer, M.A. Delorit, and M.A. Lee, "Physicians' Experiences with the Oregon Death with Dignity Act," *New England Journal of Medicine* 342 (2000): 557–63; L. Ganzini, T.A. Harvath, A. Jackson, E.K. Goy, L.L. Miller, and M.A. Delorit, "Experiences of Oregon Nurses and Social Workers with Hospice Patients Who Requested Assistance with Suicide," *New England Journal of Medicine* 347 (2002): 582–88.

[a]Reported by hospice nurses, ranking the importance of reason on a scale of 1 to 5, 1 being "Not at all important in decision to request a lethal prescription" and 5 being "Very important in decision to request a lethal prescription."

[b]Reported by physicians.

symptoms.[38] Suicide is often associated with depression—in retrospective reviews of suicides, for example, researchers report that in approximately 80 percent of completed suicides by cancer patients the decedent was depressed.[39] In the decade following a suicide attempt, only 10 to 14 percent of patients complete suicide, suggesting that for most suicidal persons the desire to die is not permanent.[40] Both depression treatment and suicide prevention are effective. Depression is treatable even among elderly, medically ill patients, 60 to 65 percent of whom remain well for several years following treatment.[41] There are no well-designed, randomized clinical trials of the efficacy of depression treatment in the final months of life, but anecdotal information regarding the effectiveness of psychosocial interventions and psychostimulants is compelling.[42] Studies conducted outside of Oregon of patients with cancer and AIDS report a strong relation between depression and interest in assisted suicide or hastened death.[43]

Oregon physicians report that 20 percent of requests for assisted suicide came from depressed patients (table 11.3), but no depressed patient received a lethal prescription.[44] Given that the overall prevalence of depression among terminally ill patients is between 10 and 25 percent,[45] depression does not appear to increase the attributable risk for actually requesting assisted suicide. Oregon hospice social workers, who have expertise in recognizing depression in terminally ill patients, report that among patients who received lethal prescriptions, depression was one of the least important reasons for their request.[46] In our study of ALS patients, depression (as measured by DSM-IV criteria) was not associated with desire for assisted suicide, nor did it predict interest in assisted suicide at the end of life.[47] Furthermore, among patients who requested assisted suicide, only 11 percent who received a trial of medication for anxiety or depression or were evaluated by a mental health professional changed their minds about assisted suicide.[48]

There are striking differences between the studies inside and outside of Oregon in the role of depression in interest in physician-assisted suicide, the reasons for which are not clear. Many have proposed that health care professionals simply fail to diagnose depression—underdiagnosis of depression is common in many medical settings.[49] Whether this applies in the context of explicit requests for assisted suicide is not clear. Hospice clinical social workers would be expected to have a fair degree of expertise in the evaluation of mood disorders among those who are terminally ill. A likelier explanation stems from differences in the populations studied. Studies conducted outside Oregon have found that more than 10 percent of surveyed terminally ill patients express an *interest* in assisted suicide or desire for hastened death.[50] However, only 1 percent of Oregonians who die each year make an *explicit* request for assisted suicide, and only 0.1 percent die by assisted suicide.[51] That is, only one in one hundred terminally ill patients who might endorse interest in assisted suicide on a questionnaire would, were it legal, die by assisted suicide; risk factors for one group might not be risk factors for the other. Oregon physicians describe patients who actively pursue assisted suicide as focused, determined, strong-willed, and stubborn individuals who are single-minded and uncompromising in their approach to obtaining a lethal prescription.[52] It is possible that even though depression may increase a patient's interest in assisted suicide, the apathy and volitional impairments associated with depression make it difficult to convince others of the sincerity or authenticity of the request. Studies of patients who actually request assisted suicide are needed to clarify the role of depression.

Although the evidence seems not to support depression as a risk factor among patients who actually request assisted suicide, the hopelessness that often accompanies depression may be a factor. Hopelessness and depression are not synonymous. Depression reflects low mood and difficulty finding pleasure in the here and now. Hopelessness reflects negative and pessimistic views of the future. Among ALS patients, hopelessness was associated with desire for assisted suicide and strongly predicted continued interest over time.[53] My clinical interviews with patients requesting physician-assisted suicide indicate that many dread their future and perceive little value in going through the dying process.

Do Patients Request Assisted Suicide Because of Treatable Physical Symptoms?

Physical symptoms are modestly important in motivating requests for assisted suicide. The Oregon Department of Human Services reports that inadequate pain control was an important reason in patients' decisions to seek physician-assisted suicide in 22 percent of the 171 deaths to date.[54] Physicians surveyed report that among requesting patients, pain or fear of worsening pain was an important consideration for 43 percent, fatigue for 31 percent, and dyspnea for 27 percent (see table 11.3).[55] Hospice nurses report that 15 percent of patients who received lethal prescriptions had more pain than other hospice patients and 42 percent had less.[56] This suggests that when pain is an important factor in the request, it is not the absolute level of pain but, as Eric Cassell suggests (in chapter 5 in this volume), the meaning of the pain and the prospect of worsening pain that is of concern. Whether better symptom management would lead patients to retract their requests for aid in dying is not known. My clinical assessments suggest that many patients appear to find further symptom treatment problematic if it results in cognitive dysfunction, challenges their sense of being in control in some way, or results in greater dependence on others.[57]

Do Patients Who Request Assisted Suicide Lack Access to Palliative Care Options?

Eighty-five percent of deaths by physician-assisted suicide in Oregon occurred among patients enrolled in home hospice care, which is the most comprehensive form of end-of-life care available. Physicians have reported to the ODHS that virtually all patients who request assisted suicide are offered hospice care, but approximately 17 percent decline it.[58] Two-thirds of Oregon physicians report having responded to a request for assisted suicide by recommending a substantive intervention—pain or symptom control; hospice referral; mental health, social work, chaplain, or palliative care consultation; a trial of antidepressants; or seeking advice from a colleague—and half implemented the intervention.[59] Oregon physicians report that palliative interventions are associated with patients' changing their mind in some but not all situations; 43 percent of patients who received such an intervention later decided not to avail themselves of it, compared with 10 percent who did not change their mind. In one study of eighteen patients who did not receive a substantive intervention, eleven were already enrolled in hospice, and five additional patients had no pain.[60] Oregon physicians were significantly less likely to prescribe lethal medication to patients who were not enrolled in hospice.[61]

Has Legalization of Assisted Suicide Impeded Development of Palliative Care?

Several lines of evidence support the contention that palliative care has improved since passage of the Death with Dignity Act. In 2002, 37 percent of Oregonians who died were enrolled in a hospice program, compared with 22 percent in 1994.[62] Thirty percent of physicians report that they increased their referrals to hospice between 1994 and 1998, whereas only 2 percent report having made fewer referrals; 78 percent had made at least one hospice referral in the previous year. Among physicians who cared for at least one terminally ill patient in the previous year, 76 percent report having made efforts to improve their knowledge of the use of pain medications in end-of-life care, and 79 percent said that their confidence in prescribing pain medications had improved.[63]

Has Managed Care Promoted Physician-Assisted Suicide in Order to Save Money?

One-third of the patients we studied who requested assisted suicide were covered by a managed-care health plan or health maintenance organization, whereas 49 percent of Oregonians overall received coverage from a managed care organization over the same period of time. Managed care patients were no less likely than patients with other types of insurance to receive palliative care: approximately half of the patients in both groups who requested a lethal prescription received palliative interventions, such as referral to hospice or improved pain control.[64] These data suggest that the rate of requests for assisted suicide is not significantly influenced by type of insurance or cost containment efforts in managed health care plans.

Has Oregon Become a Destination for Non-Oregonians Requesting Assisted Suicide?

Oregon physicians report that only one of 144 requests came from a terminally ill patient who moved to Oregon to attempt to gain access to physician-assisted suicide.[65] Thus despite concerns, there seems to date not to have been significant immigration by individuals seeking assisted suicide.

What Roles Do Meaning, Control, and Independence Play in Patients' Requests for Assisted Suicide

As table 11.3 illustrates, all sources of information about Oregon patients who request assisted suicide underscore the importance to these patients of remaining in control and not being dependent on others.[66] In interviews conducted by the ODHS, physicians reported that loss of autonomy was an important reason for the request among 87 percent of patients, and loss of control of bodily functions was important for 58 percent[67] (see table 11.1). In qualitative interviews colleagues and I carried out, physicians described individuals who request assisted suicide as valuing self-sufficiency and dreading the thought of being dependent on others.[68] For these patients, the dying process represents too much risk of becoming dependent through pain, mental deterioration, institutionalization, or loss of function. Physicians use adjectives such as strong willed and stubborn to describe these patients, who are adamant in their request.

One patient was described by her physician as follows: "I think her big fear was loss of control. She wanted to control things right up to the end. She wanted to plan it. She wanted things to go the way she wanted it. And she did not want to wait. She did not want to take a chance at waiting until it would not be under her control. She was very in charge." Concerns about control and dependence on others also occur in the context of difficulty in finding meaning in life. In contrast to the energy they bring to attempting to obtain a lethal prescription, patients struggle to find value and purpose in the lives they are now living and are convinced that future moments can only be worse in quality than the present.

The Oregon Experience

To date, studies from Oregon suggest that patients who actively attempt to obtain lethal prescriptions place great value on being in control and not being or becoming dependent on others. They have pervasively negative expectations of the future and perceive little value in the dying process. They struggle to find meaning in their lives. Concerns about being a burden may reflect views about dependence rather than communications from others.

The available evidence does not bear out widely voiced concerns that physician-assisted suicide will be requested by those who are socially disadvantaged or make their requests based on lack of access to palliative care, poor social support, or financial needs. Further studies of patients themselves in the process of requesting assisted suicide are needed if we are to understand more clearly the role played by physical symptoms (especially pain) and depression in their decisions to seek physicians' aid in dying.

Notes

1. Oregon Department of Human Services, *Physician-Assisted Suicide,* www.ohd.hr .st.or.us/chs/pas (accessed December 1, 2003).

2. Ibid.

3. K. Haley and M.A. Lee, *The Oregon Death with Dignity Act: A Guidebook for Health Care Providers* (Portland, Ore.: Center for Ethics in Health Care, Oregon Health and Science University, 1998). (Also available at www.ohsu.edu/ethics/guide/.)

4. Oregon Department of Human Services, *Physician-Assisted Suicide.*

5. H.M. Chochinov, K.G. Wilson, M. Enns, N. Mowchun, S. Lander, H.M. Levi, and J.J. Clinch, "Desire for Death in the Terminally Ill," *American Journal of Psychiatry* 152 (1995): 1185–91; E.J. Emanuel and E. Daniels, "Oregon's Physician-Assisted Suicide Law: Provisions and Problems," *Archives of Internal Medicine* 156 (1996): 825–29; K. Faber-Langendoen, "Death by Request: Assisted Suicide and the Oncologist," *Cancer* 82 (1998): 35–41; K.M. Foley, "Competent Care for the Dying Instead of Physician-Assisted Suicide," *New England Journal of Medicine* 336 (1997): 54–58; H. Hendin and G. Klerman, "Physician-Assisted Suicide: The Dangers of Legalization," *American Journal of Psychiatry* 150 (1993): 143–45; H.G. Koenig, H.J. Cohen, D.G. Blazer, K.R. Krishnan, and T.E. Silbert, "Profile of Depressive Symptoms in Younger and Older Medical Inpatients with Major Depression," *Journal of the American Geriatric Society* 41 (1993): 1169–76; P.R. Muskin, "The Request to Die: Role for a Psychodynamic Perspective on Physician-Assisted Suicide," *Journal of the American Medical Association* 279 (1998): 323–28; P.A. Singer and M. Siegler, "Euthanasia: A Critique," *New England Journal of Medicine* 322 (1990): 1881–83; J. Teno and J. Lynn, "Voluntary Active Euthanasia: The Individual Case and Public Policy," *Journal of the American Geriatric Society* 39 (1991): 827–30; R.D. Truog and C.B. Berde, "Pain, Euthanasia, and Anesthesiologists," *Anesthesiology* 78 (1993): 353–60.

6. Foley, "Competent Care for the Dying Instead of Physician-Assisted Suicide."

7. A. Alpers and B. Lo, "Physician-Assisted Suicide in Oregon: A Bold Experiment," *Journal of the American Medical Association* 274 (1995): 483–87; E.D. Pellegrino, "Ethics," *Journal of the American Medical Association* 273 (1995): 1674–76.

8. Alpers and Lo, "Physician-Assisted Suicide in Oregon"; R.K. Portenoy, N. Coyle, K.M. Kash, F. Brescia, C. Scanlon, D. O'Hare, R.I. Misbin, J. Holland, and K.M. Foley, "Determinants of the Willingness to Endorse Assisted Suicide: A Survey of Physicians, Nurses, and Social Workers," *Psychosomatics* 38 (1997): 277–87.

9. E.J. Emanuel and M.P. Battin, "What Are the Potential Cost Savings from Legalizing Physician-Assisted Suicide?" *New England Journal of Medicine* 339 (1998): 167–72.

10. J.F. Drane, "Physician Assisted Suicide and Voluntary Active Euthanasia: Social Ethics and the Role of Hospice," *American Journal of Hospice and Palliative Care* 12 (1995): 3–11; Faber-Langendoen, "Death by Request"; Foley, "Competent Care for the Dying Instead of Physician-Assisted Suicide"; H. Hendin, K. Foley, and M. White, "Physician-Assisted Suicide: Reflections on Oregon's First Case," *Issues in Law and Medicine* 14 (1998): 243–70; R.M. Sobel and A.J. Layton, "Physician-Assisted Suicide: Compassionate Care or Brave New World?" *Archives of Internal Medicine* 157 (1997): 1638–40.

11. Oregon Department of Human Services, *Physician-Assisted Suicide.*

12. Ibid.

13. A.D. Sullivan, K. Hedberg, and D.W. Fleming, "Legalized Physician-Assisted Suicide in Oregon—The Second Year," *New England Journal of Medicine* 342 (2000): 598–604.

14. L. Ganzini, D.S. Fenn, M.A. Lee, R.T. Heintz, and J.D. Bloom, "Attitudes of Oregon Psychiatrists toward Physician-Assisted Suicide," *American Journal of Psychiatry* 153 (1996): 1469–75; M.A. Lee, H.D. Nelson, V.P. Tilden, L. Ganzini, T.A. Schmidt, and S.W. Tolle, "Legalizing Assisted Suicide: Views of Physicians in Oregon," *New England Journal*

of Medicine 334 (1996): 310–15; T.A. Schmidt, A.D. Zechnich, V.P. Tilden, M.A. Lee, L. Ganzini, H.D. Nelson, and S.W. Tolle, "Oregon Emergency Physicians' Experiences with, Attitudes toward, and Concerns about Physician-Assisted Suicide," *Academic Emergency Medicine* 3 (1996): 938–45; D.S. Fenn and L. Ganzini, "Attitudes of Oregon Psychologists toward Physician-Assisted Suicide and the Oregon Death with Dignity Act," *Professional Psychology: Research and Practice* 30 (1999): 235–44.

15. L. Ganzini, H.D. Nelson, T.A. Schmidt, D.F. Kraemer, M.A. Delorit, and M.A. Lee, "Physicians' Experiences with the Oregon Death with Dignity Act," *New England Journal of Medicine* 342 (2000): 557–63.

16. L. Ganzini, T.A. Harvath, A. Jackson, E.K. Goy, L.L. Miller, and M.A. Delorit, "Experiences of Oregon Nurses and Social Workers with Hospice Patients Who Requested Assistance with Suicide," *New England Journal of Medicine* 347 (2002): 582–88.

17. L. Ganzini, S.K. Dobscha, R.T. Heintz, and N. Press, "Oregon Physicians' Perceptions of Patients Who Request Assisted Suicide and Their Families," *Journal of Palliative Medicine* 6 (2003): 381–90.

18. L. Ganzini, W.S. Johnston, B.H. McFarland, S.W. Tolle, and M.A. Lee, "Attitudes of Patients with Amyotrophic Lateral Sclerosis and Their Care Givers toward Assisted Suicide," *New England Journal of Medicine* 339 (1998): 967–73.

19. L. Ganzini, M.J. Silveira, and W.S. Johnston, "Predictors and Correlates of Interest in Assisted Suicide in the Final Month of Life among ALS Patients in Oregon and Washington," *Journal of Pain and Symptom Management* 24 (2002): 312–17.

20. M.J. Silveira, A. DiPiero, M.S. Gerrity, and C. Feudtner, "Patients' Knowledge of Options at the End of Life: Ignorance in the Face of Death," *Journal of the American Medical Association* 284 (2000): 2483–88.

21. Ganzini et al., "Physicians' Experiences with the Oregon Death with Dignity Act."

22. Sullivan, Hedberg, and Fleming, "Legalized Physician-Assisted Suicide in Oregon."

23. Fenn and Ganzini, "Attitudes of Oregon Psychologists toward Physician-Assisted Suicide and the Oregon Death with Dignity Act"; L.L. Miller, T.A. Harvath, E.R. Goy, A. Jackson, M.A. Delorit, and L. Ganzini, "Attitudes and Experiences of Oregon Hospice Nurses and Social Workers Regarding Assisted Suicide," unpublished manuscript.

24. Ganzini et al., "Physicians' Experiences with the Oregon Death with Dignity Act"; Miller et al., "Attitudes and Experiences of Oregon Hospice Nurses and Social Workers Regarding Assisted Suicide."

25. Ganzini et al., "Physicians' Experiences with the Oregon Death with Dignity Act"; Miller et al., "Attitudes and Experiences of Oregon Hospice Nurses and Social Workers Regarding Assisted Suicide."

26. L. Ganzini, H.D. Nelson, M.A. Lee, D.F. Kraemer, T.A. Schmidt, and M.A. Delorit, "Oregon Physicians' Attitudes about and Experiences with End-of-Life Care Since Passage of the Oregon Death with Dignity Act," *Journal of the American Medical Association* 285 (2001): 2363–69.

27. B.K. Dobscha, R.T. Heintz, N. Press, and L. Ganzini, "Oregon Physicians' Responses to Requests for Assisted Suicide: A Qualitative Study," *Journal of Palliative Medicine,* 7 (2004): 450–60.

28. Miller et al., "Attitudes and Experiences of Oregon Hospice Nurses and Social Workers Regarding Assisted Suicide."

29. Dobscha et al., "Oregon Physicians' Responses to Requests for Assisted Suicide."

30. Oregon Department of Human Services, *Physician-Assisted Suicide.*

31. Ganzini et al., "Oregon Physicians' Perceptions of Patients Who Request Assisted Suicide and Their Families."

32. Oregon Department of Human Services, *Physician-Assisted Suicide.*

33. Ibid.

34. Ganzini, Harvath, et al., "Experiences of Oregon Nurses and Social Workers with Hospice Patients Who Requested Assistance with Suicide."

35. Oregon Department of Human Services, *Physician-Assisted Suicide.*

36. Ganzini et al., "Physicians' Experiences with the Oregon Death with Dignity Act."

37. Ganzini, Harvath, et al., "Experiences of Oregon Nurses and Social Workers with Hospice Patients Who Requested Assistance with Suicide."

38. American Psychiatric Association, *Diagnostic and Statistical Manual of Mental Health Disorders: DSM-IV* (Washington, D.C.: American Psychiatric Association, 1994).

39. M.M. Henriksson, E.T. Isometsa, P.S. Hietnane, H.M. Aro, and J.K. Lonnqvist, "Mental Disorders in Cancer Patients," *Journal of Affective Disorders* 36 (1995): 11–20.

40. R. Diekstra, "An International Perspective on Epidemiology and Prevalence of Suicide," in *Suicide over the Life Cycle: Risk Factors, Assessment and Treatment of Suicidal Persons,* edited by S.J. Blumenthal and D.J. Kupfer (Washington, D.C.: American Psychiatric Press, 1990), 533–70.

41. E. Murphy, "The Course and Outcome of Depression in Late Life," in *Diagnosis and Treatment of Depression in Late Life: Results of the NIH Consensus Development Conference,* edited by L.S. Schneider, C.F. Reynolds III, B.D. Lebowitz, and A.J. Friedhoff (Washington, D.C.: American Psychiatric Press, 1994), 81–98.

42. W. Breitbart, H.M. Chochinov, and S. Passik, "Psychiatric Aspects of Palliative Care," in *Oxford Textbook of Palliative Medicine,* edited by D. Doyle, G.W.C. Hanks, and N. MacDonald (New York: Oxford University Press, 1998), 933–54.

43. Breitbart, Chochinov, and Passik, "Psychiatric Aspects of Palliative Care"; Chochinov et al., "Desire for Death in the Terminally Ill"; E.J. Emanuel, D.L. Fairclough, and L.L. Emanuel, "Attitudes and Desires related to Euthanasia and Physician-Assisted Suicide among Terminally Ill Patients and their Caregivers," *Journal of the American Medical Association* 285 (2001): 734–35; K.G. Wilson, J.F. Scott, I.D. Graham, J.F. Kozak, S. Chater, R.A. Viola, B.J. deFaye, L.A. Weaver, and D. Curran, "Attitudes of Terminally Ill Patients toward Euthanasia and Physician-Assisted Suicide," *Archives of Internal Medicine* 161 (2001): 1117–8.

44. Ganzini et al., "Physicians' Experiences with the Oregon Death with Dignity Act."

45. M. Hotopf, J. Chidgey, J. Addington-Hall, and K.L. Ly, "Depression in Advanced Disease: A Systematic Review." pt. 1, "Prevalence and Case Finding," *Palliative Medicine* 16 (2002): 81–97.

46. Ganzini, Harvath, et al., "Experiences of Oregon Nurses and Social Workers with Hospice Patients Who Requested Assistance with Suicide."

47. Ganzini et al., "Oregon Physicians' Perceptions of Patients Who Request Assisted Suicide and Their Families"; Ganzini, Silveira, and Johnston, "Predictors and Correlates of Interest in Assisted Suicide in the Final Month of Life."

48. Ganzini et al., "Physicians' Experiences with the Oregon Death with Dignity Act."

49. S.D. Passik, W. Gugan, M.V. McDonald, B. Rosenfeld, D.E. Theobald, and S. Edgerton, "Oncologists' Recognition of Depression in Their Patients with Cancer," *Journal of Clinical Oncology* 16 (1998): 1594–60.

50. Breitbart, Chochinov, and Passik, "Psychiatric Aspects of Palliative Care"; Chochinov et al., "Desire for Death in the Terminally Ill"; Emanuel et al., "Attitudes and Desires related to Euthanasia and Physician-Assisted Suicide among Terminally Ill Patients and Their Caregivers"; Wilson et al., "Attitudes of Terminally Ill Patients toward Euthanasia and Physician-Assisted Suicide."

51. Oregon Department of Human Services, *Physician-Assisted Suicide;* Ganzini et al., "Physicians' Experiences with the Oregon Death with Dignity Act."

52. Ganzini et al., "Oregon Physicians' Perceptions of Patients Who Request Assisted Suicide and Their Families."

53. Ganzini, Silveira, and Johnston, "Predictors and Correlates of Interest in Assisted Suicide in the Final Month of Life."

54. Oregon Department of Human Services, *Physician-Assisted Suicide.*

55. Ganzini, "Physicians' Experiences with the Oregon Death with Dignity Act."

56. Ganzini, Harvath, et al., "Experiences of Oregon Nurses and Social Workers with Hospice Patients Who Requested Assistance with Suicide."

57. Oregon Department of Human Services, *Physician-Assisted Suicide.*

58. Ganzini et al., "Physicians' Experiences with the Oregon Death with Dignity Act."

59. L. Ganzini, H.D. Nelson, T.A. Schmidt, D.F. Kraemer, M.A. Delorit, and M.A. Lee, "Physicians' Experiences with Legalized Physician-Assisted Suicide in Oregon," in *Clinical and Epidemiological Aspects of End-of-Life Decision-Making,* edited by A. van der Heide, B. Onwuteaka-Philipsen, E.J. Emanuel, P.J. van der Maas, and G. van der Wal (Amsterdam: Royal Dutch Academy of Arts and Sciences, 2001), 109–20.

60. Ganzini et al., "Physicians' Experiences with the Oregon Death with Dignity Act."

61. Ganzini, Nelson, Lee, et al., "Oregon Physicians' Attitudes about and Experiences with End-of-Life Care."

62. Ganzini, Nelson, Schmidt, et al., "Physicians' Experiences with Legalized Physician-Assisted Suicide in Oregon."

63. Ann Jackson, executive director, Oregon Hospice Association, personal communication; Ganzini et al., "Physicians' Experiences with the Oregon Death with Dignity Act"; Miller et al., "Attitudes and Experiences of Oregon Hospice Nurses and Social Workers Regarding Assisted Suicide.

64. Ganzini et al., "Physicians' Experiences with the Oregon Death with Dignity Act."

65. Ibid.; Ganzini, Harvath, et al., "Experiences of Oregon Nurses and Social Workers with Hospice Patients Who Requested Assistance with Suicide."

66. Oregon Department of Human Services, *Physician-Assisted Suicide.*

67. Oregon Department of Human Services, *Physician-Assisted Suicide.*

68. Ganzini et al., "Oregon Physicians' Perceptions of Patients Who Request Assisted Suicide and Their Families."

12

The Distortion of Cases in Oregon

Peter Goodwin, M.B. Ch.B., F.R.C.S. Ed.

In their attempt to discredit the Oregon Death with Dignity Act, opponents have focused on several cases of physician-assisted death, notably those of "Helen" (not her real name) and Kate Cheney. I was closely involved with the case of Helen, a woman in her mid-eighties with breast cancer. Helen was referred to me through Compassion in Dying when I was their senior medical adviser. In *The Case against Assisted Suicide*, Foley and Hendin suggest that Helen's case reveals a team of incompetent and irresponsible physicians assisting in the death of a depressed and irrational woman.[1] Such a reading of the case insults the physicians who cared for Helen, the hospice team who made their own independent assessments, and most important, Helen and her family.

Helen had had a mastectomy in about 1975. Twenty years later, in 1995, she developed cancer in the left breast. Following a lumpectomy and, eventually, a mastectomy, in 1997 she refused further therapy. The cancer recurred in the chest wall and neck glands. Her oncologist suggested a biopsy and therapy, but she again decided against aggressive treatment. Subsequently, she talked about her desire to explore the possibility of an assisted death with her primary care physician. As the cancer spread to her lungs, breathing became difficult, and she wanted the choice of physician aid in dying.

Helen's primary care physician was of the opinion that she clearly understood the consequences of refusing further treatment. However, he was leaving primary care for a position in the field of urgent care and referred her to an internist whom he considered to be an expert in the care of the dying. Helen was under the impression that the new physician would help her access Oregon's assisted-dying law. When she realized that the new physician would not help her, she felt betrayed and, according to her children who were with her during the consultation with the new physician, cried with despair and frustration in his presence.

The new physician decided Helen was depressed. Concluding that on this basis she was ineligible for assistance in dying, he refused her request. Helen's family then contacted Compassion in Dying. After several telephone conversations with Helen, her family, and the physician who had refused to help her, I decided her situation warranted further evaluation. I referred her to a family physician whom I believed would be objective in his assessment of her request. He did not find her to be depressed. He sent her to two consultants, one a psychiatrist, who evaluated her carefully during a lengthy consultation, the other a pulmonary disease specialist. Neither of these physicians found her to be depressed. The family physician prescribed the potentially lethal medication, and was with her when she took it and died peacefully.

I have met with Helen's family and read her medical records. Six physicians were involved in her terminal care. Only one believed he saw signs of depression, and he failed to confirm his suspicion with objective testing. The others all considered her psychologically healthy and competent to make medical decisions for herself. The family is resentful of the way Helen, a fiercely independent and determined woman, has been misrepresented by opponents of physician-assisted dying. The internist's observations have been portrayed as a "diagnosis" of depression that Foley and Hendin claim "was ignored," though they acknowledge that "the opinion of one of the original doctors" prompted a full psychiatric evaluation.[2]

Criticism of this case continues with innuendo and distortion. Lacking actual familiarity with the case, commentators such as Foley and Hendin substitute personal assumptions and conjectures for data. They assume that Helen's original primary care physician did not support her decision and that Helen was in no immediate distress, hinting that "irrational motives" prompted her decision. The fact is that in addition to breathlessness, Helen was suffering paroxysms of coughing that left her gasping for air. An X-ray taken by the internist four weeks before Helen died confirmed widespread tumor involvement of both lungs and bilateral pleural effusions. A more benign example of factual flaws is the statement that Helen's husband contacted Compassion in Dying, when in fact he had been dead many years.[3]

Wesley Smith, a spokesperson for the International Anti-Euthanasia Task Force, engages in similar distortions and goes even further, labeling the medical care provided to Helen as "pure Kevorkianism." Similarly, in a column published on October 31, 1999, an assistant editor to the *Oregonian,* Oregon's statewide newspaper, who was vehemently opposed to the law quoted Smith's opinion as "rampant Kevorkianism."[4]

Opponents of the Oregon law point to a second case they claim presents evidence of abuse and coercion. Kate Cheney was an eighty-five-year-old woman, a Kaiser Permanente patient, dying of inoperable stomach cancer. Kate's daughter, Erika, who became her full-time caregiver during her terminal illness, accompanied Kate when she talked with her primary care physician about assisted dying. Although the physician considered Kate to be competent to make health care decisions for herself, he referred her to a hospice program. Erika, who is hearing impaired, misinterpreted the physician's intent and described him as "dismissive."[5] She and Kate requested a new physician.

The new physician also considered Kate competent to make health care decisions for herself and agreed to participate in her request for assisted dying. In accordance with Kaiser protocol, he referred her to a psychiatrist independent of the Kaiser organization. The psychiatrist acknowledged that assisted suicide seemed consistent with Kate's values throughout her life but questioned her capacity to understand the gravity of her request. At this point, Erika wrote a letter to the *Oregonian* describing the difficulties Kate was facing in her request for physician assistance in dying. In an act significant for its openness and objectivity, Kate and her family permitted a reporter, Erin Hoover Barnett, to follow her progress, attend physician appointments with her, and even read her confidential medical records. Thus Kate's case received full coverage in a story that ran in the *Oregonian* on October 17, 1999.[6] I have used this article, supplemented by well-documented and verifiable information from Kaiser records, as sources of information.

Kate and Erika objected to the psychiatric opinion that Kate was not mentally competent, and the psychiatrist suggested they request a second opinion. A psychologist, again independent of the Kaiser system, saw Kate at home. The psychologist decided that Kate was competent but refused Erika's request to audiotape the interview and noted that "Erika may be somewhat coercive."[7]

The medical director of the Kaiser hospice program, a pulmonary care specialist who is an assistant director and the community liaison for the Center for Ethics in Health Care at Oregon Health and Science University and a highly respected medical ethicist, visited Kate in her home. He first interviewed her alone and then in the presence of her son-in-law. He became convinced that Kate was competent to make decisions for herself. Subsequently, a well-regarded, experienced palliative care specialist, independent of the Kaiser system, also saw her at her home and reported that her care was appropriate and that she understood all options for palliative care as well as the implications of her request for the option of assisted dying. When the prolonged process to ensure compliance with the law was finally completed, Kate received the medication from the Kaiser pharmacist. Kate and her family put the medication away and did not speak of it again for more than a month.

In contrast to the impression given by Foley and Hendin, Barnett's article presents Kate as rational and steadfast in her desire for an assisted death. The loving and determined support of her family is evident. Her downhill course is well documented. Opponents, however, have fixated on one word, "coercive," used by a single psychologist who found Kate fully capable, to discredit the family, Kate's caregivers, and an entire health care system.

A few examples of the many innuendoes, unfounded conclusions, conjectures, and misstatements Foley and Hendin enlist to support their accusations suffice. "This particular case," they write, "raises the question of what real meaning or value is Oregon's prohibition of coercion if it can be circumvented so easily."[8] Rather than coercion, there is evidence of Erika's eagerness not "to influence Kate's decision," as Foley and Hendin suggest, but vehemently to support Kate against what both she and her mother perceived as unsympathetic health care providers. Foley and Hendin write that the family should have said, "We love you and want to keep you around as long as possible"—implying that Kate's loved ones failed to do so.[9] Yet that is exactly what they did. They agreed to Kate's taking her life-ending medication only when Kate insisted that the time had come.

Foley and Hendin also suggest that arranging respite care for Kate at a nursing home in the week before her death sent her "a message that she was a burden." They ask, "What other option could she choose but to hasten her death." Yet earlier they acknowledge that Kate "had considered going permanently into a nursing home but had decided against it." Foley and Hendin repeatedly describe the hospice medical director as an "administrator," though his role in Kate's care was that of a clinician and ethicist intent on clarifying whether she was competent to make health care decisions for herself. They write that Kaiser suggested obtaining a second psychiatric opinion, but it was clear from the medical record that the outside psychiatrist, not Kaiser Permanente, suggested this option.[10]

Some criticism even lacks internal consistency. For example, in his contribution to Foley and Hendin's book, Hamilton criticizes Kaiser caregivers for freely discussing Kate Cheney's case in the press (which they did at the request of the patient and her daughter), then castigates them for attempts at "secrecy." Hamilton insinuates that financial self-interest might have motivated the Kaiser physician-ethicist. Foley and Hendin do the same, writing that "the role of a single HMO administrator making the final decision in a matter in which the HMO might have a financial conflict of interest . . . was questioned."[11]

Such baseless accusations and unfounded attacks on physicians and family members do a disservice to others who also stand against assisted dying on moral grounds but do not stoop to such tactics. They ignore the safeguards mandated by the law as well as the careful judgment exercised by Oregon's hospice programs, in which both Helen and Kate (and 85 percent of all the Oregon patients who have taken medication to hasten their death) were enrolled. Hospices add another layer of thorough, interdisciplinary evaluation of the patient's mental health, family dynamics, and available palliative care alternatives. The hospices that delivered care to Helen and Kate do not agree with assertions that the system somehow failed these two independent women in their final days.

Since passage of the Death with Dignity Act, the Oregon Health Division has published an annual summary of its oversight of the law. Foley and Hendin claim that the restrictions imposed by the Oregon Health Division to protect the confidentiality of patients and their families appear to be "extraordinarily secretive."[12] The abuse heaped on Kate and her family, as well as her medical attendants, when they went public seems to support the need for stringent restrictions on public access to confidential information. Hamilton's and Foley and Hendin's criticisms suggest the lengths to which opponents of the Oregon law are willing to go to advance their moral objection to and biases about legalization of physician-assisted death. Attempts to discredit patients, families, and caregivers based on incomplete, misleading information and innuendo is repugnant and intellectually unforgivable when careful and objective analysis should be the norm.

Notes

Editors' note: From the 1997 enactment of the Oregon Death with Dignity Act until 2003, 171 terminally ill Oregonians used the statute to secure assistance from their physicians in ending their lives. Under the statute, the Oregon Department of Health is charged with collecting information about these cases; these data are discussed by Linda Ganzini in chapter 11 of this volume. However, opponents of physician-assisted dying repeatedly claim that two of these cases in particular contain evidence of abuse or the potential for abuse. We asked Peter Goodwin, an Oregon physician knowledgeable about these cases, to assess the critiques of them.

1. K. Foley and H. Hendin, "The Oregon Experiment," in *The Case against Assisted Suicide: For the Right to End-of-Life Care,* edited by K. Foley and H. Hendin (Baltimore: Johns Hopkins University Press, 2002), 144–74, esp. 146–57.

2. Ibid., 148, 153.

3. Ibid., 146.

4. W.J. Smith, "Storm Warnings over Oregon," *Western Journal of Medicine* 171 (1999): 220–21; D. Reinhard, "In the Dark Shadows of Measure 16" (editorial), *Oregonian,* October 31, 1999, D5.

5. E. Hoover Barnett, "Is Mom Capable of Choosing to Die?" *Oregonian,* October 17, 1999, G2.

6. Ibid., G1–3.

7. Ibid., G2.

8. Foley and Hendin, "The Oregon Experiment," 157.

9. Ibid.

10. Ibid., 156, 157.

11. N.G. Hamilton, "Oregon's Culture of Silence," in *The Case against Assisted Suicide: For the Right to End-of-Life Care,* edited by K. Foley and H. Hendin (Baltimore: Johns Hopkins University Press, 2002), 175–91; Foley and Hendin, "The Oregon Experiment," 186–87.

12. Foley and Hendin, "The Oregon Experiment," 157; Hamilton, "Oregon's Culture of Silence," 186–87.

13

A Model That Integrates Assisted Dying with Excellent End-of-Life Care

Barbara Coombs Lee, B.S.N., J.D.

In April 1993 a group of Seattle residents formed a nonprofit organization called Compassion in Dying (Compassion). The stated purpose was to provide information, consultation, and emotional support to terminally ill, mentally competent adults who wished to hasten death in the face of intolerable suffering. The AIDS epidemic played some role, as several founders knew at least one AIDS patient who had ended his life violently in the absence of a more humane option. By 1993 communities affected by AIDS had produced many witnesses to prolonged, agonized deaths, including terminal symptoms of dementia, profuse diarrhea, and open sores. Some of those witnesses vowed not to endure the same.

The lack of open, honest guidance and support to those who wished not only to exhaust medical options to relieve symptoms but also to consider hastened death as an option of last resort struck the founders of Compassion as a great disservice to dying patients.[1] Failure to meet this need can propel the person who consciously anticipates profound bodily disintegration toward desperate options that are both violent and inhumane—death by hanging is most common in these circumstances in Europe, while in the United States self-inflicted gunshot predominates.[2] Perhaps most disturbing, some patients see a jump from a tall building as their only option.[3] These choices are cruel in their violence and devastating in their impact on survivors. And they have nothing to do with medicine as a helping profession.

The Interface with Medical Care

The founders of Compassion in Dying included a physician, a hospice nurse, members of the clergy, several social workers, and other social service professionals. In addition to offering compassionate services, they intended their work to be "a demonstration that mentally competent, terminally ill adult patients can hasten death in a voluntary, safe, and humane manner."[4]

With the goal of meeting the perceived need in a responsible manner, the founders issued eligibility guidelines and practice safeguards as a framework to create, to the extent possible, a situation in which the patient might receive both excellent end-of-life care and the choice of assisted dying with self-administered medication. This document, which presaged the structure ultimately codified as the right to assisted death in Oregon, outlines the following eligibility criteria:

- A medical evaluation has determined the patient's condition is, in reasonable medical judgment, likely to result in death within six months.
- The patient is an adult who is competent to make health care decisions and does not exhibit pathologic depression or other mental impairment that affects judgment.
- The patient's condition causes suffering that is severe and intolerable to the patient.
- The patient's suffering does not result from inadequate comfort care, especially inadequate pain management.
- The patient has a firm understanding of the diagnosis, prognosis, and available interventions in palliative care.
- The patient has originated the request for information about assisted dying, put it in writing or on videotape, and repeated it over time. The request is voluntary, rational, and enduring. Inadequate health insurance or economic concerns do not motivate the request.
- Requests may not be made through an advance directive or surrogate decision maker.
- There is no expressed disapproval from any member of the immediate family.[5]

Compassion adopted this last requirement to protect the organization, given the uncertain legal status of assisted dying in Washington state. It is clinically advisable to talk with the patient's family and evaluate the family dynamics and the level of support for a patient's request for aid in dying. Doing so can illuminate confounding factors and ease the family's bereavement. Family consensus and support is a fundamental goal. However, there would be no *legal* reason to disenfranchise a competent adult by bestowing veto power on any disapproving family member.

These initial practice guidelines took their cues from models of careful medical and social service practice and have matured over the past ten years. Defining characteristics include the following:

- assessment of the client's physical and mental condition and informed action based on that assessment
- advocacy integrated into, rather than set apart from, accepted standards of care
- coequal goals to optimize end-of-life care and support patient choice and control
- interdisciplinary teams of volunteers and staff that include nurses, physicians, psychologists, social workers, and members of the clergy
- regular continuing education for volunteers and staff and systematic quality assurance reviews
- consultation and collaboration with a client's care providers, helping to address all aspects of care, from pain and symptom management to emotional, social, and spiritual well-being
- the offer, through volunteer medical experts and professional staff, of peer-to-peer education and advice on challenging palliative care problems
- referral to local hospice and palliative care specialists
- sharing of information about medication for assisted dying only in the context of the supportive relationship with an eligible client
- limitation of assistance to exclude either providing or administering the means of assisted dying
- file notes on every client throughout the course of illness until death or discontinuation of the supportive relationship, records and client information being subject to confidentiality policies and procedures
- procedures for case closure and data management

An example may serve to illustrate these principles. Margaret, a middle-aged woman with amyotrophic lateral sclerosis (ALS), called Compassion from a small midwestern town, concerned that as her disease progressed, breathlessness would bring intolerable suffering. She wanted the means to hasten her death if that occurred. During the intake interview we learned she was not under hospice care and her husband was the primary caregiver. She was able to walk with a walker, feed herself, and bathe with some help. She did not currently have symptoms of breathlessness. During a long conversation Margaret received assurance that she would have several options to achieve a peaceful, humane death when the time came. For now, she could be assured that we would serve as a resource and companion as her disease progressed. We sent Margaret basic materials about Compassion and a booklet, "A Gentle Death," addressing end-of-life options and patients' rights and responsibilities.[6]

The team discussed Margaret at its next meeting and decided she probably was not terminal by our criteria but that we would continue a supportive relationship. Margaret talked with Helen, her primary contact at Compassion, about once a week. Because Margaret lived in a distant city, these conversations were all by telephone. Although Compassion's preferred model is one of community-based volunteer teams, our clinical staff often serves clients through phone conversations and written materials.

When Margaret's disease appeared to enter a terminal phase, Helen suggested that she ask her physician to enroll her in the local hospice. Hospice enrollment went smoothly, but soon afterward Margaret had her first episode of air hunger. The hospice staff seemed unfamiliar with the use of morphine in small doses to address this symptom in ALS, and Helen asked if the hospice medical director would be willing to talk with a palliative care specialist in that state. Helen facilitated a telephone consultation that resulted in the hospice's providing Roxanol and instructing Margaret and her husband in its use.

When Margaret became so disabled that she needed more assistance than her husband could provide, he hired a daytime caregiver. Margaret continued to request information about medications to hasten her death, and after reviewing the eligibility criteria once again Helen consulted with a medical adviser and sent Margaret a protocol for accumulation and self-administration of medication. Margaret derived great comfort from having this information, which she shared with her husband and her caregiver. Helen became Margaret's confidant and friend. They talked frequently, and Helen helped Margaret come to some closure of her life experience. Margaret said she depended on Helen's support to feel calm and in control. Helen continued to discuss Margaret's situation and her own supportive role at monthly team meetings.

Over the next four months Margaret experienced more frequent anxiety related to her breathing. Her husband and caregiver learned that a small dose of

Roxanol, and sometimes a call to Helen, quickly eased Margaret's anxiety. As Margaret's condition deteriorated further, she lost the ability to self-administer medication. Helen and the caregiver talked frequently and speculated that Margaret had made a transition out of a desire to hasten her death, without expressly saying so. Margaret's breathing capacity continued to decline, and she required the small Roxanol doses more frequently. Eventually hospice initiated continuous opiate administration with a skin patch. The caregiver often talked with Helen and relayed the conversation to Margaret, who seemed to enjoy staying in touch even when she could not speak. Margaret died peacefully in her sleep about one year after her first conversation with Helen.

Access to the means to a humane, hastened death appears to have eased Margaret's suffering and provided much-needed assurance. By addressing her fears and giving her a sense of control, it may also have prolonged her life.

A Decade of Experience

In ten years, Compassion has received many thousands of individual inquiries about end-of-life options. Cases handled by Compassion's national office and by its chapters in the states of Washington and Oregon produce our most complete data. Together, these three offices have had sustained working contact with 2,992 clients. The experience reflects service to clients in environments in which physician-assisted dying was legal and those in which it was not. Of those individuals who met criteria for terminal illness, 1,490 subsequently died. The mean time from initial contact to death was 243 days.[7]

Either detailed consultation or the kind of ongoing and extensive contact we call "case management," as illustrated in the case of Margaret, was provided to 952 clients. To date, 291 clients (92 women and 109 men) have hastened their deaths with support and consultation from Compassion. Among early cases, AIDS was the dominant condition, but in later years it gave way to cancer as the most common diagnosis.

Compassion's client service follows a health care model, and we take seriously an obligation to collect data and keep it confidential. Volunteers and staff record information on an intake form that includes data fields we feel would be important to an investigation of patients who ask about assisted dying and of their decision-making process. Compassion keeps a chronological record in progress note format and documents each contact or attempted contact. A case closure form that includes information about the mode of death and twenty-

six other variables completes the data collection at the time of death or termination of the relationship. The information is transferred to an electronic
database to enable statistical queries.

Clients' ages have ranged from twenty-five to ninety-four, with a mean of
just under sixty-six (65.8 years). These clients have been overwhelmingly Cau-
casian, with one each of Asian, Latin American, and Native American descent.
Most list their religion as Protestant or "other"; Buddhism, Islam, and Catholi-
cism are also represented. Many who answered "none" or "other" to the question about religion responded "yes" to the question of whether they consider
themselves "spiritual." Most are educated at the college or graduate school level,
although six clients have had only a primary education. Most received prescriptions from physicians who either openly acknowledged or appeared to
understand how the client intended to use them. In Oregon, of course, open
acknowledgment is the rule.

We ask clients to describe their suffering and tell us which aspects would make
them want (or choose) to hasten death. The most common determining elements mentioned are loss of control and fear of the loss of control, loss of autonomy, loss of control of bodily functions, and physical discomfort other than
pain. Of the 201 clients who hastened death, only twenty-three named pain,
though thirty-one named the side effects of pain treatment as a source of suffering sufficient to cause them to hasten death. Ingested medication was effective in causing a peaceful death in all 201 cases. The time from ingestion to
coma is usually very short, and from ingestion to death less than two hours.
We prepare family members for the possibility that the period of coma might
be lengthy, and neither we nor the families considered prolonged coma a "complication" when it occurred.

The story of "Paul" (not his real name) illustrates the integration of medical
care and assisted dying in an environment without legal physician-assisted dying. Paul, a thirty-two-year-old man, had a ten-year history of treatment for
AIDS. His brother also has AIDS, and the parents have called on enormous reserves of love and strength to maintain close relationships with both their sons.
For years Paul talked about wanting assistance in dying if he ever faced intolerable suffering, but he never acted on his desire, assuming he could make those
plans when he really needed them.

Paul received his care from specialists in both neurology and oncology. Their
treatment options had run out, as all available medications had failed to slow
a recent rapid progression of illness. Cytomegalovirus infected Paul's central

nervous system, and he lost so much weight his frame carried no fat and barely any muscle. He was bed bound and on intravenous morphine, but he remained mentally clear and acutely aware of what lay ahead.

Paul asked his physicians to write a prescription for medication to hasten his death. With no curative options and meager palliative ones, both agreed to support his wish, but neither knew an effective, available medication they might prescribe. One of Paul's friends called Compassion in Dying. Our assessment indicated that Paul met our eligibility criteria, so we willingly shared our knowledge and experience with his family. Paul's friend brought our assessment to the physicians, who were pleased to receive a carefully considered protocol and evidence of its efficacy.

Paul took medication to hasten his death with his family, friends, and physicians in attendance. As sad as the occasion was, that he was able to escape the final deterioration he so abhorred gave some solace to those who loved him.

Patients like Paul often consider violently ending their lives. Struck by how many Compassion clients talked about violent means, we began to probe this issue during our intake interviews. We consider violent suicide a substantial risk when the client has made a concrete plan and obtained the means to carry it out. Since 1998, Compassion of Oregon has identified fifty-nine such clients who qualified for legal assisted dying and began the request process. Of these, thirty-nine eventually died of their underlying disease, and twenty died peacefully with medication under the provisions of the law. Independent anecdotal evidence indicates that hospices in Oregon have seen fewer of the violent suicides that occasionally occur among hospice patients.[8] Acknowledging rational decisions to hasten death and integrating them into medical care with a careful and legitimate process may avoid the tragedy of premature, violent suicide among terminally ill patients.

Fully Integrating Palliative Care and Assisted Dying in Oregon

Complete integration with excellent end-of-life care can occur only in a jurisdiction that recognizes assisted dying as part of legitimate medical practice. The Oregon Death with Dignity Act specifies that only the "attending physician" who has "primary responsibility for the care of the patient and treatment of the patient's terminal disease" may provide a prescription for medication to hasten death.[9] The drafters intended that assisted dying be considered in the context of a physician-patient relationship, end-of-life care, and symptom management.

They appear to have succeeded. In 2003 forty-two physicians wrote sixty-seven prescriptions for medication to hasten death.[10] Two of the state's largest health care systems, Kaiser Permanente and Oregon Health and Science University, have procedures and ombudsmen in place to ensure that a patient who requests assisted dying does not inadvertently lose access to other options in the continuum of end-of-life care. Hospices across the state have adopted procedures to ensure that no patient is denied hospice care because he or she has requested assisted death. Similarly, they take steps to guard against any compromise in the level of care after a request has been made.[11]

Legalization enables open consideration of assisted dying along with palliative care modalities, open discussion of the patient's request by the health care team, and open dialogue about treatment alternatives that might attenuate the specific suffering that is motivating the patient to consider hastened death. An open process may, in part, account for the low number of assisted deaths that have occurred in Oregon over the past six years.

Some barriers to full integration still exist, but they can be overcome. For example, patients who learn their physician will not participate in assisted dying can choose either to forgo the option or to transfer care to a doctor who will both deliver palliative care and consider a request for assisted dying. Problems arise only when doctors are not forthright about refusing to participate in assisted dying.[12] Some physicians may try to avoid a confrontation by misrepresenting the prognosis or, worse, giving the patient false reassurance on which they later renege. Several Compassion patients have been disappointed to learn that their physician's pat on the knee or the promise to "not let you suffer" did not, in fact, reflect a willingness to fulfill the duties of an attending physician under Oregon's assisted-dying law, as they had assumed. Several clearly terminal patients have been told their requests were premature.[13] Occasionally, physicians who oppose assisted dying have appeared to allow their moral view to cloud their assessment of the patient's mental or physical condition.

A nonparticipating physician who is honest and forthright can refer the patient without compromising the quality of end-of-life care. Nonparticipating hospices can and do make arrangements for a patient support organization like Compassion in Dying to counsel the patient and monitor compliance with the law. Hospice continues to provide the full range of its services until the moment of death, whether or not the patient chooses assisted dying. In Oregon, hospice nurses often attend the hastened deaths of their patients. The proportion of those hastening death who were simultaneously enrolled in hospice climbed substantially in the six years of implementation of the Death with

Dignity Act, reaching 93 percent in 2003.[14] This contrasts sharply with our experience in other states, where hospice enrollment among those who choose assisted dying is less than 50 percent. We believe legalization of assisted dying greatly facilitates the provision of hospice care while patients pursue the choice of a hastened death.

Newspapers have carried several personal patient stories, and critics believe they have discovered abuses between the lines. Often repeated, critics' observations have progressed from a stated "concern" to an assumption that serves their argument to specific hypotheses derived from these false assumptions. Arguments often finish with the sort of provocative question or innuendo that is more often seen in propaganda than in academic publications. Authors who oppose Oregon's Death with Dignity Act rely on these techniques heavily in their descriptions of the cases of "Helen" and Kate presented in chapter 12.[15] Among the "urban myths" thus created are that patients who choose assisted dying are not offered palliative care and that demented or depressed patients, or those who are being coerced, qualify under the law.

Accusations of this type malign not only the patients, families, and physicians involved but also the hospices in which patients were enrolled, the Oregon Hospice Association, and officials at the Oregon Department of Human Services charged with oversight of the law. Eighty-six percent of all patients who have used Oregon's assisted dying law were enrolled in hospice, and it is well recognized that hospice delivers excellent palliative treatment and routinely addresses the mental health of its patients with a multidisciplinary team approach. If physicians respond that they offered no additional palliative care options after the patient's request, that is most likely because all feasible palliative care was already in place.[16] The Oregon Hospice Association, the Oregon Department of Human Services, and in one case, local police have all investigated critics' charges and found them to be without merit. No credible neutral source repeats these misrepresentations. Critics who press these arguments rely on articles from a newspaper known for its opposition to the Oregon law as their primary source.[17] Yet even the reporter who conducted the interviews and wrote the stories disagrees with the conclusions critics draw from her writings.[18]

A Medical Establishment Out of Step with Its Patients

Although attitudes toward self-determination in dying are changing rapidly, the organized medical community is responding slowly. The plight of suffering patients affects many individual physicians and nurses, and even without organizational support many physicians—especially those who have had experience similar to that of Paul's physicians—occasionally incorporate assisted death into their medical practice.[19] Evidence of widespread covert assisted dying, compared with Oregon's experience with regulation, suggests that legally recognizing physician-assisted death as legitimate medical practice might have the unexpected effect of reducing its incidence.[20]

With few exceptions, however, organized medicine promulgates an inflexible doctrine that assisted dying is "fundamentally incompatible with the role of healer."[21] This seems to reflect an outmoded view not only of the importance of relieving suffering as a form of healing but also of the relationship between physician and patient. The comment of one physician opposed to legal assisted dying illustrates an archaic perspective. Dr. Kenneth R. Stevens, president of Physicians for Compassionate Care, has said, "I was taught that a prescription is an order from a doctor to a patient. [In assisted death,] you're not pulling the trigger but you're giving the patient the loaded gun."[22] Today, patients are more likely to regard their physician's prescription as an educated recommendation than a dictatorial order.

The Importance of Having a Choice

Dying patients deserve the best we can offer in symptom management, adaptive technology, psychosocial support, and spiritual comfort. They also deserve a sense of control over the degree and duration of deterioration and suffering they endure. The choice of assisted dying gives patients that sense of control. Many never exercise the choice, but they all can experience a heightened sense of autonomy and peace of mind from knowing that it is theirs to make. Compassion in Dying's experience in Oregon and elsewhere suggests that suffering may be more tolerable when it is endured voluntarily. Peace of mind, endurance, patient autonomy—these are worthy goals for a healing profession. Integrating the choice of assisted dying into excellent end-of-life care helps achieve them.

Notes

1. T.E. Quill and C.K. Cassel, "Nonabandonment: A Central Obligation for Physicians," *Annals of Internal Medicine* 122 (1995): 368–74.

2. Martine Cornelisse, psychologist, Dutch Association for a Voluntary End of Life, personal communication, May 28, 2003; see also F. Casadebaig, D. Ruffin, and A. Philippe, "Suicide in the Elderly at Home and in Retirement Homes in France," [translated title]

Revue d'Epidemiologie et de Santé Publique 51 (2003): 55–64; A. Poleske, F. Bolechala, E. Skupien, F. Trela, and A. Ziebe, "Completed Suicide and Depression in the Elderly," [translated title] *Przeglad Lekarski* 59 (2002): 295–97; J. Hallifax, "Murder-Suicide 'Epidemic' in Florida," *Miami Herald,* July 29, 2001, 6B.

3. C. Carmichael, "Last Right," *New York Times Magazine,* May 20, 2001, 97.

4. T.A. Preston and R. Mero, "Observations Concerning Terminally Ill Patients Who Choose Suicide," *Journal of Pharmaceutical Care in Pain and Symptom Control* 4 (1996): 183–92.

5. Compassion in Dying, "Guidelines and Safeguards"; at www.CompassionInDying .org/guidelines.php (revised April 9, 1997).

6. Compassion in Dying Federation, "A Gentle Death: Freedom to Choose at Life's End (1998). Excerpts available at www.CompassionInDying.org/gentle_death.php.

7. Compassion in Dying of Oregon database; five years accumulated experience through 2002.

8. Ann Jackson, executive director, Oregon Hospice Association, personal communication, April 28, 2003.

9. Oregon Death with Dignity Act, *Oregon Revised Statutes,* secs. 127.800 and 127.995(2) (1995).

10. Oregon Department of Human Services, *Fifth Annual Report on Oregon's Death with Dignity Act* (Portland, Ore.: Oregon Department of Human Services, March 6, 2003), 12.

11. A. Jackson and B. Coombs-Lee, "Hospice and Choice: Working Together in Oregon," paper presented to the Washington State Hospice and Palliative Care Organization, April 28, 2003.

12. M.P. Battin, "Is a Physician Ever Obligated to Help a Patient Die?" in *Regulating How We Die: The Ethical, Medical, and Legal Issues Surrounding Physician-Assisted Suicide,* edited by L.L. Emanuel (Cambridge: Harvard University Press, 1998), 21–47.

13. Case reports relayed in Compassion in Dying case management team meetings and documented in file notes.

14. Oregon Department of Human Services, *Fifth Annual Report on Oregon's Death with Dignity Act,* Table 4, page 23.

15. K. Foley and H. Hendin, "The Oregon Experiment," in *The Case against Assisted Suicide: For the Right to End-of-Life Care,* edited by K. Foley and H. Hendin (Baltimore: Johns Hopkins University Press, 2002), 144–74, 146, 157.

16. Ibid., 153–54.

17. Ibid., 145–49, 156–58.

18. Erin Hoover Barnett, personal communication, October 5, 2000.

19. L.R. Slome, T.F. Mitchell, E. Charlebois, J.M. Benevedes, and D.I. Abrams, "Physician-Assisted Suicide and Patients with Human Immunodeficiency Virus Disease," *New England Journal of Medicine* 336 (1997): 417–21.

20. See chapter 7 in this volume; Oregon Department of Human Services, *Fifth Annual Report on Oregon's Death with Dignity Act.*

21. American Medical Association, *Code of Medical Ethics, Current Opinions* (Chicago: American Medical Association, 2002), Opinion 2.211, 42.

22. Quoted in D. Colburn, "Assisted Suicide Numbers Surge," *Oregonian,* March 6, 2003, A1, A11.

14

Thirty Years' Experience with Euthanasia in the Netherlands

Focusing on the Patient as a Person

Johannes J.M. van Delden M.D., Ph.D., Jaap J.F. Visser, L.L.M., and Els Borst-Eilers, M.D., Ph.D.

Although the Netherlands is an extremely flat country, it appears to have slopes that can be skied down when it comes to euthanasia.[1] At least, that is what many authors commenting on the Dutch experience with euthanasia would have their readers believe. We have argued elsewhere that most such comments lump together different types of end-of-life decisions based on unacceptable simplifications.[2] Rather than repeat our critique, here we further the discussion by analyzing the Dutch situation.

The Importance of Context: The Netherlands and the Dutch

Why was the Netherlands the first country to pass euthanasia legislation—that is, legislation permitting voluntary active euthanasia? This question is hard to answer in a way that explains everything. Nevertheless, some relevant observations can be made. First, one could hold that although their response was unique, the Dutch were responding to the very same developments that were occurring in many other countries. At the end of the 1960s there was a shared feeling that medicine's propensity to prolong life had perhaps gone too far. In several countries these perceptions fueled debates about nontreatment decisions and euthanasia, inspired by the idea that patients should be recognized as persons in control of their own lives, including the end of their lives.

The focus of debate, however, differed much across countries. Some, such as the United States, concentrated on nontreatment decisions (the famous case of Karen Ann Quinlan being a prime example), whereas in the Netherlands the primary focus was on euthanasia—a difference probably best explained by differences in culture, legal system, and health care.[3] The Netherlands has become home to a wide variety of beliefs. Over the centuries it served as a refuge to dissidents and religious groups who were oppressed or expelled from elsewhere— French Huguenots, free thinkers such as Spinoza and Descartes, Sephardic Jews from Portugal, and Ashkenazi Jews from eastern Europe, among others. Despite a predominantly Calvinist religious tradition, though one with a large Roman Catholic minority, tolerance in religious matters and freedom of thought prevented a single dominant view from taking hold. This resulted in, among other things, a long tradition of public theological debate. The Dutch can argue for hours about every aspect of good and evil. At the same time, they have learned over the centuries to live with one another in an atmosphere of tolerance, despite some major theological differences, and to respect one another's beliefs.

The Netherlands was certainly not the first country to debate euthanasia. The debate began in the middle of the nineteenth century, when drugs became available to physicians with which they could influence the way people died. At that time, euthanasia was discussed in England, Germany, and the United States but not in the Netherlands. In fact, the first proposal to legalize euthanasia was made in 1906 in the state of Ohio.[4]

In more recent decades, however, Dutch society has rapidly become more secular and less divided along religious lines, and this has placed decisions about life and death in another perspective. Responsibility for one's life, once safely in the hands of the church or the medical profession, shifted back to the individual. Many Dutch people believe that they must be free to make their own decisions about their lives, including when and how their lives should end. These ideas have gradually gained ground, even among practicing Christians. At the same time, the Dutch have great respect for human life. The Netherlands has no death penalty, individuals are not allowed to own firearms, and the abortion rate is one of the lowest in the world. A large majority of the population is of the opinion that abortion and euthanasia must be possible but sees both as last resorts.

Another reason for the Netherlands' response to the issue of euthanasia is its legal system. The Dutch system of criminal justice is based not on a principle of legality, which holds that all cases should be prosecuted, but rather on a principle of expediency. The principle of expediency holds that there can be cases in which prosecution of a possible criminal act would not serve the public interest; it thus creates room for public policy in the area of criminal justice. This, together with the recognition of necessity (*force majeure*) in the penal code, have made it possible to keep euthanasia within the purview of criminal law yet accept it under certain circumstances. (Of course, the law of 2001 has changed all this, a matter to which we return later in this chapter.)

Finally, the Dutch have a freely accessible and affordable system of health care. Everyone is assured of care from the cradle to the grave, including long-term nursing care for the elderly and those who are chronically ill. Thus a patient who needs expensive care for several years has no financial incentive to end his or her life. All these elements have played a role in the debate of the past thirty years on euthanasia and other medical decisions at the end of life.

The Debate

In 1973 the whole country was suddenly forced to confront the issue of euthanasia. In that year, the district court in Leeuwarden heard a case involving a doctor who had ended the life of her seriously ill mother, who had made repeated and explicit requests for euthanasia. The daughter wanted to spare her mother pointless suffering and loss of personal dignity. She felt that her mother —who was experiencing intolerable pain and suffering, knew that she was near death, and had made it clear that she did not want go on living—should not continue to suffer to the bitter end. The court held that the doctor had committed a criminal offense. In fact, formally speaking, she had committed murder.

However, the court also said that a doctor is not always obliged to keep alive against his or her will a patient who is suffering severely, without hope of a remedy. The doctor ultimately received a short, suspended sentence.

Like all doctors, Dutch physicians are trained to cure patients. But they also learn that they shouldn't allow people to suffer needlessly. A doctor may therefore end up with conflicting responsibilities in the case of a patient who is suffering unbearably without prospect of improvement and is asking for euthanasia. In the years that followed the Leeuwarden case, debate on this dilemma continued. Initially divided, the medical profession later moved toward developing criteria for euthanasia, and in 1984 the Royal Dutch Medical Association codified the emerging professional consensus in five requirements that can still be recognized in the law discussed below. From the beginning, the association also emphasized that doctors should report every case of termination of life. It was also the Royal Dutch Medical Association that persuaded the minister of justice in 1990 to establish a formal notification procedure to harmonize regional prosecution policies and to eliminate those practices that discouraged physicians from reporting cases, such as interrogation of relatives and physicians by uniformed police officers.

Politicians, lawyers, doctors, and ethicists struggled for years to find a way to enable doctors to accede to a patient's request for euthanasia without laying themselves open to prosecution. Members of the medical profession wanted to be certain that they were acting within the law, as did their patients. The courts, however, refused to recognize a "medical exception" to homicide law, an option explicitly rejected in 1984 by the Supreme Court, which found that euthanasia could not be regarded as a normal medical procedure. Nonetheless, the Court did open the way to allowing nonprosecution of physicians who performed euthanasia.

In 1982 the government asked a state commission to consider the question; the commission's report was published in 1985. Looking back, it is clear that its findings had considerable impact on later developments. The commission established a definition of euthanasia that has been in use in the Netherlands ever since: actively terminating the life of another person on the explicit request of that person.

The commission also drew up a series of "due care" criteria to be met in every case of euthanasia and proposed that new legislation be passed. Although this suggestion initially had little impact, it later became enormously influential. The commission's recommendation was, in fact, that under certain conditions euthanasia should no longer be regarded as a criminal offense.

In 1984 a ruling by the Supreme Court, the Netherlands' highest court, led to a breakthrough. The Court held that a doctor who ends a patient's life at the patient's request because his or her suffering is unbearable and without prospect of improvement faces a conflict of obligations. On the one hand, the doctor has the duty to try to cure the patient and to relieve the suffering. On the other, he or she cannot allow the patient to suffer unnecessarily if no remedy is available to relieve the suffering. In such a situation, a physician who ends a patient's life can invoke the legal defense of necessity (*force majeure*). In practice, this meant that a court could decide that a doctor who had complied with a number of specific due care criteria in making the decision and in carrying out the action was not criminally liable.

The core of the due care criteria set out in the Court's decision were the very same ones described by the Royal Dutch Medical Association and the state commission. Over the years, these criteria have been refined by the medical profession and in case law, but essentially they have not changed. With the recently passed act that legalizes euthanasia, the set of due care criteria has been embedded in law.

Empirical Studies of the Practice of Euthanasia

The Dutch government and Parliament spent years struggling to establish a legal framework, but it was only after the Supreme Court ruling and the commission report that both sides finally came up with a draft bill. In the course of time it had become clear that the Dutch population was broadly in favor of legislation on euthanasia. Before the first legislation was passed, however, in 1990 the government (a coalition of Social Democrats and Christian Democrats) commissioned empirical research into the incidence of euthanasia and other medical decisions at the end of life,[5] which was repeated in 1995 and again in 2001.[6] All three studies attracted considerable international attention. It is, after all, unique to have such a sensitive subject researched in an objective manner, through questionnaires and interviews with doctors whose anonymity is guaranteed. We present the main findings in table 14.1.

The first point to be noted is the stability of the euthanasia practice: Although there has been a slight increase in the incidence of euthanasia over the years, the incidence of active termination of life as a whole hardly changes. The second point is the continuing presence of life-terminating acts without explicit request of the patient. We return to these cases in the next section.

These studies show in considerable detail which doctors and which patients are involved in the decisions to actively terminate life. In interviews conducted in 2001, 57 percent of doctors said that they had performed euthanasia or assisted suicide. A further 32 percent said they could conceive of situations in which they would be prepared to do so.[7] General practitioners were involved in 77 percent of euthanasia cases and nearly all cases of assisted suicide. About 21 percent of euthanasia cases were performed in hospitals.

With respect to the patients involved, the studies demonstrate that in two-thirds of cases of euthanasia or assisted suicide the patient was in the terminal stages of illness, usually cancer (77 percent). The estimated shortening of life was less than one week in 46 percent of cases; only 13 percent of patients had a life expectancy of more than one month. Euthanasia occurs relatively infrequently among vulnerable groups, such as the oldest old and residents of nursing homes.

The studies also reveal that physicians do not comply with most requests for euthanasia. In 2001, for instance, ninety-seven hundred patients explicitly asked

Table 14.1. Incidence of Active Termination of Life in the Netherlands, Various Years

	1990	1995	2001
Annual number of deaths	128,824	135,675	140,377
Cause of death (percentage)			
Euthanasia	1.8	2.4	2.5
Assisted suicide	0.3	0.3	0.2
Life-terminating acts without explicit request			
of the patient	0.8	0.7	0.7
Total	2.9	3.4	3.4

Source: Data from B. Onwuteaka, A. van der Heide, D. Koper, I. Keij-Deerenberg, M.L. Rurup, A.M. Vrakking, J.J. Georges, M.T. Muller, G. van der Wal, and P.J. van der Maas, "Euthanasia and Other End-of-Life Decisions in the Netherlands in 1990, 1995, and 2001," *Lancet* 362 (2003): 395–99.

their physicians to end their lives. The data summarized in table 14.1 show that euthanasia was performed in response to thirty-five hundred of these requests and assisted suicide in three hundred—that is, only approximately two out of five requests for euthanasia were met. In the remaining cases, the patient's request led neither to euthanasia nor to assisted suicide. In about half of these, the patient died before a final decision to perform euthanasia had been made. In the other half, the physician refused to honor the patient's request. The most frequently mentioned reasons for refusing a request were that the patient's suffering was not unbearable (35 percent), that there were still alternatives available for alleviating the suffering (32 percent), and that the patient was depressed or had psychiatric symptoms (31 percent).[8] In these cases, the doctor took steps other than euthanasia or assisted suicide to relieve the patient's suffering.

Life-Terminating Acts without Explicit Request by the Patient

Cases of life-terminating acts without explicit request of the patient were described in all three reports. The absolute numbers were 1,000 cases in 1990 and 900 in both 1995 and 2001. In a number of cases the decision had been discussed with the patient, or in a previous phase of the illness the patient had expressed a wish for euthanasia if suffering were to become unbearable without explicitly requesting euthanasia; this was true of 59 percent of cases in 1990,

53 percent in 1995, and 36 percent in 2001. In all other cases, patients were incompetent. In 95 percent of the cases, the physician discussed the case with colleagues, nursing staff, or the patient's relatives (on average, with persons in two of these categories). In two-thirds of cases, morphine was the only drug administered.

The percentage of patients with cancer who died from life-terminating acts without explicit patient request is considerably less than that for euthanasia—40 percent (data from 2001 study).[9] The patients involved were also closer to death, compared with patients whose request for euthanasia or assisted suicide was granted. In 42 percent of cases of life-terminating acts without explicit request of the patient, life was shortened by at most twenty-four hours, and in a further 35 percent by at most one week. Only in 18 percent was life shortened by a longer period. These characteristics are largely the same for the 1990 and 1995 cases. The 2001 study also indicates that about one-third of the life-terminating acts without explicit request of the patient can also be described as terminal sedation—that is, cases in which high dosages of sedatives were given without hydrating the patient. However, in these cases physicians had described their own acts as intended to shorten life.

The publication of data on life-terminating acts without explicit request of the patient introduced a new dimension in the Dutch euthanasia debate. Since the mid-1980s, this debate had been focused on euthanasia and assisted suicide in which the patient's explicit request was a central feature. In part the discussion had been deliberately narrowed in this way because it was felt that consensus was closest for these cases. As noted earlier, the Dutch even changed their definition of euthanasia to specifically include only cases in which there was an explicit request by the patient.

The description of life-terminating acts without explicit request of the patient has broadened the discussion once again. But what does their appearance in the reports mean? Does this prove the existence of a slippery slope? Before 1991, Dutch commentators on euthanasia talked exclusively about cases that fell within the narrow definition of acts carried out at the patient's request. Only later did the existence of the cases of acts *without* explicit request of the patient become known, giving the impression that the Dutch had begun with hastening death on request and had ended up doing so with nonvoluntary cases.

This, however, is not necessarily true. We simply do not know whether life-terminating acts occurred without the patient's request less or more frequently in the past. What we do know is that the occurrence did not increase in the decade between 1991 and 2001.

We also know that the prevalence of such practices is much higher in other countries, such as Australia and Belgium, that only briefly permitted euthanasia and could not have "slid down the slope" by tolerating it for years.[10] The Belgian numbers for 1998 merit a little more attention. The percentages for euthanasia, physician-assisted suicide, and life-terminating acts without explicit requests of the patient in that year are 1.1, 0.1, and 3.2 percent, respectively. One thing is striking: the ratio of cases on request of the patient versus those not on explicit request in Belgium—one in three—is the reverse of that in the Netherlands.

A study was carried out in Belgium, Denmark, Italy, the Netherlands, Sweden, and Switzerland using the same design as previous studies in the Netherlands and in Belgium, the results of which were recently published.[11] In all countries other than the Netherlands and Switzerland, the incidence of life-terminating acts without explicit request of the patient was higher than the incidence of physician-assisted death (combination of voluntary euthanasia and physician-assisted suicide) on request of the patient. Perhaps an open debate and a tolerant policy are not that bad after all.

Nonetheless, though they do not prove the existence of a slippery slope in the Netherlands, the cases of nonvoluntary euthanasia do pose a serious problem. They are obviously not justified by the principle of respect for patient autonomy and therefore can only be tolerated (if at all) in extreme situations in which termination of life is absolutely the last resort. Legally, these cases remain a criminal offense.

Reporting Euthanasia

To accept euthanasia in an individual case is one thing; to accept it as a matter of public policy is quite something else. It is often argued that proposals to legalize euthanasia can never contain absolute safeguards. We think this is true; there is no rule that cannot (and will not) be broken. However, the same can be said for the prohibition of driving drunk. The question is whether the fact that safeguards can or might be ignored justifies prohibiting euthanasia in an individual case. The Dutch at first tried to have it both ways by creating a public policy based on individual cases. This resulted, at the very least, in an unsatisfactory situation of accepting and prohibiting at the same time, thereby creating uncertainty and vagueness both for patients and physicians and no doubt contributing, to some extent, to reports critical of the Netherlands.

Persuading physicians to bring cases of euthanasia to the knowledge of the authorities is a problem for any euthanasia policy. The Dutch notification procedure helped to raise the notification rate from 18 percent in 1990 to 41 percent in 1995.[12] The 1995 study revealed that doctors who had not reported cases of euthanasia usually had acted according to the criteria. Why, then, did they fail to report their actions to the public prosecutor? The main reason was that they felt they were being treated as criminals precisely because, though they had exercised due care, they had to report to the Public Prosecution Service and then face long periods of uncertainty during which they were technically murder suspects.

In response to this circumstance, the government tried to further diminish the number of unreported cases by developing a new notification procedure, in which much of the assessment was done outside the legal system. To this purpose, in 1998 five regional multidisciplinary assessment committees were created to assess all reported cases of euthanasia. The committees consist of a lawyer (who serves as chair), a physician, and an ethicist. They meet approximately once every three weeks to discuss thirty to forty cases per meeting. The outcome of these discussions can be one of three things. In most cases the committee will conclude (in 6 percent after receiving further information from the reporting physician) that the physician has acted carefully and has met the standards. If the committee feels that the physician has not acted in a careful way, the case is handed over to the prosecutor, who then starts a legal investigation. To date, only 0.1 percent of all cases assessed have proceeded to investigation. In other cases in which legal standards were met but the doctor did not exercise sufficient professional care, the medical inspector is alerted.

The effect of this procedural change on the notification rate is not completely clear yet, but the first results can be given. In 1996, 1,700 cases of euthanasia were reported; in 1997, 1,900. In the first ten months of 1998, authorities were notified of 2,241 cases. These cases were all handled under the old regulations. Since the assessment committees started with their work, the number of reported cases has dropped. The last two months of 1998 yielded 349 cases (resulting in 2,590 for the whole of that year). Subsequent years have consistently shown fewer reported cases each year. The number of reported cases for 2002 (1,882) has not reversed this trend.[13]

Interpreting these declining numbers is not without difficulty; one cannot simply deduce a percentage for the reporting of euthanasia in one year, because these numbers represent only the numerator. To generate percentages, one would need also to know how many cases occurred in that year, including unreported cases. The most recent nationwide study indicates that in 2001 there were 3,800 cases of euthanasia and assisted suicide. Of these, 2,054, or 54 percent, were reported. This response is clearly less than was hoped for. Somewhat paradoxically, the new study also finds that doctors in general were satisfied with the new procedure.[14] Yet still the reporting rate lags behind.

Another development may be more successful in raising physicians' willingness to report cases of euthanasia or assisted suicide. A network of general practitioners and other physicians (Support Consultation Euthanasia the Netherlands [SCEN]) has been set up to assist doctors facing decisions about euthanasia or assisted suicide. These consultants have had special training in palliative care and in all aspects of the law on euthanasia. They are also available to help physicians with existential questions that might arise—most physicians find it a heavy task to perform euthanasia. Attending physicians dealing with requests for euthanasia should preferably confer with one of these consultants. There is reason to believe that cases in which a SCEN consultant has been involved are reported more frequently.

A New Law on Euthanasia

As noted earlier, the government wanted to create an assessment system that did not call for the public prosecutor to be involved in every case. This wish was in accordance with the outcome of the 1995 interviews in which doctors had said they would rather be judged by a broader committee, containing at least one physician. The coalition parties therefore developed a proposal to grant immunity from prosecution to those doctors whose cases had come before a review committee that decided the doctor had acted with due care. This immunity from prosecution was to be regulated by law. The cabinet adopted this proposal in 1998, and so was born the Euthanasia Act that came into force in April 2002.

The act states that although euthanasia remains in principle a criminal offense, a medical doctor who has reported to the committee and been found to have acted with due care in the hastened death of his patient will not be prosecuted. In such a case, the Public Prosecution Service is not notified, and the doctor cannot be prosecuted. Only if the review committee finds that the doctor has not acted with due care will it contact the Public Prosecution Service, which then decides whether to press charges. The review committees are obliged to report the number of cases of euthanasia they have assessed in their annual report.

The review committees have authority to judge cases of euthanasia or assisted suicide only, both of which require there to have been a voluntary, well-considered request on the part of the patient. In all cases in which there was no request of the patient or in which it can be doubted that the patient would have been able to make a well-considered request (for example, in the case of a psychiatric patient), the committee is not entitled to pass a final judgment. The coroner must report such cases directly to the public prosecutor.

The Dutch government has thus tried to regulate these matters in a transparent way, combining openness and legal certainty. Doctors know what they have to take into account in coming to a decision and can report what they have done without anxiety. They know that if they act with due care they will not be prosecuted.

What are these "due care" criteria? According to the Euthanasia Act, the doctor must

- be satisfied that the patient's request is voluntary and well considered
- be satisfied that the patient's suffering is unbearable and that there is no prospect of improvement
- have informed the patient of his or her situation and further prognosis
- have come to the conclusion, together with the patient, that there is no other reasonable alternative
- have consulted at least one other independent physician, who must have seen the patient and stated in writing that the attending physician has fulfilled the criteria listed in the previous four points
- have exercised due medical care and attention in terminating the patient's life or assisting in the patient's suicide

In addition there is an article stating that a written request for euthanasia drawn up by the patient in advance may be effective should the patient no longer be able to express his or her will when the time comes. The physician may consider such a document as a form of guidance in his decision making.

It is clear from the criteria what a crucial role the doctor plays. The patient must make a voluntary and well-considered decision, and certainly the doctor will consult with the patient at every step. Ultimately, however, it is the doctor's actions that are under scrutiny, and it is the doctor who bears final responsibility. This sets a limit on a patient's right to choose. Patients have no right to euthanasia in the Netherlands, and doctors are not obliged to grant a request for euthanasia.

Doctors must decide for themselves whether they can meet the due care criteria in specific situations. The decision must be genuinely voluntary, so they have to be sure that a patient's request is not the result of family pressure. Whether the suffering is unbearable is, of course, a subjective judgment. Every individual has his or her own limits in terms of how much pain and suffering and loss of dignity is bearable. The prospect of improvement, however, can be assessed more objectively in medical terms. Recent advances in palliative care have made it even more relevant to discuss alternative options with the patient. The obligation to consult a second, independent physician, preferably a consultant from the SCEN network, is an essential part of the review system. The second physician must see the patient in person and submit his or her opinion, in writing, to the review committee. The committee then studies the case to determine whether the attending physician exercised due care in reaching the decision and in his or her actions. Finally, the review committee must render an opinion on each case submitted.

Euthanasia: A Last Resort

The Dutch medical profession itself believes that euthanasia must always remain an exception. Euthanasia may be the conclusion to a careful medical process, but it must always be the last resort. Many requests are driven by fears of pain, of loneliness, of becoming a burden on others, or of dying an undignified death. So a request for euthanasia should in the first place be seen as a cry for help, and only when other ways of relieving suffering have been exhausted should such a request be granted.

Two characteristics of the Dutch health care system provide reasons to believe that this describes reality rather than just being the socially acceptable thing to say. First of all, the Dutch health care system is accessible to all and guarantees full insurance coverage for end-of-life and palliative care. This insurance is mandatory for all except those with incomes over a stipulated high level. We can safely conclude, therefore, that patients will be under no financial pressure to end their lives.

Second, the Netherlands now has a good level of palliative care. In the past, the Netherlands was often criticized for its presumed lack of palliative care. The existence of only a few hospices, for example, was interpreted as proof of a neglect of palliative care. Although much of this criticism was based on a misunderstanding of the Dutch health care system (in the Netherlands, most palliative care takes place at home, in the nursing home, or in special hospital departments), it is also fair to say that in the beginning of the euthanasia debate, palliative care did not get the attention it deserved. In more recent years, however, much effort has been made to improve palliative care, partly in response to the international critique.

At present, a broad range of palliative care is available in the Netherlands.[15] There are many options for obtaining palliative care at home. The care that terminally ill patients need can also be provided in nursing homes, hospitals, and hospices. In mid-2002 there were hospice units in thirty-seven nursing homes and in twenty-six homes for the elderly. In addition, there were sixteen independent, professionally staffed hospices and twenty-one volunteer-run hospices. Most palliative care, however, is provided by the Netherlands' seventy-eight hundred general practitioners, since 65 percent of the forty thousand people who die of cancer each year die at home. More and more, general practitioners receive support from hospital-based (so-called transmural) palliative care teams.

As has been noted, the physician must always look for reasonable alternatives to euthanasia. Moreover, the second physician must determine whether the options for palliative care have been sufficiently explored. Thus efforts are made to ensure that euthanasia remains a last resort. Once a patient has received optimal palliative care, the question of euthanasia may not arise again. Even the best palliative care, however, cannot always prevent a patient from deciding that his or her suffering and loss of dignity have gone far enough. For such situations we need the possibility of euthanasia, within a context of careful decision making and openness.

Persons at the End of Life

The Dutch debate on euthanasia was the Netherlands' response to medicine's increasing ability to prolong life. It was inspired by the idea that patients should be treated as persons. What have thirty years of experience with euthanasia brought the Netherlands? We think the main result of the national debate is a well-developed framework for decision making in individual cases, now embedded in law. Physicians who must decide whether to comply with a patient's request for euthanasia know what they must take into account and can report what they have done without fear of being prosecuted, as long as they have acted with due care. The debate has also contributed to a certain peace of mind among patients. They can be sure that they will be treated by physicians who respect them as persons and have no intention of prolonging life as long as possible, without regard to the quality of that life, against a patient's will. Moreover, maybe somewhat paradoxically, the euthanasia debate has given a strong impulse to the development of palliative care.

There is no empirical evidence to support the suggestion that the Netherlands is on a slippery slope (let alone one that can be skied down) when it comes to physician-assisted death. At the same time, the number of cases of life-terminating acts without explicit request of the patient has not decreased.

Having said this, we certainly do not want to imply that a solution has been found for all individual cases. Requests from elderly people who are tired of life and for whom life has lost all meaning, but who do not suffer from any serious illnesses, cannot be complied with under the present framework. This was confirmed in the 2002 ruling of the Supreme Court. In addition, physicians remain reluctant to follow advance directives containing a written request for euthanasia for patients who are no longer competent. In both cases the Dutch debate has met its own limits. By emphasizing the role of the physician in the normative framework for euthanasia, cases that are more or less exclusively grounded in the patient's evaluation of his or her life fit in less well.[16]

On the societal level, we in the Netherlands now have a law that is supported by a large majority of the population and is grounded in a thorough knowledge of what is going on in medical practice. In spite of this, physicians still seem insufficiently prepared to be transparent. The frequency with which cases of euthanasia are reported clearly lags behind the expectations. It is not yet clear what steps can be taken to improve this response. We doubt, however, that the necessary steps can be found in new regulations. There will have to remain room for discretionary power of both the physician and the public prosecutor to judge what is best in individual cases. Only then can the debate on euthanasia serve its real end: to treat the patient as a person.

Notes

1. J.J.M. van Delden, "Slippery Slopes in Flat Countries," *Journal of Medical Ethics* 25 (1999): 22–24.

2. J.J.M. van Delden, L. Pijnenborg, and P.J. van der Maas, "Dances with Data," *Bioethics* 7 (1993): 323–29.

3. L. Pijnenborg and P.J. van der Maas, "The Dutch Euthanasia Debate in International Perspective," in *End-of-Life Decisions in Dutch Medical Practice*, edited by L. Pijnenborg (Rotterdam: Erasmus Universiteit, 1995), 119–32.

4. H.Y. Vanderpool, "Doctors and the Dying of Patients in American History," in *Physician-Assisted Suicide*, edited by R.F. Weir (Bloomington: Indiana University Press, 1997), 33–66.

5. P.J. van der Maas, J.J.M. van Delden, and L. Pijnenborg, *Euthanasia and Other Medical Decisions Concerning the End of Life* (Amsterdam: Elsevier, 1992); also published as a special issue of *Health Policy* 22 (1992).

6. G. van der Wal and P.J. van der Maas, *Euthanasia and Other Medical Practices at the End of Life* [in Dutch] (The Hague: SDU Uitgevers, 1996); P.J. van der Maas, G. van der Wal, I. Haverkate, C.L. de Graaff, J.G. Kester, B.D. Onwuteaka-Philipsen, A. van der Heide, J.M. Bosma, and D.L. Willems, "Euthanasia, Physician-Assisted Suicide, and Other Medical Practices Involving the End of Life in the Netherlands, 1990–1995," *New England Journal of Medicine* 335 (1996): 1699–1705; B. Onwuteaka, A. van der Heide, D. Koper, I. Keij-Deerenberg, M.L. Rurup, A.M. Vrakking, J.J. Georges, M.T. Muller, G. van der Wal, and P.J. van der Maas, "Euthanasia and Other End-of-Life Decisions in the Netherlands in 1990, 1995, and 2001," *Lancet* 362 (2003): 395–99.

7. G. van der Wal, A. van der Heide, B.D. Onwuteaka-Philipsen, and P.J. van der Maas, *Medical Decision Making at the End of Life: The Practice and the Evaluation Procedure* [in Dutch] (Utrecht: Uitgeverij de Tijdstroom, 2003).

8. I. Haverkate, B.D. Onwuteaka-Philipsen, A. van der Heide, P.J. Kostense, G. van der Wal, and P.J. van der Maas, "Refused and Granted Requests for Euthanasia and Assisted Suicide in the Netherlands," *British Medical Journal* 321 (2000): 865–86.

9. G. van der Wal et al., *Medical Decision Making at the End of Life: The Practice and the Evaluation Procedure.*

10. H. Kuhse, P. Singer, P. Baume, M. Clark, and M. Rickard, "End-of-Life Decisions in Australian Medical Practice," *Medical Journal of Australia* 166 (1997): 191–96; L. Deliens, F. Mortier, J. Bilsen, M. Cosyns, R. Vander Schicle, J. Vanoverloop, and K. Ingles, "End-of-life Decisions in Medical Practice in Flanders, Belgium: A Nationwide Survey," *Lancet* 356 (2000): 1806–11.

11. A. van der Heide, L. Deliens, K. Faisst, T. Nilstun, M. Norup, E. Paci, G. van der Wal, P.J. van der Maas, and EURELD Consortium, "End-of-Life Decision-Making in Six European Countries: Descriptive Study," *Lancet* 362 (2003): 345–50.

12. Van der Maas et al., "Euthanasia, Physician-Assisted Suicide and Other Medical Practices Involving the End of Life in the Netherlands," 13.

13. Regionale toetsingscommissies voor euthanasia, *Jaarverslag 2002* (The Hague: Ministry of Health, 2003).

14. Van der Wal et al., *Medical Decision Making at the End of Life.*

15. A.L. Francke, *Palliative Care for Terminally Ill Patients in the Netherlands* (The Hague: Ministry of Health, 2003).

16. J.J.M. van Delden, "The Unfeasibility of Requests for Euthanasia in Advance Directives," *Journal of Medical Ethics* (2004), forthcoming.

15

The Death of My Father

Herman H. van der Kloot Meijburg, D.Div., C.T.

Dear Friends,

I want to share with you the death of my father, Fritz van der Kloot Meijburg.

On Saturday evening, January 13, 2001, my father died in his sleep. It was at his request. At last he was at peace. This was what he had hoped for: to die in his sleep.

Five years ago, at the age of eighty-five, my father was diagnosed with amyotrophic lateral sclerosis (ALS). My parents had just moved to a home for the elderly, but for another reason: my mother had been diagnosed with Alzheimer's disease. It was a reasonable solution, and it provided my parents with some degree of support. So ALS came as a surprise to my father and the family. Ever since my father's diagnosis, this disease has been slowly eating away at his physical condition.

I have known my father as a real organizer and planner, even to the extent that what had been planned or arranged in his agenda ruled his day. At times, if the barber did not show up to do his hair, he would get annoyed because the appointment was on his agenda—although sometimes the barber didn't even know he had an appointment with my father! If I promised him that I would visit with him at some time during the day, he always asked me the exact time I would come, and he would write that down in his agenda.

What may sound like a weakness may also be perceived as a sign of strength: ALS wasn't planned for; it was not on his agenda, and therefore he closed the door to this disease. He even ignored his disease to such an extent that he would try to continue life's routines as best he could despite his diminishing condition. Sometimes I told him that it wouldn't bother me if he decided to stay in his apartment and save his energy instead of insisting on taking me downstairs to the entry hall to say good-bye.

It came as a great shock to my father that the home physician advised him to look for a place for my mother in a nursing home. He had hoped that he would be able to look after his wife in the home for the elderly, but the effort was wearing him out. When my mother was moved to the nursing home, five miles down the road, he felt guilty that he was the cause of her being there. Consequently, he set up a scheme of visiting her on a daily basis seven days a week. At first he used his electric scooter; later, he became dependent on others to take him there.

Amyotrophic lateral sclerosis is a rude disease and is, at an earlier age—let us say, with people in their fifties—known for a relatively fast kill. Over time, the nerve system withers away, no longer activating the muscles. The muscles, being unused, atrophy. In the process, the speech is also affected and, at the end, the muscles of the breathing system, as well. Patients with ALS fear suffocation.

But my father, as I have said, had no place in his life for ALS. For different reasons, he ignored it in a way that kept him alive over a longer period of time.

Looking back, I admire him for the way he took the blows—for example, the physiotherapist telling him at a certain stage in his illness that the therapy was no longer required because it no longer helped to improve or stabilize his physical condition, or the time he had to accept that he could no longer make it to the toilet on his own. In 1997 he signed a euthanasia form and asked his home physician whether he would be willing to put him out of his misery if a time came when he could bear it no longer. The physician agreed not to abandon him if that time were to come.

In the years since then we have been negotiating with him about life and death. I became very cunning in offering alternatives when he said it had been enough. When can one say he is truly suffering? What is unbearable? If you can no longer walk, you can compensate by using an electric wheelchair. If you can no longer make phone calls, I can call people for you, I argued. And there was always something to look forward to: his sixtieth wedding anniversary in 2000; he and my mother would not want to miss the visit of the town mayor! A birthday of one of his grandchildren. And how about me, his son? I could not go on without him. I offered to put him in a nice hot bath every week and did so, with the help and companionship of a friend. We stepped up the frequency of our visits to him and ended up visiting him every day. My sister and I challenged his determination and nurtured his ambivalence. Part of this was done unconsciously.

In September of 2000 he was transferred to the nursing home where my mother had been taken five years earlier. He was terribly uncomfortable about this move; but the care he now required was of such a nature that he needed nursing home assistance. I told him that there were some advantages, too: now he need no longer put in all the effort to get to see his wife every day. They would be together again most of the time. However, it was a shock to see what happened: from the day he entered the nursing home he was totally disoriented. While he was living in the home for the elderly he had managed to find his way to my mother. In the nursing home he got lost every time he tried to go to her ward. In the end, we decided to bring my mother upstairs, to where he was staying. It was then that I finally realized my father had set one of his feet in another world, and that it was not the world of the living. It was the first time I was able to take his "Herman, enough is enough" seriously. I suddenly realized that he hadn't taken any of his beer for months in a row, and he used to drink a can of beer with his dinner every day. I noticed his appetite had diminished; he lost weight. It was as if the illness were making up for lost time because up until then my father had not allowed the illness a place in his agenda. There was a noticeable loss of speech. I was alarmed to see him saying good-bye to those who visited with him, and telling me over and over again how much he appreciated my looking after his things. I was alarmed when he asked me every time I visited him whether I had sorted out the "mess" on his table. It was in December that the attending nursing home physician called my sister and me into her office to share her concerns about my father's physical and mental condition.

After the New Year she called me again to say that my father had again asked her to put an end to his misery. Wouldn't it be possible for him to die in his sleep, and couldn't she provide him with the means? Would she be so kind as not to abandon him this time? She promised and told my father that afterward she would report the case to the coroner because she considered his request to die in his sleep without the risk of accidentally waking up again as a form of euthanasia. My sister and I also had a long talk with my father. He was of such a clear mind about what he wanted for himself that we did not dare to challenge him again, as we had done before. Enough was really enough now. We had no option but to respect what our father was sharing with us. He had now written his own death in his agenda, and we knew him well enough to know that none of us could blot it out. He asked us to promise him that we would look after "Mamma," his wife. Our promise was a great relief to him.

In the days that followed, we rallied his grandchildren. They all came and sat down with him, knowing the end would come soon.

Early in the evening on Thursday, January 11, my father took three pills out of the hands of the attending physician and swallowed them with a little water. I do not think that physician had ever been thanked before in the way my father thanked her. We sat around with him for about half an hour and talked about the big and small things of family life. At a certain moment, while dozing, he lifted his eyes and looked at me and my sister, saying, "Have you passed your examinations alright, and did you bring your diplomas?" Yes, he was ready; he was organized and had prepared himself well for the journey he was about to take. He died peacefully in his sleep two days later, just as he had wanted.

In the middle of the night we took our mother to see him. She was well aware of what had happened and held his hand for a while, saying that although it sometimes came in disguise, the good in the person she had loved all her life had always prevailed, even to the very end.

Herman H. van der Kloot Meijburg
Voorburg, January 2001

16

Assisted Death in the Netherlands
Physicians at the Bedside When Help Is Requested

Gerrit K. Kimsma, M.D., M.A., and Evert van Leeuwen, Ph.D.

The medical role of a physician in the Netherlands always entails providing the best available care for a patient. In addition, most physicians support legal acceptance of the role helping a patient die. Assisting death in no way precludes giving the best palliative care possible but rather integrates compassionate care and respect for the patient's autonomy and ultimately makes death with dignity a real option.

Here, based on interviews with physicians who have assisted in suicide or carried out euthanasia, we develop a conceptual framework regarding the relationship between physicians and patients who have requested aid in dying.[1] What values are realized when patients request aid in dying? How do physicians respond emotionally to the experience of participating in assisted suicide or euthanasia? What do available data tell us about how families cope with this form of dying?

First, however, we must answer some of the criticisms that have been raised about the Dutch experience with physician-assisted death.[2] Based on critics' views of the qualities and deficiencies of the American medical system in the area of end-of-life care, we provide an outsider's perspective on the American debate concerning physician-assisted death.

American Criticism of Dutch Practice

In seeking to understand the Dutch experience with physician-assisted death, it is necessary to note some of the major differences between the medical cultures of the United States and the Netherlands.[3] First, there is almost universal coverage of health care in the Netherlands. Except for a few very wealthy patients, no one pays for needed medical care out of his or her own pocket. Economically disadvantaged patients qualify for standard care, including advanced cancer and palliative care paid for by insurance, on the basis of equal rights to health care. Long-term home care and institutionalized care are provided through legislated state funds, and free, round-the-clock, intensive home care at the end of life is available on the basis of need. Palliative care advisory units for physicians are available by telephone, and personal consultation is available at virtually any hour of the day.[4]

Contrary to concerns raised in the U.S. context, in the Netherlands there is no rationale for opposing assisted suicide on the grounds that basic care is denied to so many. Economic motives do not dictate the availability of care, including palliative care and the option of assistance in dying.[5] Of course, as elsewhere, there is in the Netherlands continuous debate over the use of scarce resources; but this debate does not compromise the availability of need-based care.

There is also no discrimination on the basis of age, sex, or race in delivery of health care in the Netherlands, especially not as far as physician-assisted death is concerned.[6] (Immigrants from other European countries and from Africa and Asia make little use of the present option of assistance in dying, although the reasons have not been investigated.) Nor has there ever been any protest by organizations for the handicapped in the Netherlands in the thirty years that euthanasia has been practiced in an open atmosphere.

In contrast, although the high quality of technological medical interventions available in the United States is impressive, we are troubled by the deficiencies of the American health care system. Disparities in care between the rich and the poor, ethnic groups, and those who have insurance and those who do not are difficult to justify in a society with economic resources as deep as those of the United States.

End-of-life care in the United States is an area of special concern, as the 1995 "Study to Understand Prognosis and Preferences of Outcomes and Risks of Treatment" makes clear.[7] Much of the criticism of assisted suicide and euthanasia —notably, that by Foley and Hendin—rests on fear that once "assisted suicide or euthanasia is sanctioned . . . those who are depressed, disabled, economically disadvantaged, or elderly, are especially vulnerable."[8] What is suggested is that social or economic pressure to hasten death, expressed in patients' concerns about being or becoming both social and economic burdens, raises fears that the lives of disadvantaged patients may be terminated without their request. Such a development would, of course, be criminal in any system of health care that is worthy of the name. We agree that physician-assisted suicide and euthanasia should never be an easy way out for physicians who practice in an imperfect health care system. However, the absence of a perfect system of health care delivery is not, in itself, sufficient reason to deny aid in dying to patients who seek a dignified death.

Wrong Readings and Wrong Interpretations

Concerns about euthanasia and assisted suicide in the Netherlands have focused on questions of whether there can be adequate safeguards and on doubts as to the voluntariness of patients' decisions, the adequacy of responses to suffering, including palliative care, and whether depression or other psychiatric issues are adequately addressed among patients who request aid in dying. We must respond briefly to these concerns, particularly as they have been set out by Foley and Hendin.

Safeguards

Assisted dying should be protected by adequate safeguards, including palliative care and appropriate public and medical evaluation procedures, rather than be disallowed altogether because of the apparent failings of the health care system. In the Netherlands, those safeguards and state-financed public evaluations have been developed over the past twelve years. Granted, the procedures are not perfect. Yet imperfect safeguards and procedures do not make it impossible to assess the authenticity of patients' requests for assistance in dying.

We agree with Zylicz, a Dutch opponent of assistance in dying, when he writes, "We will not eliminate euthanasia in the Netherlands, but we can go a long way toward making it not seem necessary by providing better care."[9] Despite evidence that the number of euthanasia cases has stabilized over the past six years with improvements in palliative care, twelve years of research on issues of end-of-life care indicate no increase in the number of physicians who believe that "adequate treatment of pain and counseling the dying" can eliminate the need or desire for euthanasia. Nor is it appropriate to question, as many critics do, the professional integrity of physicians who participated in assisted dying. Data showing that only one of every three patients who request it receive assistance in dying attest to the prudence of Dutch physicians in these matters.[10]

Safeguards for assistance in dying are complex because assistance in dying is not only a legal issue but also a medical, ethical, and political matter. We invite both opponents and supporters of physician-assisted suicide and euthanasia to discuss the failures and weaknesses of the present system in the Netherlands and to propose new procedures.

Voluntariness

Doubts have also been raised about the voluntariness of patients' requests for euthanasia, based on data from 1992 indicating that, as Hendin argues, "more than 50 percent of the physicians considered it appropriate to suggest euthanasia to patients."[11] This interpretation is misleading. In fact, physicians are inclined to wait—perhaps too long—for patients to initiate discussion of the issue. In his 1992 dissertation, van der Wal finds that the physicians he surveyed prompted dialogue about euthanasia in only 10 percent of cases; in 80 percent of cases, patients themselves raised the matter, and families did so in 6 percent of cases.[12]

We believe it is important for a physician to know a patient's position on the issue of assistance in dying. If a patient believes he or she might well make such a request in the future, an intensive discussion about the motives and consequences for both parties can begin. This discussion results in agreements between the patient and the physician about the appropriate and possible actions that may be taken in the future, when the disease takes an expected course. It furthermore enables the physician to prepare himself or herself when an actual request for assistance in dying is expressed. The recommended way in which end-of-life decisions are introduced is to leave the question entirely open while offering the patient an opportunity to initiate discussion—for example, by saying, "If you wish to discuss your feelings about the end of life and your ideas and expectations, I am open to this, but I will wait for your move, unless you want me to talk about the various options." From the start of any such exchange it should be clear that physicians are hesitant and ambivalent about discussing the option of assisted dying.

Many physicians may be theoretically in favor of an early discussion of euthanasia, though in practice there is still a high threshold of reluctance to start such a discussion. We believe that talking about death with patients in a realistic way always entails a kind of ambivalence, a heightened awareness, and that this experience is significant through the entire process of providing assistance in dying.

Suffering and Palliative Care

Critics also argue that Dutch practice does not adequately address suffering. For example, drawing on data published in 1992 by van der Maas and colleagues, Hendin contends that fear of future suffering or loss of dignity was deemed a sufficient criterion to end life in a quarter of requests for euthanasia.[13] Such a sweeping statement is misleading. Hendin apparently has no knowledge of the often long and exhausting process by which a decision is made about assisted dying, one in which fears and anxieties are discussed from the start in order to distinguish between real possibilities of future suffering and fears based on patients' experiences with the deaths of family or friends, which often leave deep scars. For any given disease, what is at stake for the patient is the kind of additional suffering or further loss of dignity that could reasonably be expected. In thinking about suffering, it is particularly important to take into account the patient's life expectancy at the time of physician-assisted death: These are usually patients who have exhausted all medical options and are literally at the end of their capacity to endure further suffering. More specifically, we are speaking of one or two weeks, sometimes a month—rarely longer—depending on the characteristics of the disease in question. Moreover, physician-assisted dying takes place mainly in the home, where family physicians often call on a daily basis and closely follow patients and their families.

Fear and anxiety about future suffering are in themselves not sufficient grounds to initiate physician-assisted death under the procedures required in the Netherlands. Time and again, in courses, publications, and assessments made by Regional Euthanasia Evaluation Committees, future suffering is deemed to be insufficient in itself to justify assisted dying unless the patient is presently suffering unbearably or his or her suffering is imminently expected to become intolerable and unrelievable.[14] Behind many requests for assisted suicide there are other requests, and interviewing patients to find out the how and why of their fears is normal medical and nursing practice.

Nor is it appropriate to suggest, as Hendin does, that a significant percentage of patients receive euthanasia or assisted suicide even when there are palliative care alternatives that could reasonably be expected to meliorate their suffering.[15] Patients clearly have the right to refuse even palliative treatments. Dutch physicians are legally required to take a prudent approach in cases of treatment refusal that involve psychic suffering and are professionally advised to do so by the Royal Dutch Medical Association in cases of somatic suffering, but they cannot simply override patients' refusals.

What is essential in cases of patients' refusal of available treatment is the measure and degree of a potential benefit. An element of *proportionality in benefit* is at stake in palliative care. Ultimately, in our view, when beneficial medical options for cure and for palliative care diminish, the patient, after being properly informed, increasingly becomes the final arbiter in accepting or rejecting these options. The possible alternatives are discussed in the interaction between patient and physician, and such discussion continues. In the end it may happen that doctor and patient reach a mutual conclusion that reasonable options are no longer available—one of the criteria for legitimate requests for assisted death under the new euthanasia law.

That some patients accept palliative treatments in comparable situations does not constitute sufficient ground to override a particular patient's refusal if it is based on understandable reasons. Just as physicians will not initiate the process to hasten death simply because a patient rejects effective medical interventions with few or acceptable side effects, physicians also respect a patient's refusal of interventions that for that patient will add little benefit but potentially much discomfort.

Psychiatric Issues

Concerns have also been raised that Dutch safeguards fail to adequately protect terminally ill patients who are suffering from depression or other psychiatric conditions by making euthanasia too readily available to them. Citing the similarities between depressive traits of physically healthy suicidal patients and terminally ill patients, Hendin argues that the similarities between these two groups are not well recognized and that "these patients need assurance that they are still wanted; they also need treatment for depression." Moreover, he and Foley contend that even when patients are not depressed, "they are usually ambivalent about their desire to die and are often expressing an anguished wish for help," and "when this ambivalence is not heard . . . an assisted suicide can occur with the patient in a state of terror."[16]

Hendin bases his argument on the Brongersma case, in which the Dutch Supreme Court upheld the conviction of a physician whom the lower court decided had acted "outside of the medical domain."[17] In this particular case of assisted suicide, the family physician, who correctly followed procedure and obtained two consultations supporting his decision, helped end the life of an elderly man whose suffering encompassed complaints ranging from physical deterioration to social isolation and existential anguish. The Amsterdam Appellate Court found the physician guilty because the patient's suffering was not the result of an incurable illness, as medically defined, but by the combined effects of old age and various physical complaints. Thus the court judged the patient's situation not to fall within the domain of a medically defined disease with concurrent unbearable suffering.

Hendin suggests that the suffering of a terminally ill patient with a strong wish to die is the same as that of a suicidally depressed patient. We beg to differ, based both on our experience and on the notion of respect for patients. Most patients who request euthanasia are alert, competent persons who are very much aware of the impact their deaths will have on their families and of how much they will be missed. In most cases, relatives learn to accept the patient's wishes as part of their own process of letting go. They learn to accept that such wishes are consistent in the light of the available options and the values that have guided the patient's life.

Feeling sad in the face of death and the loss of life is a normal response. Whenever signs of a clear and consistent clinical depression are present, however, the advice is to have a psychiatric evaluation, before any further steps are taken. That consultation is available to every patient, without exception, regardless of whether the patient is hospitalized or at home.

Critics like Hendin and Zylicz have also argued that requests for euthanasia or assisted suicide can mask depression and anxiety among terminally ill patients who have an excessive need for control. Some terminal patients do, indeed, have such a need, but to claim that in such cases the effort to determine the circumstances of one's death "provides an illusory sense of regaining control" seems to us unduly judgmental.[18] Such an attitude seems to judge irrelevant the stages of grieving, identified by Kübler-Ross and her "death awareness movement," that lead to the acceptance of impending death.[19] To accept that death is imminent, that one's life will end in the near future, has a completely different meaning for terminally ill patients. Wong, Reker, and Gesser, for instance, conclude that acceptance of death among elderly, terminally ill patients is more prominent than anxiety about death. They predict that "those who find life devoid of meaning because of an incurable disease may be high in escape acceptance and low in fear of death and death avoidance."[20]

This "escape acceptance" at the end of life, when one's life is full of pain and misery and death may be a welcome alternative, is not the same as suicidal feelings caused by depression. Patients who pursue assisted death are adult human beings confronting the gravest decision of their lives and choosing against dependence on medications that will dull their consciousness and against becoming a victim of the progressive symptoms of a disease. How much respect is shown to these patients if their final struggle for some sense of control is called "illusory"? The suggestion lurking here is that because normal, competent human beings do not wish to die, patients who want to die are not to be taken seriously. There seems to us a real risk that such a perspective will restore a taboo against death: death will become something that should not be looked at directly but should be dealt with by sedation or antidepressants instead of honest communication between competent human beings.

The certainty and conviction shown by many patients who ask for assisted death may even be startling to the physician: Patients ask for assistance not as victims but with the goal of being the directors of whatever measure of life they have left. In fact, many patients with this strong conviction realize that their physicians actually need to grow in the acceptance of such a request. Patients sometimes wait, out of respect for their physicians, until the physician can share in the mutuality of the process.

Physicians at the Bedside

Although Dutch practice in regard to medical interventions at the end of life is by far the most extensively studied of any country, the emphasis of most research has been to gather data about procedures, decisions, conditions, and diseases. Little has been published on the actual process and the emotions of both patients and physicians, and most of the available information is still limited to anecdotal accounts of personal experiences. In the remainder of this chapter, we fill out the empirical evidence with a description of the process at the bedside, drawing on in-depth interviews with physicians who include assisted dying within their practice published in *Asking to Die,* as well as data from a retrospective analysis of physicians' experiences and views by Haverkate and colleagues.[21]

Anecdotes and interviews are not in themselves moral justifications of physician-assisted death, nor do retrospective evaluations of that act constitute moral arguments. What such information can provide, however, is a perspective on moral and legal issues connected with the dying process that reflects the experience of practitioners and society struggling with these issues. Before we address these concerns, however, some preliminary remarks are in order.

Following an initial period of debate about the moral status of euthanasia within medicine, since the late 1970s Dutch practice has evolved in the supportive environment created by legal recognition of euthanasia as a medical option. The moral debate has given way to social policy and practice that supports individual choice while respecting religious and personal objections to assisted death. The present rules and regulations seek to integrate physician-assisted death within the range of accepted professional medical practices. They represent attempts to find reasonable solutions to the social, legal, and ethical concerns that arise with such a complex and sensitive intervention.

Moreover, that for the most part physician-assisted dying involves patients for whom there are no further treatment options, who choose to die at home under the care of their family physician (more than 80 percent of the reported cases), has been fundamental to the development of the current practice of assisted death in the Netherlands. In 85 percent of the cases reported to the Regional Euthanasia Evaluation Committees, patients are suffering from symptoms of late-stage terminal cancer. These patients often have long-term relationships with their family physicians, who may remain their primary provider of health care. Only 15 percent of the 2,054 cases reported for 2001 took place within either a hospital or a nursing home.[22] In what follows, we describe the practice and experience of euthanasia in the Netherlands as a matter of law, a matter of clinical practice, and a matter of interpersonal relationships—the story of physicians, patients, and families.

Legal Requirements of Euthanasia Law

As a matter of law, after thirty years' evolution in medical ethics and jurisprudence in the Netherlands, the Dutch euthanasia law that took effect in April 2002 set down legal conditions under which criminal charges in cases of euthanasia or assisted suicide will be dismissed.[23] The law requires, first, that there be a request by the patient, who has been fully informed about the medical situation, is suffering unbearably, and for whom there are no acceptable medical alternatives. An independent consultant must evaluate the request, and the physician's participation in ending a patient's life must be "medically careful." The context within which these conditions apply—agreement by the physician to fulfill the patient's request for help in ending his or her life—is simply not comparable to any other chain of events in medicine. The law itself acknowledges the uniqueness of euthanasia in defining it as a criminal act that will, nonetheless, not be prosecuted if it has been carried out according to the stipulated conditions. Euthanasia is recognized to be outside normal medical practice insofar as the intervention must be reported to the legal authorities. Yet the fact that the euthanasia law sets out conditions of practice brings it into harmony with other laws regulating health care, and the very existence of rules and regulations determining how it should be carried out in effect "normalizes" physician-assisted dying.

The Process of Euthanasia

As a matter of clinical practice, euthanasia involves a series of steps taken by the patient and physician. Over the course of his or her illness, a patient asks a physician for help in achieving a death with dignity and without unnecessary suffering. Most physicians do not welcome this conversation but, upon request, will discuss the conditions under which they would be willing to assist. When the patient comes to find his or her circumstances intolerable and feels that the time has come to end life, the physician who has agreed to provide the help requested seeks a consultation from an independent colleague unfamiliar with the case, a colleague whose role it is to determine that the required legal conditions have been met. Today, most of the physicians who consult in euthanasia cases have received special training for this purpose and meet regularly with other consultants and members of a support network.

When all the conditions for physician-assisted death have been fulfilled, a time is set, good-byes are said, and the physician ends the life of a patient either by injection or oral administration of a toxic substance. After the patient has died the physician reports the act to the local health care authorities. A physician representing the health care authority reviews the physician's report of the case to confirm that legal requirements have been met and confers with the prosecutor, who allows burial or cremation and then sends the official forms and reports to a Regional Euthanasia Evaluation Committee. The committee then has six weeks within which to decide whether the physician exercised due care in carrying out the assisted death.

Relationships at the End of Life

Finally, with regard to interpersonal relationships at the end of life, the practice of euthanasia is intense, deeply moving, and complex, filled with ambivalence and paradox. The process that unfolds before and especially after a patient has requested assisted death must be carefully spelled out and undertaken with great prudence and care.

Our experience, one as a physician and both as members of Regional Euthanasia Evaluation Committees, and the experiences reflected in our interviews with physicians, have brought home to us how central ambivalence, prudence, and connection with the patient are to all that takes place, from the moment a discussion about assisted death is initiated to the death itself. When practiced in institutional settings, such as nursing homes or hospitals, euthanasia necessarily involves more persons (given the size and complexity of such organizations) and may be less intimate than in the home care setting. One oncologist, who provided assistance in ending the life of a patient at home, describes the experience of performing euthanasia in the institutional setting as "colder and more impersonal than when it is done at home." The same oncologist notes that "in the hospital euthanasia must be scheduled like other appointments, which sounds very cold." A nursing home physician describes the need to initiate safeguards and protect the privacy of patients or persons within institutions almost as a conspiracy to prevent other patients from knowing what happened.[24]

What we know about the unfolding process is colored further by the home care setting and by our discussions with family physicians. We wish to stress the procedural aspect that implies a constant hands-on approach as opposed to suggestions of decisions that are based on incidental encounters with patients.

Euthanasia is a process that is filled with emotions, which arise with the initial request for assisted death and evolve as the physician's relationship with the patient and family changes over time. The act itself is approached with utmost apprehension. Physicians' emotional reactions of anxiety, resistance, and uncertainty are balanced by rational convictions not to abandon one's patient. One physician was representative in stating outright, "I dread each time a patient raises the issue of euthanasia." Another noted, "The tension drains and exhausts me."[25] This sort of reaction has different origins. Being involved with dying patients is always emotionally charged, and the prospect of having to let a patient die is always difficult. The counterintuitive act that is requested when a patient seeks assisted death has a shattering effect in itself: the knowledge that when worst comes to worst, one may have to end the life of a person one has come to know. Additionally, one walks a tightrope with respect to the law and will have to submit oneself to legal scrutiny. These emotions are *and should remain* integral to the process of assistance in dying because they forestall development of routine reactions and attitudes of callousness. From our discussions with many physicians we are convinced that they are keenly aware of the precarious circumstances in which a request for assistance in death places them. Cases of euthanasia or assisted suicide stay with a physician for the rest of his or her life.

Yet physicians also realize that they must preserve an adequate professional distance. They need time to think and reflect as they move toward such a momentous decision. As one of the physicians we interviewed stated, "I need the time, not only to make sure the patient is consistent, but also to prepare myself and the patient's family." Another noted, "I spend months pondering details of the situation before I ever come to a decision. My patient's plight invades every aspect of my thinking." This resistance to entering the process of assisted death—"because physicians do not like to perform euthanasia. It is a terrible job"—is countered by "feelings [that one has abandoned one's patient] for not having done it."[26] The physician must remain responsible for the process, but as medical options diminish and chances for alleviating the patient's suffering exhaust themselves, the burden of that responsibility increases.

As the physician and patient move toward assisted death—over days, or weeks, or months—both feel the need for a personal relationship among the physician, patient, and family. The physicians we interviewed commonly mentioned several aspects of that relationship, but especially its uniqueness and how it brings physicians to confront their own mortality. These features, which lie at the limits of typical physician-patient relationships, might almost justify recognizing a distinct, separate physician-patient relationship for the process of assisted dying, especially in the cases of euthanasia and physician-assisted suicide.

First, there is the experience of uniqueness, which is echoed by most physicians we interviewed: "Each euthanasia is so unique and personal, and is really a reflection of both the patient and the physician." Part of that uniqueness relates to a deep confrontation with, as one physician states, "my own mortality."[27] This experience will be familiar to any physician who has helped people die.

There is an additional quality in the relationship when a physician's willingness to assist in dying has been explored. The physician's confrontation with personal mortality seems to translate into a need to develop a personal relationship with the dying patient, to know the patient better and to open oneself as a fellow human being. One consultation began with the patient's expressed need to have a more personal relationship with the person who would end his life; in a certain sense, he wanted to restructure the physician-patient relationship. Family physicians spend more time with terminally ill patients and their families than they do with other patients. They are expected to make house calls at night, during weekends, and at other times outside of normal office hours.

The change in the content of the dialogue at the sickbed is even more important. Monitoring changes in the patient's mental and physical symptoms and discussing options and side effects takes place within a context of narratives about the patient's life, and often similar stories about life events are solicited from and offered by the physicians. It has become resoundingly clear from our interviews that physicians need this deepened relationship to be able to perform assisted death. With all due respect to the depth of medical relationships at the end of life in other contexts, we hold the conviction that in the case of a request for physician-assisted dying, one may speak of a specifically distinct relationship.

We believe that the most appropriate term for this type of relationship is *medical friendship,* a term coined by Lain Entralgo in his classic description of the medical relationship in ancient Greece and recently taken up again by Clark and Kimsma. One physician interviewed in *Asking to Die* stated, "Perhaps love is too sentimental a word, but I had such a deep sympathy for him; he influenced me beyond what I could have imagined."[28]

By adopting Lain Entralgo's term we do not intend in any way to demean medical relationships outside the realm of a request assisted dying. Opponents of assistance in dying usually also profess a deeply felt, genuine commitment to their patients. Nevertheless, we think there are differences that matter. Consider Zylicz's description of the physician-patient relationship: "We have a duty . . . to those who cannot be treated anymore, who do not respond to the treatment, or who are damaged by it—a duty of care like that of a mother who cares, who comforts, who suffers with her child."[29] We agree with the physician's commitment and enlivened suffering with the patient that Zylicz describes. However, the physician-patient relationship at issue is not one of an adult with a child but one between adults, a key difference. A relationship between adults expresses itself in a certain mutuality, such as the patient's respect for the physician putting him- or herself ethically and emotionally at risk in agreeing to help the patient hasten death.

Most patients are fully aware what it means for a physician to provide assistance in dying. Most physicians see that process as one of "joint decision making"[30] in which each participant plays a substantial part and needs time to come to grips with the imminent future. Often, a unique interaction can be observed, in which the patient realizes that the physician needs time before the decision is really shared. One patient, in a case in which one of us acted as the legally required independent consultant, literally said of his physician, "He is a good physician. But I see that I need to give him time to learn to accept that he will help me to end my life." Similarly, an elderly physician remarked, "I had to conclude 'If he remains steadfast in wanting to die, the moment will come that I can only love him by killing him.'" When he told his patient that an "internal restriction was holding me back and I probably would not dare do it," the patient said, "If that is the case, then I will have to wait until you dare."[31] That expression of respect for the physician's turmoil took away the last barrier to giving the patient the rest he sought.

"Waiting for the physician" is not a passive act. Often, before he or she comes to realize that there are no further interventions or palliative care available, the patient has willingly submitted to medical interventions that may or may not have alleviated the suffering. It is important that these measures be attempted so that the physician can be convinced that all available options have been exhausted and can support the decision to take the step of ending a life. After all, the physician's professional duty is first and foremost to alleviate suffering and to protect life, even when a patient at the end of life sees no further meaning and value in staying alive.

Family and friends have a special place and meaning. In the home care setting, the primary caregivers, usually family members and friends, are often as involved as the patient and the physician in the process of assisted dying. In the daily routine at the sickbed, these caregivers must deal with emotions as well as with cognitive and spiritual questions. Even more, caregivers must learn to cope with losing a spouse, parent, sibling, friend, or neighbor. The physician not only has to reconcile his or her own personal feelings, he or she also must lead others and help them to cope with their issues and feelings.

When a patient has requested help in dying, his or her close associates face distinct issues. It is one thing to learn to accept the patient's death as inevitable when it is the "natural" outcome of disease. It is quite another to learn to accept death as inevitable when a family member or friend chooses to die because his or her life has become unbearable. The patient's choice to die confronts the family as a whole, a system in which the patient is irreplaceable. For the family, the part the patient has played in its collective story, its biography, may be more important than the medical story of the patient's illness. Individual family members and caregivers are sometimes not ready to let go because there are unresolved hurts and issues that need to be addressed. Yet there is a certain urgency when confrontations take time to resolve, even though the willingness to reconcile has been expressed, because time is running out.

For the family physician, attention to the family's grieving process and acceptance of a request to die is important because the family will usually remain in the physician's care after the patient's death. Guiding them along the process of acceptance now is a precondition for helping them cope with the death later. Sometimes physicians organize family meetings, followed by separate therapeutic sessions with individual family members, in which their feelings of abandonment and their resistance to letting go are discussed before the process to end a life can take its course. Patients who have decided to end their suffering by choosing death need the support of the people with whom they have close relationships.[32] Ultimately, however, the patient and physician must focus on the patient's choice, whatever the response of the family as a whole or its individual members.

Our in-depth interviews have shown that for partners and families, physician-assisted death is, in the end, a positive experience. Without exception the eleven family members who spoke with us told deeply moving stories of dying that bear witness to a process that is looked on with gratitude and a conviction that this was the best available option.[33] (Short descriptions of these interviews were published in 1993 and 1994.)[34] As moving as they are, because the stories are so few in number they are not necessarily representative or convincing. Accumulated quantitative data recently published by Swarte and colleagues give them additional weight, however.[35] These data come from a retrospective comparative study of 189 family members and friends of cancer patients who died at the Utrecht Academic Clinic after euthanasia (72 percent response rate) between 1992 and 1999 and 316 family members and friends of cancer patients who died a natural death (66 percent response rate) in the same period. Individuals whose family member or friend died after euthanasia showed significantly lower scores on the inventory of traumatic grief and impact of event score than individuals whose loved one died a "natural" death. These effects may be attributed to a single overriding factor: the opportunity for anticipatory grieving and comfort with the patient who has decided to ask for assistance. After such a request, family and friends can focus on closure in direct communication with the patient who has regained a sense of control. The accumulated data suggest that assisted death gives patients and families a greater chance to bring closure to relationships, more time to prepare for the death of a loved one, and more interaction with medical and nursing staff, all of which may derive from greater opportunity to talk openly about death and dying.

The Final Steps of Physician-Assisted Death

Deciding to accept the patient's request to provide aid in ending his or her life is often stressful and exhausting, but once made, that decision can bring tranquility. More often than not the patients themselves are a source of strength, the resoluteness of their choice helping others to realize that they must follow in this acceptance of death.[36] Once he or she has accepted the patient's decision, the treating physician must seek a formal consultation from an independent consultant. The function of this consultant, who is not connected to the case and is independent of the physician who will perform euthanasia, is to ensure that the treating physician is acting with due care and to advise him or her whether the case meets the requirements of the law with regard to the patient's request (that it is voluntary and well considered) and suffering (that it is un-bearable, without hope for improvement). A complete consultation considers information from the treating physician, from medical records, and from an interview with the patient and the family or other caregivers. The consultant's written report will later be sent to the Regional Euthanasia Evaluation Com-mittee. If necessary, the consultant can halt the procedure in order to imple-ment additional measures, such as a change in palliative treatment.

The consultant can be any physician, but nowadays often it is a member of a network of consultants organized under the auspices of the Royal Dutch Medical Society. This network, Support Consultation Euthanasia Netherlands (SCEN), provides individual support through information, advice, and guid-ance on all aspects of assisted death as well as on specific procedures. This in-cludes evaluating the circumstances to ensure that palliative care alternatives have not been overlooked, with the further option to consult a palliative care organization in case of uncertainty or when there are questions.

The consultant checks with the physician in charge as to the reasoning be-hind fulfilling the patient's request for assisted death—specifically, why in this particular case the physician and the patient have concluded that suffering is unbearable and hopeless. The consultant then speaks with the patient and the family. Special care must be taken to adequately introduce the consultant so that the patient does not feel he or she must submit to some form of a test.

The act of assisted death itself takes place after a date and a time has been set. The physician discusses the available options with the patient: lethal injec-tion or oral administration of barbiturates. Official guidance from the Royal Dutch Medical Association recommends that the patient, if able to do so, drink the toxic substance. When the time arrives, the physician obtains the barbitu-rates from the pharmacy and makes the final, awaited visit. After a last check to confirm the patient's wishes, the physician administers the deadly drug.

The enormity of this act is reflected in physicians' descriptions of their emo-tions and responses: "It is very difficult to prepare myself for that moment. My inner responses are a telling measure of the emotional weight I am carrying. I sleep badly. My scope narrows to focus in on the details that must be attended to." Assisting death weighs heavily not just on the physician but on his or her close associates as well. As one physician noted,

> I am not the only one who is under great stress during this time. My family shares my discomfort. I am not mentally "there" with them. I am consumed with thoughts of my patient. Inevitably family relationships suffer. This is always the case when I am involved in a [case of] euthanasia. I am irritable, and it is most pronounced on the day of the euthanasia appointment. When the date for the appointment arrives, I have a hard time concentrating during the day. I also sleep very badly during the first few nights after the event. For me these are very familiar feelings; they happen each time I am involved in a euthanasia.

An oncologist stated, "The worst moment of my life occurs when I must perform euthanasia. . . . Personally, I do not tolerate the stress very well and I cannot sleep afterwards. At the moment I administer the drug I always wonder if I have done the right thing. Although the patient wants euthanasia and there is support from everyone—the family, the staff, the consulting physician—I nevertheless feel horrible."[37]

However representative interviews and anecdotes may be, many nonetheless will not find such qualitative data convincing evidence of the emotional struggle inherent within the act of assisted death. Data reported by Haverkate and colleagues provide a more quantitative account. These data are drawn from a retrospective nationwide survey investigating the emotional responses of 405 Dutch physicians (both family physicians and institutional practitioners) who performed euthanasia, assisted suicide, or ended a patient's life without his or her explicit request. In this study, physicians reported feelings of both comfort (satisfaction, relief) (52 percent) and discomfort (burdensomeness, emotional drain, heavy responsibility) (42 percent), with family physicians showing the highest percentages in both instances, probably because of their greater personal involvement in dealing with patients and families on a one-to-one basis. Physicians' comfort with assisted death was directly related to the gender of patients (female), life expectancy (mostly less than one or two weeks, often only days), and the severity of patients' suffering. Feelings of discomfort were related to younger age, male sex, a diagnosis of cancer, and relatively longer life expectancy (more than a month). Feelings of discomfort were increased in physicians who had accepted hastening death without an explicit request with the aim of alleviating pain and symptoms.[38]

Of the 110 physicians who had performed euthanasia more than once, 45 percent found their last case just as difficult as previous cases, 26 percent found it less difficult, and 29 percent reported that it had been more difficult. For assisted suicide ($n = 14$) the proportions were, respectively, 38, 23, and 40 percent; for ending a life without an explicit request of the patient ($n = 45$), 55, 34, and 10 percent, respectively. An overwhelming majority, 95 percent, indicated they would be willing to perform euthanasia or assisted suicide again. Five percent had regrets but no doubts that euthanasia or assisted suicide had been an appropriate course of action for the patient. Neither did they doubt that they had exhausted possible treatment alternatives and that patients had been given adequate time to make genuine and free decisions, because of the duration of the decision-making process. They were also satisfied with dealing with the issue of the choice between assisted suicide and euthanasia and with the nature of families' involvement. In 85 percent of the cases of euthanasia, the physician considered the euthanasia to have significantly improved the quality of dying for the patient, while 12 percent reported that it had improved this quality "somewhat." With respect to cases in which the physician ended life without explicit request, these figures were 67 percent and 26 percent, respectively.[39] While it is true that these data may represent rationalized judgment on the part of respondents, they show at least that physicians are convinced that beneficence was bestowed in the practice of assisted death.

Goals of Care at the End of Life

The evidence for the emotional impact of assisted dying on physicians shows that euthanasia and assisted suicide are a far cry from being "easier options for the caregiver" than palliative care, as some critics of Dutch practice have suggested.[40] We wish to take a strong stand against the separation and opposition between euthanasia and assisted suicide, on the one hand, and palliative care, on the other, that such critics have implied. There is no "either-or" with respect to these options. Every appropriate palliative option available must be discussed with the patient and, if reasonable, tried before a request for assisted death can be accepted. Although the home care setting might preclude some special measures that could be taken within the setting of hospice or nursing home care, a patient's wish to die at home might still be fully acceptable.

Opposing euthanasia to palliative care in the way critics have suggested fundamentally disregards the wishes of the patient in the face of death. Doing so neither reflects the Dutch reality that palliative medicine is incorporated within end-of-life care nor the place of the option of assisted death at the request of a patient within the overall spectrum of end-of-life care.[41]

Ultimately, what is at stake are the goals of medicine in caring for patients at the end of life. Medical care might aim to prolong life at any cost. If so, the development of advanced technology and special treatments will prevail until social and economic standards halt them. We think that this option can easily lead to dehumanizing death within hospitals or special care settings. Medical care should support the patient in the final phase of life. Medicine in the end should consist in a relationship aimed at helping us all toward a fully human and dignified life. Various care settings are available to reach this goal: hospices, nursing homes, hospitals, and other institutions. Nevertheless, a large portion of terminally ill patients in the Netherlands choose to die at home, with their families and amid familiar surroundings. In either setting, but mostly in home care, patients ask to be relieved of the burden of life when no hope remains. It is neither a medical error nor an easy decision to grant that request. On the contrary, assisting in death acknowledges the difficult and complex fact that all the medical treatments will eventually have to stop, not because of socio-economic constraints or a lack of technology and knowledge but because life is a grand yet finite and fragile thing.

Notes

1. D.C. Thomasma, T. Kimbrough-Kushner, G.K. Kimsma, and C. Carlucci-Ciesielski, eds., *Asking to Die: Inside the Dutch Euthanasia Debate* (Dordrecht: Kluwer, 1998).

2. K. Foley and H. Hendin, eds., *The Case against Assisted Suicide: For the Right to End-of-Life Care* (Baltimore: Johns Hopkins University Press, 2002).

3. T. Quill and G.K. Kimsma, "End-of-Life Care in the Netherlands and the United States: A Comparison of Values, Justifications and Practices," *Cambridge Quarterly of Healthcare Ethics* 6 (1996): 189–205.

4. K.W. Schuit, P.E. Post, C. Budde, F.E. van Heest, and C. Rolff, "Calling a Consultant Is Effective in Terminal Care" [in Dutch], *Huisarts en Wetenschap* 46 (2003): 388–91.

5. G. van der Wal, A. van der Heide, B.D. Onwuteaka-Philipsen, and P.J. van der Maas, *Medical Decisions at the End of Life: The Practice and the Evaluation Procedure* [in Dutch] (Utrecht: Uitgeverij de Tijdstroom, 2003), 69–70.

6. M.T. Muller, G.K. Kimsma, and G. van der Wal, "Euthanasia and Assisted Suicide: Facts, Figures and Fancies," *Drugs and Aging* 13 (1998): 183–91; G.K. Kimsma, "Assisted Death in the Netherlands and Its Relationship with Age," in *Aging: Decisions at the End of Life,* edited by D. Weisstub, D.C. Thomasma, S. Gautier, and G.F. Tomossy (Dordrecht: Kluwer, 2001), 49–67.

7. SUPPORT Principal Investigators, "A Controlled Trial to Improve Care of Seriously Ill, Hospitalized Patients: The Study to Understand Prognoses and Preferences of Outcomes and Risks of Treatment (SUPPORT)," *Journal of the American Medical Association* 274 (1995): 1591–98; B. Lo, "Improving Health Care Near the End of Life: Why Is It So Hard?" *Journal of the American Medical Association* 274 (1995): 1634–46.

8. K. Foley and H. Hendin, "Changing the Culture," conclusion to *The Case against Assisted Suicide: For the Right to End-of-Life Care,* edited by K. Foley and H. Hendin (Baltimore: Johns Hopkins University Press, 2002), 311–32, 312.

9. Z. Zylicz, "Palliative Care and Euthanasia in the Netherlands: Observations of a Dutch Physician," in *The Case against Assisted Suicide: For the Right to End-of-Life Care,* edited by K. Foley and H. Hendin (Baltimore: Johns Hopkins University Press, 2002), 122–43, 143.

10. Van der Wal et al., *Medical Decisions at the End of Life,* 101, 52.

11. H. Hendin, "The Dutch Experience," in *The Case against Assisted Suicide: For the Right to End-of-Life Care,* edited by K. Foley and H. Hendin (Baltimore: Johns Hopkins University Press, 2002), 97–121, 103.

12. G. van der Wal, *Euthanasia and Assisted Suicide by Family Physicians* (Rotterdam: Wyt Uitgeefgroep, 1992), 28–35.

13. Hendin, "The Dutch Experience," 103.

14. Support Consultation Euthanasia Netherlands (SCEN), course materials to qualify for independent consultant for physician-assisted dying, available to course participants; G.K. Kimsma, "Assessing Suffering: A Proposal for a Conceptual Frame" [in Dutch], *Medisch Contact* 55 (2000): 1757–59.

15. Hendin, "The Dutch Experience," 103.

16. Ibid.; Foley and Hendin, "Changing the Culture," 313.

17. T. Schalken, "Commentary on the Dutch Supreme Court/Hoge Raad's verdict 00797/02, December 24, 2002," *Tijdschrift voor Gezondheidsrecht* 3 (2003): 237.

18. Ibid.; Zylicz, "Palliative Care and Euthanasia in the Netherlands," 133–35; Foley and Hendin, "Changing the Culture," 314.

19. E. Kübler-Ross, *On Death and Dying* (New York: Simon and Schuster, 1969); M.C.G. Chaban, *The Life Work of Dr. Elisabeth Kübler-Ross and Its Impact on the Death Awareness Movement* (Lewiston, N.Y.: Edwin Mellen, 2000).

20. P.T.P. Wong, G.R. Reker, and G. Gesser, "Death Attitude Profile–Revised: A Multidimensional Measure of Attitudes toward Death," in *Death Anxiety Handbook: Research, Instrumentation and Application,* edited by R.A. Neimeyer (Washington, D.C.: Taylor and Francis, 1994), 121–48, 195.

21. Thomasma et al., *Asking to Die;* I. HaverKate, A. van der Heide, B.D. Onwuteaka-Philipsen, P.J. van der Maas, and G. van der Wal, "The Emotional Impact on Physicians of Hastening the Death of a Patient," *Medical Journal of Australia* 175 (2001): 519–22.

22. Ministry of Health, Welfare, and Sports, *2001 Annual Report of the Regional Euthanasia Evaluation Committees* (The Hague: Ministry of Health, Welfare, and Sports, 2002), 15.

23. *Law on Evaluation of Ending Life after a Request and Assisted Suicide* [in Dutch], Staatsbad 1002: 194: 1–8 (April 12, 2002).

24. Thomasma et al., *Asking to Die,* 342, 349, 299.

25. Ibid., 289, 272.

26. Ibid., 297, 313, 276, 291.

27. Ibid., 291.

28. P. Lain Entralgo, *Doctor and Patient* (London: World University Library, 1969), 17; C.C. Clark and G.K. Kimsma, "'Medical Friendships' in Assisted Dying," *Cambridge Quarterly of Healthcare Ethics* 13, no. 1 (2004): 61–67; Thomasma et al., *Asking to Die,* 297.

29. Zylicz, "Palliative Care and Euthanasia in the Netherlands," 142.

30. Thomasma et al., *Asking to Die,* 338.

31. Ibid., 295.

32. Ibid., 323.

33. Ibid., 409–84.

34. G.K. Kimsma and C. Carlucci-Ciesielski, "Euthanasia: To Report or Not to Report. Interviews with Next of Kin" [in Dutch], *Medisch Contact* 48 (1993): 328–32; C. Carlucci Ciesielski and G.K. Kimsma, "The Impact of Reporting Cases of Euthanasia in Holland: A Patient and Family Perspective," *Bioethics* 8 (1994): 151–58.

35. N. Swarte, M.L. van der Lee, G.J. van der Bom, J. van den Bout, and A.P.M. Heinz, "Effects of Euthanasia on the Bereaved Family and Friends: A Cross-Sectional Study," *British Medical Journal* (2003): 327–32.

36. Thomasma et al., *Asking to Die,* 283.

37. Ibid., 331, 339.

38. HaverKate et al., "The Emotional Impact on Physicians of Hastening the Death of a Patient," 520.

39. Ibid., 521.

40. E.D. Pellegrino, "The False Promise of Beneficent Killing," in *Regulating How We Die: The Ethical, Medical, and Legal Issues Surrounding Physician-Assisted Suicide,* edited by L.L. Emanuel (Cambridge: Harvard University Press, 1998), 71–92, 76.

41. Van der Wal et al., *Medical Decisions at the End of Life,* 101.

𝕯 Political and Legal Ferment

17

Political Strategy and Legal Change

Eli D. Stutsman, J.D.

Oregon has experienced unprecedented legal and political reform since the 1994 passage of the Oregon Death with Dignity Act.[1] The significance of the *legal* reform in Oregon is demonstrated by the very existence of the act, the only law of its kind in the United States. No other state provides its citizens with a comprehensive list of statutory criteria that, once satisfied, permit a physician to openly assist a competent terminally ill adult patient seeking to hasten his or her impending death.[2]

The significance of the *political* reform in Oregon is demonstrated by a remarkable measure of voter and institutional support for the act. The Oregon Death with Dignity Act is supported by nearly seven out of ten Oregon voters and by key statewide officials, including Governor Ted Kulongoski, former governor John Kitzhaber (a physician whose tenure from 1994 to 2002 overlapped the critical period for reform in Oregon), Oregon secretary of state Bill Bradbury, and Oregon treasurer Randall Edwards.[3] When faced with threats from Congress, the Oregon law has been rigorously defended by six out of seven members of the Oregon congressional delegation.[4] Although Oregon attorney general Hardy Myers does not personally support the state's novel law, he too has mounted a strong defense against federal challengers.[5] Finally, in a 2002 survey that asked candidates their position on the Death with Dignity Act, twelve of the thirty state senators and twenty-five of the sixty state representatives serving in the 2003 Oregon legislature supported the law in writing.[6]

Support for Oregon's new law cuts across party, faith, and gender lines. Polling conducted after the 1997 campaign revealed that a majority of both Democrats (72 percent) and Republicans (51 percent) supported Oregon's new law, with the strongest support coming from nonaffiliated independents (83 percent). The same survey also showed strong support across gender lines (60 percent of women and 70 percent of men) and faith affiliations (56 percent of Catholics, 60 percent of Protestants, and 89 percent of those professing no religion).[7] Such strong support from lay Catholics may come as a surprise given that most of the money spent in opposition to death-with-dignity legislation comes from the political arm of the Catholic Church.

If you want to hold public office in Oregon, you will be expected to announce your position on death with dignity, and your position will matter. Indeed, in Oregon today, an elected official's position on death with dignity is arguably the single most important political litmus test. During the 2002 gubernatorial primary, all three Democratic candidates and all three Republican candidates pledged their support for the Oregon Death with Dignity Act.[8] That all six candidates felt compelled to announce their position in favor of death with dignity during a primary race for the votes of their own party is both extraordinary and yet expected. During the same 2002 election cycle, in a statewide survey for the U.S. Senate race, 45 percent of Oregon voters sampled responded that Republican senator Gordon Smith's effort to overturn the Oregon Death with Dignity Act was a "very convincing" reason to vote him out of office;[9] when measuring voter sentiment on a social issue, 45 percent is a huge number. In comparison, 41 percent of respondents believed that Senator Smith's effort to overturn *Roe v. Wade,* the landmark decision that permits legal abortion, was a "very convincing" reason to vote against him. All other issues tested in that same survey, including gun control, social security, minimum wage, tax cuts, environmental pollution, and toxic waste cleanup, were of less importance to Oregon voters. Any issue that is so demonstrably important to voters will draw the attention of every serious political candidate, pollster, and strategist, friend or foe.

In the ten short years from 1993 to 2002, an extraordinary legal and political transformation has occurred in Oregon but not elsewhere. Indeed, outside of Oregon, although popular support remains high, there is no vestment of public authority and little political legitimacy for death with dignity. What makes Oregon so different? How did a social issue like death with dignity become a political litmus test?

Popular Support at the National Level

Oregon voters are not unique in their support for death with dignity. Strong popular support has been demonstrated in public opinion polls since the early 1970s. Whether the question is posed in a national or state survey or is framed as a matter of an individual's right or the federal government's attempts at intervention, public opinion consistently supports death-with-dignity reform.

It was not always so. In 1947, 54 percent of respondents to a Gallup survey answered no when asked, "When a person has a disease that cannot be cured, do you think doctors should be allowed by law to end a patient's life by some painless means if the patient and his family request it?"[10] At that time, only 37 percent of respondents were in favor, and 9 percent responded either "don't know" or "no answer." Twenty-six years later, however, when the exact same question was posed again, these numbers were nearly reversed: 53 percent in favor of allowing a hastened death, 34 percent opposed, and 7 percent "don't know" or "no answer."[11]

From that point forward, national surveys established a record of steadily increasing support for death with dignity, climbing rapidly in the mid-1980s, roughly coinciding with advances in medical science that extended end-of-life dilemmas beyond anything possible just a few generations ago. Surveys conducted between 1988 and 1993 show a 15 percent surge in support for death-with-dignity reform during this short period of time. In 1998 fully 58 percent of those asked, "When a person has a painful and distressing terminal disease, do you think doctors should or should not be allowed by law to end the patient's life if there is no hope of recovery and the patient requests it?" said it should be legal; 27 percent said it should not, and 14 percent said either "don't know" or "no answer."[12]

In 1990 Gallup repeated the question asked in 1947 and 1973; this time, 65 percent supported legalizing physician-assisted dying, 31 percent opposed, and only 4 percent said "don't know" or "no answer."[13] A 1993 Harris poll asked the question slightly differently: "Do you think that the law should allow doctors to comply with the wishes of a dying patient in severe distress who asks to have his or her life ended, or not?" Seventy-three percent of respondents to this survey were in favor of assisted dying, 24 percent were opposed, and 3 percent answered "don't know" or "no answer."[14] The upward trend didn't stop in 1993. In 1996, two years after voters in Oregon approved the first-in-the-nation law permitting a physician-assisted death, Gallup recorded its highest numbers ever to the same question it asked in 1947, 1973, and 1990 when respondents said they favored such laws by a margin of 75 percent to 22 percent, with 3 percent saying "don't know" or "no opinion."[15]

Popular Support at the State Level

Public opinion surveys confined to statewide voter samples have produced results similar to those obtained from the national surveys canvassed above. As has been noted, popular and institutional support for death with dignity within Oregon is at an all-time high. Surveys fielded in other states, including Maine in 1998, Hawaii in 2002 and 2003, Vermont in 2003, and Arizona in 2003, all indicate, as in Oregon and the nation as a whole, a high level of popular support for death-with-dignity reform. In a 1998 survey of Maine voters, for example, 63 percent of the respondents answered yes when asked, "Do you want Maine to allow terminally ill adult patients the voluntary informed choice to obtain a physician's prescription for drugs to end life?" Thirty-one percent opposed the statement, and 5 percent were not sure.[16]

In a 2002 survey of Hawaii voters, 72 percent of respondents answered in favor of legalizing physician-assisted death when asked, "Would you favor or oppose legislation giving terminally ill persons of sound mind the right to have physician assistance in dying, if the bill included appropriate safeguards to protect against potential abuse?" Only 20 percent opposed, and 7 percent were not sure.[17] This same question received 71 percent support in Hawaii in 2003 and 68 percent support in Vermont.[18]

Also in 2003, Arizona voters were asked, "When a person has a disease that cannot be cured and is living in severe pain, do you think doctors should be allowed by law to assist the patient to commit suicide if the patient requests it? Or not?" Respondents supported the concept of assisted dying by 57 percent; 32 percent opposed, and 6 percent said it "depends on circumstances." Five percent said "don't know" or refused to answer.[19]

Popular Opposition to Government Intrusion

Although it is more common to pose questions that solicit a respondent's level of support for an idea or cause, sometimes it is more useful to rephrase the question to reflect the work at hand. In a 1998 national survey, fielded during the first of two congressional attempts to nullify Oregon's law, respondents were asked, "Do you favor or oppose Congressional legislation that would prohibit physicians from prescribing medications that terminally ill patients could take to end life?" Respondents nationwide opposed such legislation almost three to one, with 72 percent opposed, only 26 percent in favor, and 2 percent not sure.[20] That same survey asked a generic question about support for death-with-dignity legislation by asking respondents to agree or disagree with the following statement: "People in the final stages of a terminal disease that are suffering and in pain should have the right to get help from their doctor to end life, if they so choose." Seventy-four percent of respondents agreed with the statement, 25 percent disagreed, and 1 percent were not sure.[21] This study was conducted in response to the 1998 Lethal Drug Abuse Prevention Act, which, had it passed Congress, would have nullified the Oregon Death with Dignity Act. The failed Lethal Drug Abuse Prevention Act was followed by the Pain Relief Promotion Act of 1999, a similar law targeted at Oregon that also failed to pass Congress.

Opponents of Oregon's Death with Dignity Act seized new opportunities in 2001 with the advent of the second Bush administration and the arrival of Attorney General John Ashcroft. In his former role as a U.S. senator from Missouri, Ashcroft had cosponsored the federal legislation against Oregon's death-with-dignity law. In his first year as attorney general, and just weeks after the September 11, 2001, terrorist attacks, Ashcroft issued an enforcement directive to the Drug Enforcement Administration, over which he now presides, directing DEA agents to prosecute Oregon physicians practicing in accord with the Oregon Death with Dignity Act. Soon thereafter, a national survey revealed that Americans continued to support physician-assisted dying and were also overwhelmingly opposed to Attorney General Ashcroft's efforts in Oregon. After hearing a description of Oregon's law in a previous question, respondents were asked, "This proposition, allowing physician-assisted suicide, was approved by a majority in Oregon. Attorney General Ashcroft recently moved to overrule [Oregon's law], which he says is now illegal. Do you think Attorney General Ashcroft was right or wrong to do this?" A strong majority, 58 percent, opposed the attorney general's intervention, 35 percent supported it, and 7 percent were not sure.[22]

In sum, support for death with dignity is consistently strong within and outside of Oregon and still trending upward. Although Oregon has advanced death-with-dignity reform like no other state, it would be wrong to attribute that development primarily to characteristics of the Oregon voter.

Converting Public Support into Public Policy

The challenge of any political effort is to leverage popular support, using it as a driving force to shape new public policy. Although the polling technique offers a valid measure of public support, its limitations are often misunderstood. Public opinion surveys offer only a snapshot, fixed in time, of public sentiment under carefully limited circumstances. Political campaigns attempt to replicate the polling experience but in a vastly different setting. Statewide public opinion surveys pose carefully controlled questions to a small sample of voters, usually four hundred to six hundred respondents, during a fifteen- to twenty-minute interview. In sharp contrast, political campaigns often last a year or longer, consume vast amounts of human and financial resources, and are spread across an entire state in what may best be described as a protracted battle for a majority of dollars and then votes. In this real-world setting, defenders of the status quo fight mightily to control the debate while enjoying the benefits of tradition, money, organization, inertia, fear, and influence within the stakeholder community. Popular support alone is no match for the well-organized, well-funded defender of the status quo. An early lead in the polls that is unprotected by smart, well-funded political strategies will quickly be lost. This is particularly true when dealing with sensitive issues that affect law, medicine, and religion at once. Armed with this understanding, it is possible to briefly assess the various wins and losses involving death-with-dignity reform in and outside of Oregon.

Campaigning for Death with Dignity

Legal reformers have utilized both the citizen-sponsored initiative process available in twenty-four states and the traditional legislative process available in all fifty states.[23] For purposes of this chapter, however, useful data are gleaned from the six initiative campaigns fought in Washington (1991), California (1992), Oregon (1994 and 1997), Michigan (1998), and Maine (2000) and one legislative effort waged in Hawaii (2002). The two victories in Oregon and the recent near victories in Maine and Hawaii have much in common; the larger losses in Washington and California, and particularly Michigan, represent a different type of animal.

Washington's Initiative 119

The first significant initiative campaign occurred in 1991 in the state of Washington, where proponents of Initiative 119 sought to revise state law to allow euthanasia by lethal injection. Although Initiative 119 failed 46 to 54 percent because proponents' paid advertising campaign, or "media buy," was too short, too sparse, and too soft, this campaign was significant because it nonetheless provided skilled observers with the first professional statewide political contest involving death with dignity. Much has been and still can be learned from this first mature political effort.

California's Proposition 161

The second significant initiative campaign occurred in 1992 in California, where proponents sought to pass Proposition 161, a lengthy proposal also designed to allow euthanasia by lethal injection. Unlike the Washington campaign, the California campaign was a true grassroots effort that depended almost exclusively on volunteers, political handbilling (passing out literature), and free media. Opponents were anything but grassroots, however, invoking the toughest political strategies and outspending proponents significantly.

Although the California campaign was a very different campaign waged in a very different state, it failed by the same margin as the Washington initiative the year before, 46 to 54 percent, leading many to conclude that the expensive polling and paid media used during the Washington campaign added nothing to the eventual outcome. The more accurate view, however, is that opponents in California had to shift more voters (using 1990 figures, California's population was six times that of Washington) out of the "yes" column and into the "no" column—hard work that is accomplished with paid media, a costly endeavor in California's far more expensive, diverse, and numerous media markets.[24] But with sufficient funds, it is relatively easy to prevail over a defenseless grassroots campaign. In the end, owing to the sheer size of the voting population, far more "yes" voters were converted into "no" voters in California than in Washington; yet the election-day margin, expressed as a percentage, turned out the same, masking the true nature of the California defeat.

Oregon's Measure 16

The third and certainly most significant campaign occurred in 1994 in Oregon, where proponents succeeded in passing Measure 16, the Oregon Death with Dignity Act, by a margin of 51 to 49 percent. Unlike Washington's Initiative 119 or California's Proposition 161, Oregon's Measure 16 expressly prohibited "lethal injection, mercy killing [and] active euthanasia," causing many to erroneously conclude that Oregon's success was derived from little more than a political compromise or, as characterized by some right-to-die activists, a political sellout.[25]

The Oregon campaign was also notable because its political strategies were informed by the earlier defeats in Washington and California. While it is true that strategists in Oregon offered a fresh policy proposal—a "prescribing only" bill that prohibited lethal injection—they also inoculated Measure 16 by building in numerous safeguards that were crafted in direct response to the political rhetoric espoused by opponents during the 1991 and 1992 Washington and California campaigns.

Oregon's Measure 51

The fourth and equally significant campaign also occurred in Oregon when, during the 1997 legislative session, the Oregon Catholic Conference successfully lobbied the state legislature to place a repeal measure, House Bill 2954, later named Measure 51, on the November ballot. Measure 51 was designed to repeal Oregon's Death with Dignity Act, which was still tied up in litigation in federal court and had not yet been implemented. The measure was referred to the ballot because Governor Kitzhaber signaled the legislature that he would veto a direct repeal. By placing Measure 51 on the 1997 ballot for voter approval or rejection, the legislature avoided the governor's veto pen. Measure 51 went down to a stunning defeat when voters turned out 60 to 40 percent against repeal of Oregon's new law. By election day 1997, Measure 51, which began as a Catholic Conference lobbying effort in the opening days of the 1997 legislative session, had become a major political blunder. After two statewide elections, the will of the voters could not have been clearer, and the tired argument that Measure 16 was passed by too slim a margin in 1994 became irrelevant.

Michigan's Proposal B

The fifth significant initiative campaign occurred in 1998 in Michigan, where grassroots proponents, attempting to take a page from the Oregon playbook, introduced Proposal B, a prescribing-only bill modeled after Oregon's new law. Although support started out quite high, Proposal B met a stunning defeat when voters turned out 71 percent against it. The essential lesson for the political novice was that the Oregon victories could not be explained simply as the fruit of a narrow, prescribing-only bill that prohibited lethal injection and euthanasia. Although some have surmised that the antics of Dr. Jack Kevorkian doomed Proposal B from the start, an Oregon-style death-with-dignity law would have eliminated the legal loopholes exploited for years by Dr. Kevorkian, and a skilled political strategist would have painted Dr. Kevorkian as the target of reform. For skilled political observers, the loss in Michigan came as no surprise at all—a grassroots campaign is defenseless against the politically experienced, well-organized, and well-funded opponents of death-with-dignity reform.

Maine's Question 1

The sixth significant initiative campaign occurred in 2000 in Maine, where a small coalition sponsored Question 1, a proposal modeled closely after the Oregon law. This campaign was significant because it was the first attempt to replicate not only the Oregon law but also the now-proven political strategy developed in Oregon. Question 1 nearly passed, failing by a narrow margin of 51 to 49 percent. Although the effort to replicate Oregon's political strategy was incomplete, particularly the free-media and litigation strategies, and the paid political advertising was uninspiring and ultimately ineffective, it was a close race, and this was the first time proponents experienced near success outside of Oregon.

Hawaii's House Bill 2487

The final campaign occurred in 2002 in the Hawaii legislative assembly. Hawaii House Bill 2487 was also modeled closely after the Oregon law. Sponsored by Governor Ben Cayetano, the Hawaii Death with Dignity Act passed the House Judiciary Committee ten to one (with three excused), a near consensus, and the House floor thirty to twenty, revealing a remarkably high level of support from a state legislature.[26] From there, the Hawaii proposal moved to the Senate Judiciary Committee, where the committee chair held the bill hostage, refusing to bring it to a vote. Soon, however, a majority of senators sidestepped the committee chair when the Senate voted fifteen to ten to pull the bill from committee. That same day, the Senate voted thirteen to twelve to approve the bill and send it to a final vote by the full Senate.[27] It is worth noting that the same number of votes necessary to pull the bill from committee and then to authorize a full senate vote (that is, a simple majority) was all that was needed to pass the proposal out of the senate and on to the governor, who had requested the bill in the first place and was by now lobbying for its passage and ready to sign it into law. In the end, however, the Catholic Church marshaled its resources, and two senators had changed their position by the time the full Senate voted fourteen to eleven against passage.[28] A near success, the Hawaii Death with Dignity Act was only two Senate votes away from becoming the second death-with-dignity law in the nation, a significant accomplishment. Until this time, no death-with-dignity proposal had come within striking distance of success in a state legislature.

A Portal to the Modern Era

The period between 1990 and 2003 was pivotal for the death-with-dignity movement in three key respects. First, the political balance within the movement shifted to a centrist position, with the 1991 and 1992 Washington and California campaigns marking the end of the "euthanasia era" in this country. There have been no serious (that is, well-funded or well-organized) efforts to pass euthanasia legislation since. Until 1992, movement leadership had always been in favor of euthanasia by lethal injection, and debate had focused on whether a proposed initiative should be long or short on clinical details (compare Washington's short Initiative 119 to California's lengthy Proposition 161) or whether euthanasia should be limited to the competent terminally ill adult patient or extended to those who are chronically ill, incompetent, or not yet adults. Today, these ethical debates may provide useful teaching tools in academic settings, but they have become irrelevant in mainstream political discussions and, perhaps, always were.

Second, the disastrous loss in Michigan in 1998 dispelled the notion that grassroots reformers, relying almost entirely on high popular support and an Oregon-style prescribing-only law, have any chance of success against well-funded, well-organized defenders of the status quo. The modern political treatment of the issue that began in Oregon in 1992 and later led the way to victories there in 1994 and 1997, together with the near wins in Maine in 2000 and Hawaii in 2002, contains certain key elements and has much to teach. One lesson is that popular support for death-with-dignity reform is no substitute for political money, skill, and organizing. The political tactics adopted by the reformers must be up to the challenge of defeating the political tactics of the defenders of the status quo.

Third, the shift away from a focus on voluntary euthanasia called for new "ownership," which is often necessary to rehabilitate a hot-button social issue and make political success possible. It is difficult, if not impossible, for someone who has long advocated voluntary euthanasia to sustain political credibility when he or she suddenly asserts that the political balance is properly struck with a prescribing-only bill. Moreover, advocates of voluntary euthanasia have occasionally put themselves harshly at odds with organized medicine, refusing to acknowledge that there are a myriad of competing interests that, in the end, must balance. As the discussion at the beginning of this chapter demonstrates, community stakeholders and public officials will rigorously support death-with-dignity reform so long as political strategists make the issue "safe"—by abandoning euthanasia proposals and hapless campaign strategies, to name two examples.

Political Tactics

The Oregon strategy has at its core a steadfast commitment to rebalancing the competing interests at play in death with dignity to assuage the concerns held by the larger stakeholder community and in so doing to reposition the death-with-dignity issue on the political spectrum, complete with new ownership and sophisticated, well-organized, well-funded political strategies. Oregon has relied on this approach during a decade of success. The recent near wins in Maine and Hawaii are the direct result of invoking the Oregon strategy.

Framing the Issue

Among the politically minded, political work begins with framing the issue, something that we all do at one level or another throughout our lives. When young children formulate a carefully worded question and then present that question to one parent rather than the other, they have both framed the issue and selected a target audience, the goal being to sway a yes vote. By obtaining a yes vote from the easy parent, they have won an endorsement with which to lobby the more difficult parent. The child is now coalition building, working to obtain majority support. The same strategy is at the core of political work, although the questions are much more complicated and the voters far more numerous and varied, as are the institutional stakeholders whose endorsements may be needed in order to win and, if not to win, to succeed with the new policy after the initial political victory.

Although political strategies differ markedly between ballot measure campaigns and legislative campaigns, the issues that arise are often remarkably similar. This is because in a ballot measure campaign the people raise their concerns directly, whereas in a legislative campaign, the same or similar concerns emerge from the people through their elected representatives. In either case, however, the political sides frame the arguments and the institutional stakeholders ultimately confer the persuasive and often necessary endorsements on one side or the other. In other words, because the same stakeholders are involved, similar competing issues arise, the primary difference being who gets to vote and what strategies will succeed in persuading that vote.

When framing the issue, it is also good to remember that a certain percentage of voters or legislators will support reasonable death-with-dignity reforms and a certain percentage will not. These two voting segments provide the base of support for and against. The goal when framing the issue is to maintain current levels of support while simultaneously persuading soft or undecided voters in the middle to swing your way, thus creating a majority. Framing the issue is important not only because a well-framed issue encourages support but also because, as the Oregon experience demonstrates, when it is done well, it balances competing policy interests, resulting in a law that is both operationally feasible and politically defensible for years to come, despite the sensitive nature of the subject matter. The Oregon Death with Dignity Act serves as an example of successful framing with respect to several issues—particularly the prohibition against euthanasia, the restriction of assisted death to cases of terminal illness, and age and competency requirements.

Despite some popular enthusiasm for Dr. Kevorkian, the Netherlands, or euthanasia, such people, places, and activities help to make the case *against* death-with-dignity reform. As a matter of public policy in the United States, physicians should not practice as mavericks without boundaries, public laws should not be loosely defined, and it is not possible to balance the competing public interests to make euthanasia politically feasible. Consequently, successful legislation will necessarily outlaw such activity in no uncertain terms. This is one of the hallmarks of the Oregon Death with Dignity Act. It is a prescribing-only bill, expressly prohibiting "lethal injection, mercy killing or active euthanasia."[29] Moreover, the Oregon law establishes a comprehensive standard of care, leaving no room for the antics of a Dr. Kevorkian.

To qualify under the Oregon law, a patient must be suffering a terminal disease and have less than a six-month life expectancy.[30] This restriction has led some to complain that the Oregon law discriminates against patients suffering from debilitating chronic disease. There is, however, little public support for such unrestricted reform, and no campaign will succeed if it must defend permitting a hastened death for those who are chronically ill.

Adulthood and competency are both required under the Oregon law.[31] This has prompted a few activists to urge that the option of a hastened death be extended to an incompetent adult or a competent juvenile facing a terminal illness with a life expectancy of less than six months, but again, no campaign will succeed if such activity must be defended.

These brief examples reveal tough, calculated decisions about what is politically feasible. Depending on one's perspective, these political compromises may be attacked as a political sellout or praised as good public policy. For Oregonians, these political compromises provide safe and sensible death-with-dignity reform. They also codify (legalize) what many will acknowledge as the existing covert practice of hastening a difficult death.[32]

Other provisions of the Oregon law serve to remove the uncertainty that would otherwise prevail. For example, the attending and consulting physician requirements, the informed decision requirement, and the written request, waiting periods, and witness requirements not only facilitate the standard of care but also ensure good decision making.[33] Similarly, the statutory charting requirements, combined with the public disclosure requirements, ensure public oversight.[34] In sum, the law is both good medicine and good politics, making the practice safe while simultaneously inoculating against political attack.

Other examples taken from the Oregon law are more purely political. For example, in an honest debate, a residency requirement for a private-pay patient seeking care from an Oregon physician serves no medical purpose. Nevertheless, observations made during the Washington and California campaigns uncovered the overheated political argument that without such a requirement Oregon would become a "suicide destination state," so the Oregon law contains a residency requirement.[35]

Defining Ownership of the Issue

Who "owns," or sponsors, an issue is every bit as important as how it is framed. At the end of the political day, the task of every campaign is to deliver a well-framed message through well-chosen messengers. A well-framed issue sponsored by the wrong people is immediately suspect. When an issue is advanced by the wrong owners, institutional stakeholders may stand back and watch, but they are more likely to quickly oppose reform. For this reason, it is not helpful for the death-with-dignity issue to be owned exclusively by the so-called right-to-die groups, particularly those that champion voluntary euthanasia. It was no coincidence that the Oregon Death with Dignity Act was publicly sponsored by a nurse, a physician, and a surviving spouse. Public opinion research consistently demonstrates that, with respect to death-with-dignity reform, voters find the opinions of nurses to be most persuasive, physicians and family members coming in a close second. That both sides have polled and proved this fact is apparent from mirror-image political strategies that have placed nurses, physicians, and family members at the front line of the political debate. This is also why the political arm of the Catholic Church, although leading and funding the opposition campaigns, prefers to remain behind the scenes.

Defining the Opposition

It is not enough merely to define the issue and the message. It is further necessary to define the opposition, for they are sure to be employing the same strategies. With respect to the death-with-dignity debate, when a few layers of political resistance are peeled back, it becomes clear that the well-organized, well-funded political arm of the Catholic Church is the primary political opponent. Exposing the role of the Catholic Church is problematic for many and, even when it is handled well, may lead to claims of Catholic-bashing by the church, a church that has at times been victimized by social movements but also has a blemished record of its own in this regard. Fear of political reprisal has led some to shrink from the challenge.

To be successful, however, reformers cannot be timid but must earnestly expose the true nature of the political opposition so that the policy debate can be cast in accurate terms. For example, most people are surprised to learn that during the six initiative campaigns and the one legislative campaign that took place from 1991 to 2002, most of the opposition's money and political expertise came from the Catholic Church. Indeed, organized medicine had relatively little to do with the defeats in Maine and Hawaii, whereas the church had almost everything to do with them. The public record bears this out. The Catholic Church provided

- $745,951 (64.5 percent of the opponents' budget) in Washington state in 1991,[36]
- $2,199,986 (60.6 percent) in California in 1992,[37]
- $968,806 (59.3 percent) in the first Oregon campaign in 1994,[38]
- $1,677,699 (73.6 percent) in Oregon in 1997,[39]
- $2,173,330 (38.0 percent) in Michigan in 1998,[40] and
- $1,288,894 (fully 73.9 percent) in Maine in 2000.[41]

Even during the 2002 Hawaii legislative campaign, where expenditures for political advertising played a far smaller role than in a statewide ballot measure campaign, the Catholic Church nonetheless emerged as the primary opponent.[42]

What is perhaps most surprising about these expenditures is that they *under-state* the total Catholic contribution in that these figures include only what can be gleaned from public contribution and expenditure reports. In other words, these totals represent Catholic contributions that are easily recognizable in the public record from the name of the donor alone—for example, the Arch-diocese of Portland—but they do not reflect political contributions from indi-vidual Catholic donors, who may be making contributions at the behest of their church or because they are Catholic. That these percentages represent only institutional contributions is all the more telling. Politically speaking, death-with-dignity reform faces one primary political opponent, the political arm of the Catholic Church.

Consider the political impact. The Catholic Church provided nearly three-quarters of the opposition budget during the 2000 campaign in Maine, where proponents held on to a steady lead for more than a year. Both sides ran six-week advertising campaigns, and it was a close race, a cliff-hanger too close to call for much of election night. By the next morning, however, the final vote was reported at 48.5 percent in favor, 51.5 percent opposed. A shift of 9,727 no votes, out of 633,561 total votes cast, would have turned the election. In a close contest like the Maine campaign, had the Catholic Church's contribution been any-thing less than the astounding 73.9 percent of the opponents' budget, the ballot measure would most likely have passed.

What Makes Oregon Different?

The answers to the questions raised at the beginning of this chapter—Why is Oregon so different? Why did death-with-dignity reform succeed in Oregon but fail in other states?—are manifold. Oregon's experience shows that popular support, in and of itself, does not guarantee success. As the foregoing discus-sion reveals, the Oregon Death with Dignity Act is first and foremost a politi-cal document, one that effectively balances competing public policy concerns in ways that have allowed it to retain high percentages of popular support while simultaneously recruiting mainstream institutional support.

A well-crafted document, however, is not enough. The politics of social re-form is a race to define the issue, its proponents, and its opponents. Political success demands a well-framed message delivered by well-chosen messengers against a well-defined opponent. Reform efforts elsewhere cannot simply copy the Oregon law and expect to succeed.

If the goal is to win a political contest, then one must accurately assess the opponents' strengths, weaknesses, and preferred political tactics. Death-with-dignity reformers have too often adopted the wrong policy or political strategy without due regard to the task at hand, thereby losing the race before it begins. In California, for example, reformers were advised that they had the benefit of strong public support, which was true, and that the primary task therefore was to collect enough signatures to put Proposition 161 on the ballot so that the people could vote on it,[43] which was naive. Once the proposal was on the ballot, the opposition campaign spent its money, ran its political advertisements, and won without much resistance. Michigan's Proposal B was defeated even more spectacularly, for similar reasons. Both these campaigns were lost as soon as they were begun because of the political strategies adopted early on by reformers who failed to foresee the effectiveness of the opposition campaign.

Moreover, to harness the power of popular support, it is necessary to organize and raise money—lots of it. Although the mechanics of day-to-day political campaigning are well beyond the scope of this chapter, suffice it to say that during the twelve to eighteen months after a campaign goes public but before paid media advertising starts, it is necessary to engage all the professional political strategies to preserve, if not expand, support among voters and institutional stakeholders—all of which is expensive work.

Finally, paid media was a factor in every reform campaign discussed in this chapter. The Catholic Church has funded opposition campaigns wherever death-with-dignity reform has been proposed, including in Oregon in 1994 and 1997. To skilled political observers, this should come as no surprise. The church's preferred strategy is to fund efforts to oppose reform but remain behind the scenes. At the height of any statewide ballot campaign, the church will rely on the hardest-hitting and at times most misleading political advertising imaginable,[44] rendering an underfunded, poorly organized, media-poor grassroots campaign defenseless.

Seen in historical perspective, the current reform movement is making steady progress, but it is still in its infancy. The ten years between the first effort to legalize physician-assisted death with Washington's Initiative 119 in 1991 and the defeat of Hawaii's House Bill 2487 in 2002 is emerging as a pivotal time, during which there has been a sea change in the approach to death-with-dignity reform. The 1994 and 1997 victories in Oregon are very real, and the data emerging from Oregon rebut every political and clinical argument advanced by opponents of physician-assisted death. When the Oregon success is combined with the near successes on the Maine ballot in 2000 and in the Hawaii legislature in 2002, one can see the potential of the current movement toward reform. With the right ownership of the issue, proper balancing of the competing public policy concerns, and smart political strategies, death-with-dignity reform can and will succeed in the years to come.

Notes

1. Oregon Death with Dignity Act, *Oregon Revised Statutes,* secs. 127.800–127.995 (1995).
2. See, for example, ibid., sec. 127.815.
3. P. Goodwin, "Findings from Post-Election Survey," GLS Research memorandum, Post-election survey of 600 Oregon voters, January 7–12, 1998; Oregon Death with Dignity State PAC Endorsement (2002), on file at Oregon Death with Dignity Political Action Fund, Portland; D. Hamilton, "Election 2002: Back Talk—Talk Back," *Portland (Ore.) Tribune,* October 4, 2002, A4; Oregon Right to Die PAC Endorsement (1996), on file at Oregon Death with Dignity Political Action Fund, Portland; J. Kitzhaber, "Congress's Medical Meddlers," *Washington Post,* November 1, 1999, A21; S. Wolfe, "Candidate Bradbury Stumps in Ashland," *Daily Tidings* (Ashland, Ore.), October 1, 2002, 1; R. Edwards, telephone interview with author, Salem, Oregon, September 19, 2003.
4. Oregon Right to Die PAC Endorsements (1998), on file at Oregon Death with Dignity Political Action Fund, Portland; "David Wu on Health Care: Voted No on Banning Physician-Assisted Suicide," On the Issues, www.issues2000.org/House/David_Wu_Health_Care.htm (accessed March 4, 2004); "Blumenauer Testifies Against Proposed Legislation on Assisted Suicide," press release, July 14. 1998, www.house.gov/blumenauer/press_releases/pr051.htm (accessed March 4, 2004); "Walden Opposes Effort to Overturn Will of Voters: Keeps Commitment to Uphold Oregon Law on Assisted Suicide," press release, October 26, 2000, walden.house.gov/press/releases/2000/oct/pr102600.html (accessed March 4, 2004); "Darlene Hooley on Health Care: Voted No on Banning Physician-Assisted Suicide," On the Issues, www.issues2000.org/House/Darlene_Hooley_Health_Care.htm (accessed March 4, 2004); "DeFazio Blasts House Vote on Assisted Suicide: Remains Hopeful About Chances for Defeat in Senate," press release, October 27, 1999, www.house.gov/defazio/102799HCRelease.shtml (accessed March 4, 2004); "Standing Alone, Senator Wyden Kept the United States Senate from Overturning Oregon's Twice-Passed Ballot Measure Legalizing Physician-Assisted Suicide," wyden.senate.gov/meet/bio/pas.html (accessed March 4, 2004); S. Power, "Smith Backs Suicide Repeal," *Statesman Journal* (Salem, Ore.), April 26, 2000, 1A.
5. Oregon Right to Die PAC Endorsement (2000), on file at Oregon Death with Dignity Political Action Fund, Portland; "Attorney General Hardy Myers to Take Legal Action to Protect Oregon's Physician-Assisted Suicide Law," State of Oregon Department of Justice media release, November 6, 2001, www.doj.state.or.us/releases/rel110701.htm (accessed March 4, 2004).
6. See 2002 candidate surveys, on file at Oregon Death with Dignity Political Action Fund, Portland.

7. P. Goodwin, "A Survey of Voters in Oregon on Issues Related to Measure 16," GLS Research memorandum (on survey of six hundred registered Oregon voters conducted April 20–27, 1997); memo dated "April, 1997."

8. J. Lyon, "Gubernatorial Candidates Tackle Issues at Forum," *Bulletin* (Bend, Ore.), April 18, 2002, A1; N. Budnick, "For GOP, Suicide Ain't Painless," *Willamette Week* (Portland, Ore.), December 5, 2001, 11.

9. Mellman Group, "Oregon Statewide Survey," February 2002, 5, on file at Oregon Death with Dignity Political Action Fund, Portland.

10. Gallup Poll, survey of approximately fifteen hundred U.S. adults, June 6–11, 1947, Gallup Organization.

11. Gallup Poll, survey of 1,544 U.S. adults, July 6, 1973, Gallup Organization.

12. Roper Organization Poll, survey of 1,982 U.S. adults, February 1998, Roper Center for Public Opinion Research.

13. Gallup Poll, survey of 1,018 U.S. adults, November 15–18, 1990, Gallup Organization.

14. Harris Poll, survey of 1,254 U.S. adults, November 11–15, 1993, Harris Interactive.

15. Gallup Poll, survey of 1,010 U.S. adults, April 9–10, 1996, Gallup Organization.

16. P. Goodwin, "Key Survey Findings," GLS Research memorandum (on survey of four hundred Maine voters, June 3–7, 1998), June 17, 1998.

17. QMark Poll, survey of four hundred Hawaii voters; "Death with Dignity 2002", February 1–4, 2002.

18. QMark Poll, survey of five hundred Hawaii residents, "Omnibus Study" January 28–February 1, 2003; Macro International Poll, survey of four hundred Vermont voters; "Vermont Poll", results reported February 28, 2004.

19. F. Solop, "Grand Canyon State Poll," Social Research Laboratory, Northern Arizona University, March 14, 2003 (survey of four hundred Arizona voters, March 6–11, 2003).

20. P. Goodwin, "National Voter Research Findings: Attitudes Regarding the Terminally Ill," GLS Research memorandum, July 17, 1998 (on survey of one thousand U.S. adults, July 8–13, 1998).

21. Ibid.

22. H. Taylor, "2-1 Majorities Continue to Support Rights to Both Euthanasia and Doctor-Assisted Suicide," Harris Interactive, January 9, 2002 (survey of 1,011 U.S. adults, December 14–19, 2001).

23. The Initiative and Referendum Institute provides a thoughtful explanation of the initiative process at www.iandrinstitute.org.

24. Roughly two months before the November ballot, 59.5 percent of California voters answered yes to the following question: "From what you have seen, read or heard about Proposition 161, would you be inclined to vote yes or no on Proposition 161?" *The California Poll 92-06*, Field Institute, September 1992 (survey of 1,067 California voters, September 8–15, 1992).

25. Oregon Death with Dignity Act, sec. 127.880.

26. Hawaii State Legislature, 2002 sess., HB 2487 HD1, February 23, 2002, www.capitol .hawaii.gov/session2002/status/HB2487.asp (accessed March 4, 2004); Hawaii State Legis-

lature, 2002 sess., HB 2487 HD1, March 7, 2002, www.capitol.hawaii.gov/session2002/status/HB2487.asp (accessed March 4, 2004).

27. Hawaii State Legislature, 2002 sess., HB 2487 HD1, April 30, 2002, www.capitol.hawaii.gov/session2002/status/HB2487.asp (accessed March 4, 2004).

28. K. Rosati, "Physician Assisted Suicide—Victory for Now," *Hawaii Family Forum* 2, no. 5 (2002): 1–3, hawaiifamilyforum.org/newsletters20020510.pdf (accessed March 4, 2004); L. Benoit, "State Senate Rejects Physician-Assisted Suicide Bill on Final Day of Session," *Hawaii Catholic Herald,* May 10, 2002; E. Christian, "Legislative Report: Defeat of Physician Assisted Suicide a Victory for Conference," *Hawaii Catholic Herald,* June 7, 2002; Hawaii State Legislature, 2002 sess., HB 2487 HD1, May 2, 2002, www.capitol.hawaii.gov/session2002/status/HB2487.asp (accessed March 4, 2004).

29. Oregon Death with Dignity Act, sec. 127.880.

30. Ibid., sec. 127.805.

31. Ibid.

32. D.E. Meier, C.A. Emmons, S. Wallenstein, T.E. Quill, R.S. Morrison, and C.K. Cassel, "A National Survey of Physician-Assisted Suicide and Euthanasia in the United States," *New England Journal of Medicine* 338 (1998): 1193–1201.

33. Oregon Death with Dignity Act, secs. 127.815, 127.820, 127.830, 127.840, 127.850, 127.810, 127.897.

34. Ibid., secs. 127.855, 127.865.

35. Ibid., sec. 127.860.

36. Contribution data collected from public records held by the Washington State Public Disclosure Commission, 1991 Washington State Initiative 119 (election date November 5, 1991).

37. Contribution data collected from public records held by the State of California Fair Political Practices Commission, 1992 California Proposition 161 (election date November 3, 1992).

38. Contribution data collected from public records held by the Oregon Secretary of State's Office, 1994 Oregon Measure 16 (election date November 8, 1994).

39. Contribution data collected from public records held by the Oregon Secretary of State's Office, 1997 Oregon Measure 54 (election date November 4, 1997).

40. Contribution data collected from records held by the Michigan Secretary of State's Office, 1998 Michigan Proposal B (election date November 3, 1998).

41. Contribution data collected from public records held by the Maine Commission on Governmental Ethics and Election Practices, 2000 Maine Question 1 (election date November 7, 2000).

42. Rosati, "Physician Assisted Suicide—Victory for Now"; Benoit, "State Senate Rejects Physician-Assisted Suicide Bill on Final Day of Session"; Christian, "Legislative Report"; Hawaii State Legislature, 2002 sess., HB 2487 HD1, May 2, 2002.

43. This conclusion is based on a 1992 conversation with grassroots volunteer Jean Gillett.

44. M. Goad, "HMO Protests Prompt TV Stations to Pull Ad," *Press Herald* (Portland, Maine), November 2, 2000, 1A.

18

Legal Advocacy to Improve Care and Expand Options at the End of Life

Kathryn L. Tucker, J.D.

Increasingly, and largely as a result of modern medicine, dying patients want more control over the timing and manner of their deaths and want to have the option of a humane, physician-assisted death.[1] A substantial majority of citizens believe that competent, terminally ill patients should have the option of receiving medication that patients could self-administer to bring about a humane and peaceful death if pain and suffering becomes intolerable, and a majority of physicians believe such patients should have this option.[2] However, most states have statutes prohibiting assisting suicide.[3] Although it is unclear that such laws were intended to reach the act of a physician prescribing medication that a dying patient could take to bring on a humane death, it is clear that the laws deter many physicians from doing so. Despite that, there is a widespread underground practice of physician-assisted dying.[4] Thus in the debate now raging regarding physician-assisted dying, the question is not really whether the practice should occur but rather whether the practice should proceed clandestinely and unregulated or openly and regulated to protect patients and accommodate legitimate state interests.

The Federal Constitutional Claim to Physician-Assisted Dying

Patients, physicians, and the public interest group Compassion in Dying challenged the assisted suicide laws in New York (in *Vacco v. Quill*) and Washington (in *Washington v. Glucksberg*) to the extent that they prohibited physicians from providing medications that competent dying patients could use to hasten their own deaths, if they so chose.[5] Liberty and equality guaranteed by the Fourteenth Amendment of the U.S. Constitution formed the basis of the claims. Two federal courts of appeals, including the Ninth Circuit Court of Appeals sitting en banc, agreed that statutes preventing patients from exercising this option were unconstitutional.[6] In 1996 the U.S. Supreme Court reversed these appellate decisions but left the door open to both a future successful federal constitutional claim and to legislative reform.

The Court rendered unanimous decisions upholding the laws challenged in *Glucksberg* and *Quill*. The decisions were plainly influenced by the lack of information on how a legalized program for physician-assisted dying would work, since at the time the cases were presented no state had legalized this option.[7] Five justices, a majority of the Court, wrote or joined concurring opinions that limited the scope of the majority's ruling and carefully reserved issues for future cases. These five concurring justices have left the question of federal constitutional protection of the choice at issue very much open to future developments.

The majority decision, written by Chief Justice Rehnquist, did not actually resolve the narrow question posed by those challenging the states' laws; instead, the Court answered a more general and easily resolved question, one on which the parties were not in dispute: "whether the 'liberty' specially protected by the Due Process Clause includes a right to commit suicide which itself includes a right to assistance in doing so."[8] The Court recognized that the more difficult question, whether a dying suffering patient has a protected right to choose physician assistance in dying, was not foreclosed by its ruling on the more general question.[9]

Justice O'Connor, in casting the deciding vote, revealed in her concurrence that she joined the majority only on the understanding that the question decided by the majority was the "easy" question: "The Court frames the issue in this case as whether the Due Process Clause of the Constitution protects a 'right to commit suicide which itself includes a right to assistance in doing so.' . . . I join the Court's opinions because I agree that there is no generalized right to 'commit suicide.'"[10] Justice O'Connor went on to state explicitly that on the "difficult" question, she has reserved judgment and remains open to deciding that issue favorably in a future case: "Respondents urge us to address the narrower question whether a mentally competent person who is experiencing great suffering has a constitutionally cognizable interest in controlling the circumstances of his or her imminent death. I see no need to reach that question in the context of the facial challenges to the New York and Washington laws at issue here."[11]

Justice O'Connor and Justice Breyer, in a separate concurrence, explicitly expressed the view that a viable constitutional claim remained for a future case, specifically involving patients who could not obtain relief with palliative care.[12] Justices O'Connor and Breyer set forth the view that provision of pain-relieving medication to a patient that hastened death would not violate state laws prohibiting assisted suicide. Justice O'Connor stated that "a patient who is suffering from a terminal illness and who is experiencing great pain has no legal barriers to obtaining medication, from qualified physicians, to alleviate that suffering, even to the point of causing unconsciousness and hastening death."[13] She further wrote, "There is no dispute that dying patients . . . can obtain palliative care, even when doing so would hasten their deaths."[14]

Justice Breyer concurred in the judgments upholding the states' challenged laws but disagreed with the majority's "formulation of [the] claimed liberty interest."[15] Justice Breyer expressed the view that on the narrower, more difficult question, there was "greater support" in "our legal tradition" for a "right to die with dignity."[16] He explicitly reserved judgment on that question: "I do not believe, however, that this Court need or now should decide whether or not such a right is 'fundamental.' That is because, in my view, the avoidance of severe physical pain connected with death would have to comprise an essential part of any successful claim and because, as Justice O'Connor points out, the laws before us do not force a dying person to undergo that kind of pain."[17] Unfortunately, and contrary to the assumption of these justices, legal barriers to obtaining medication sufficient to adequately relieve pain do exist. Indeed, it is widely recognized that physicians fail to prescribe adequate medication for relief of pain and that legal constraints contribute to that situation.[18]

Thus Justices O'Connor and Breyer appear to have answered a question the parties had not actually posed. In so doing, they have recognized that there is a constitutional right to adequate pain medication.[19] Efforts to establish this right more firmly can be anticipated.

Justice Stevens, also concurring in the judgments, chose to write "separately to make it clear that there is also room for further debate about the limits that the Constitution places on the power of the States to punish the practice [of physician-assisted suicide]."[20] Justice Stevens emphasized that because the Court addressed only the "easy" question, its holding "does not foreclose the possibility that some applications of the statute might well be invalid."[21] Similarly, Justice Souter's concurrence reflected his reservation of decision on the narrower, more difficult question: "I do not decide for all time that respondents' claim should not be recognized."[22]

The opinions, both majority and concurring, invited legislative reform. The majority recognized that "throughout the Nation, Americans are engaged in an earnest and profound debate about the morality, legality, and practicality of physician-assisted suicide. Our holding permits this debate to continue, as it should in a democratic society."[23] Justice Souter's concurring opinion made explicit his preference for legislative action in this area: "The Court should stay its hand to allow reasonable legislative consideration"; "the legislative process is to be preferred."[24] Similarly, Justice O'Connor's concurrence demonstrated her concern that state legislatures be given the first opportunity to address the issue: "States are presently undertaking extensive and serious evaluation of physician-assisted suicide and other related issues. In such circumstances, 'the . . . challenging task of crafting appropriate procedures for safeguarding . . . liberty interests is entrusted to the "laboratory" of the States.'"[25]

Thus the United States Supreme Court invited legislative reform through state political processes.[26] To date, few state legislatures have attempted to address this issue, although commentators have proposed excellent models legislators could use to begin their debate.

Legislative Reform as the Means to Expanding Patient Choice

As of 2004, only one state, Oregon, has passed a law permitting physician-assisted suicide.[27] Implementation of that law, entitled the Oregon Death with Dignity Act and passed in 1994 through the initiative process, has been obstructed by challenges brought by right-to-life activists.[28] In a lawsuit that turned upside down the equal protection argument advanced in the *Glucksberg* and *Quill* cases, the challengers argued that a law permitting terminally ill patients to choose physician assistance in dying denied the terminally ill equal protection of the laws.[29] The case suffered from fatal threshold infirmities, however, and the Ninth Circuit dismissed it on the grounds that the plaintiffs lacked standing.[30]

Recognizing that the effort to defeat the Oregon legislation in court was doomed, right-to-life activists refocused their efforts on defeating the measure politically. They succeeded in forcing a repeal measure on the ballot for a vote in November 1997. That effort failed when 60 percent of Oregon voters rejected the repeal.[31] Following these judicial and political losses, opponents of the Oregon Death with Dignity Act sought relief from the federal government, urging the Drug Enforcement Administration to take action against Oregon physicians who act in compliance with the law on the basis that such activity would violate the Controlled Substances Act (CSA).[32]

The Drug Enforcement Administration initially opined that its agents could revoke the registrations of physicians who assisted in hastening deaths under the Oregon Death with Dignity Act. U.S. Attorney General Janet Reno, however, soon overruled this position, concluding that the CSA did not reach such conduct.[33] Opponents then sought to amend the act to expand its scope to reach the Oregon law in two successive sessions of the federal legislature.[34] Both efforts failed in the face of strong opposition from the medical community founded on the concern that the proposed measures would exacerbate physicians' fears regarding the use of controlled substances in pain management.[35]

A change in federal administration and philosophy led to a change in legal interpretation. The Bush administration's attorney general, John Ashcroft, issued a directive on November 6, 2001, advising that the Department of Justice had concluded that prescribing controlled substances under the Oregon Death with Dignity Act violated the Controlled Substances Act because "assisting suicide is not a 'legitimate medical purpose' within the meaning of 21 C.F.R. § 1306.04 (2001)" and "prescribing, dispensing, or administering federally controlled substances to assist suicide violates the CSA." In particular, "such conduct by a physician registered to dispense controlled substances may 'render his registration . . . inconsistent with the public interest and therefore subject to possible suspension or revocation under 21 U.S.C. § 824(a)(4).'"[36]

The Ashcroft directive was challenged in federal court, the plaintiffs claiming that it violated the Controlled Substances Act, the Administrative Procedure Act, and the U.S. Constitution. In April 2002 the court issued its decision, addressing only the question of whether the directive was within the scope of the CSA and concluding that the directive exceeded the authority granted under the act. A permanent injunction was entered:

> The determination of what constitutes a legitimate medical practice or purpose traditionally has been left to the individual states. State statutes, state medical boards, and state regulations control the practice of medicine. The CSA was never intended, and the [U.S. Department of Justice] and [the Drug Enforcement Administration] were never authorized, to establish a national medical practice or act as a national medical board. To allow an attorney general—an appointed executive whose tenure depends entirely on whatever administration occupies the White House—to determine the legitimacy of a particular medical practice without a specific congressional grant of such authority would be unprecedented and extraordinary.[37]

The Death with Dignity Act has now been implemented for more than six years. Each year, teams of epidemiologists from the state and federal governments review data related to implementation and issue reports summarizing the data.[38] The resounding message of these reports is that the risks opponents argued would ensue if this option were available have not come to pass.[39] Indeed, many important and measurable improvements in end-of-life care in general have occurred following implementation in Oregon.[40]

Given that risks have not been realized from the availability of a choice of a humane hastened death, and important improvements in end-of-life care have been realized in the wake of implementation of the Oregon Death with Dignity Act, efforts to overturn the act, such as the Ashcroft directive, are particularly disturbing. Opponents encourage a perverse result in seeking to nullify the Oregon law: in their zeal to prevent this end-of-life option from being available they put at risk good pain care for all patients. This is so because increasing scrutiny of physician conduct in prescribing pain medication to dying patients will unavoidably and certainly chill physician willingness to treat pain aggressively.[41]

Twenty other states have initiative mechanisms,[42] and certainly other states may follow Oregon in enacting reform legislation through the initiative process. The shortcomings of the initiative process, however, are well recognized, and it is particularly ill suited for addressing complex issues such as those related to end-of-life decision making.[43] In this complex area, a legislative process that allows for extensive fact-finding and continual refinement of proposed provisions throughout the process of development of the legislation would be preferable to the passage of a law by the inflexible procedure necessary with initiative measures.[44] In the legislative process, the concerns raised by the states and interest groups in the federal constitutional litigation could be addressed.

Numerous models have been proposed and provide a useful starting point for development of appropriate legislation. These generally include measures to ensure accurate diagnosis of terminal status; to ensure mental competency and rule out depression of a nature that would impede rational decision making; to ensure that the decision is voluntary, rational, deliberative, and enduring; and to ensure that patients have been informed of and offered alternatives such as hospice care.[45]

Although public opinion strongly favors permitting competent dying patients the right to control the timing and manner of death by having access to medications that could be used to bring about a humane and dignified death, and the U.S. Supreme Court has encouraged resolution of the issue in state legislative procedures, the powerful opposition of the right-to-life lobby, the Catholic Church, and certain factions of organized medicine may continue to make legislative reform difficult.[46] Thus a return to the courts for relief may be necessary. The U.S. Supreme Court may find a federal constitutional right in a future case. In addition, patient rights advocates have the option of seeking relief from state high courts under provisions of state constitutions.

State Constitutional Litigation

Many states have constitutions that are either more textually explicit regarding protection of individual liberties than is the U.S. Constitution or have similar text that has been construed by the state's high court as more protective of individual liberties.[47] Thus, for example, state courts have found that restrictions on the use of Medicaid funds for abortions offends state constitutions, notwithstanding that the U.S. Supreme Court has held that there is no federal constitutional right to such funding.[48] Similarly, various state courts have held that consensual homosexual activity is protected under provisions of their own state constitutions, despite Supreme Court precedent in effect at the time of the state court's consideration that there is no federal constitutional protection of such activity.[49]

State courts have often spoken in resounding terms of the greater protection of individual liberties afforded by state constitutions. A recent decision of the California Supreme Court exemplifies this: "The scope and application of the state constitutional right of privacy is broader and more protective of privacy than the federal constitutional right of privacy as interpreted by the federal courts."[50] It is now well recognized that state courts can and will actively turn to their state constitutions to reach results beyond those mandated by the U.S. Constitution.[51]

State court challenges to assisted-suicide prohibitions based on state constitutional provisions protecting individual privacy, liberty, or dignity may offer a route to reform in such states. That the Supreme Court did not definitively reject recognition of such a right under the U.S. Constitution in *Glucksberg* or *Quill* makes the prospect of a state high-court victory more likely, as it is more difficult to persuade a state high court to reach a conclusion squarely at odds with that of the U.S. Supreme Court construing a similar provision in the U.S. Constitution.

To date, the two state high courts that have considered the matter, Alaska and Florida, have determined that their state constitutions do not protect the choice of a competent terminally ill patient to choose a humane hastened death.[52] However, it is likely that as Oregon's experience yields additional data, concerns about abuse and risk, so central to state opposition, will be assuaged and defused. Indeed, even staunch opponents of assisted suicide have begun to publicly acknowledge that continued opposition to such laws cannot be justified in light of the Oregon experience.[53] A courageous high court in a state with strong constitutional protections of individual liberty, privacy, or dignity may soon recognize that the choice of a competent dying patient to hasten impending death is entitled to protection.

Recognition by a state high court that the state's constitution protects the choice of a competent dying patient to obtain medications for the purpose of achieving a humane and dignified death would be of obvious national significance. Such a decision would lead to the generation of more data on how a legalized practice of physician-assisted death actually operates. This data would help inform the debate regarding legislative reform in other states and in future cases before state or federal courts.

A Constitutional Right to Adequate Pain Medication for Dying Patients

Hastened death is not the only or the best choice for many dying patients facing severe pain and suffering, and thus advocates of excellence in end-of-life care also seek to galvanize improvements in the care of the dying and, specifically, in improving care for pain.[54] One avenue that could prompt improved care of pain is the development of challenges to laws that serve to impede or obstruct physicians from prescribing medications of a kind or quantity sufficient to relieve pain. Such challenges were suggested by the concurring opinions in *Glucksberg* and *Quill,* based on the grounds that patients have a federal constitutional right to adequate pain medication and that laws that deter access to such medications abridge that right.

Vulnerable laws would include those that discourage physicians from prescribing controlled substances. It is well documented that laws requiring that prescriptions for controlled substances be written in triplicate and laws strictly limiting the number of dosage units per prescription, for example, have the effect of deterring physicians from prescribing controlled substances.[55] Cases challenging such laws could be brought on federal constitutional grounds, asserting that to the extent the laws serve to deter physicians from prescribing controlled substances in kind and quantity sufficient to relieve the pain of a dying patient, they abridge the constitutional rights of such patients.

Undertreated Pain and Efforts to Redress the Problem

The American Medical Association has declared that "physicians have an obligation to relieve pain and suffering and to promote the dignity and autonomy of dying patients in their care. This includes providing effective palliative treatment even though it may foreseeably hasten death."[56] A great proliferation of authoritative literature has been published in the medical journals in the past decade exhorting physicians to treat pain attentively and aggressively.[57] The U.S. Supreme Court has recognized that dying suffering patients have a right to adequate pain management.[58] Nonetheless, seriously ill and dying patients in the United States are routinely undertreated for pain. In a landmark study, researchers found that 50 percent of all patients who died during hospitalization "experienced moderate or severe pain at least half of the time during their last 3 days of life."[59] At the same time, it is well established that perhaps only 10 percent of dying patients have conditions in which alleviation of pain is truly difficult or impossible.[60] Although many factors contribute to inadequate pain management, two among these stand out as most significant: physicians' fear of regulatory agency oversight and inadequate education of physicians in pain management.

The Chilling Effect of Oversight

Prescription-monitoring programs, designed to prevent diversion of strong medications to the black market, have the collateral effect of chilling physician willingness to prescribe such medications.[61] Highly publicized cases in which physicians have been investigated and punished for prescribing strong pain medications, even though the physician's conduct met established guidelines for pain management, create a climate of fear that deters appropriate prescribing.[62]

Thus it is particularly alarming to see new programs of scrutiny and sanction introduced. Most notable recently is the effort by Attorney General Ashcroft, in his zeal to overturn the will of the Oregon people who have voted—twice—in favor of a law permitting dying patients to obtain medications they can self-administer to achieve a humane hastened death, to put at risk good pain management for all dying patients nationwide. The Ashcroft directive provides that any physician who is determined to have intended to hasten a patient's death by provision of pain medications is subject to punishment under the Controlled Substances Act.

Clinicians point out that determining a physician's intent in prescribing pain medication at the bedside of a suffering dying patient is open to an investigator's after-the-fact second-guessing: Was the intent to relieve pain and suffering or to hasten death?[63] If the Ashcroft directive is permitted to take effect, the desire to avoid this sort of investigation would cause physicians to be even less willing to treat the pain of dying patients.[64] Widespread concern in the medical, hospice, and bioethics communities that the Ashcroft directive will operate in this manner to impair pain care nationwide prompted broad amicus participation opposing the directive. Similarly, state legislation ostensibly designed to prevent physician-assisted suicide will also serve to increase physician concerns that their prescribing for pain of their dying patients will bring scrutiny and sanction and will further chill physicians' already reluctant willingness to treat pain. Such a bill was introduced, but successfully opposed, in the 2003 legislative session in the North Carolina legislature.[65]

Inadequate Physician Education in Pain Management

Many physicians lack knowledge of modern pain management practices and principles. Physicians are not sufficiently educated regarding pain treatment.[66] This derives from the failure of medical schools to adequately teach pain and symptom management, as well as failure of licensing boards to require as a condition of maintaining a license to practice medicine that physicians take a minimum number of hours of continuing medical education in pain and symptom management. A number of states are addressing this by passing measures to require such training, which, one hopes, will serve as models for other states.[67]

Ineffectual Reform Efforts

The American Society of Law, Medicine, and Ethics launched an effort in 1966, titled the Project on Legal Constraints on Access to Effective Pain Management, to mitigate the problem of undertreated pain and developed a model of legislation, the Pain Relief Act. The model act creates a "safe harbor" to shelter physicians prescribing pain medications from disciplinary and criminal action as long as they "demonstrate by reference to an accepted guideline that [their] practice substantially complied with that guideline," kept appropriate records, wrote no false prescriptions, did not violate the Controlled Substances Act, and did not divert medications to personal use.[68]

Safe-harbor provisions have been widely incorporated in state laws, often called Intractable Pain Treatment Acts, but they contain a critical shortcoming that has rendered them largely ineffectual. Although the acts provide a safe harbor, an essential part of alleviating physician concerns about scrutiny for prescribing pain medications, they fail to provide a mechanism to make the safe harbor necessary. A safe harbor is sought only when the consequences of not seeking it are adverse. What is missing is an accountability mechanism for failure to treat pain adequately. Only then will the safe harbor be attractive. These acts can and should be amended to provide that when there is failure to adequately prescribe, order, administer, or dispense controlled substances, including opioid analgesics, for the relief or modulation of pain in accordance with prevailing clinical practice guidelines, a private cause of action may be brought by the patient or survivors, and recovery of attorneys' fees allowed a plaintiff who prevails. Such an explicit cause of action, with the attorneys' fee recovery provision, would make tort accountability a powerful corrective mechanism.[69]

Accountability for Failure to Treat Pain Adequately

Accountability for inadequate pain management can arise in various contexts. The most appropriate is the state medical licensing boards that are vested with authority to supervise the conduct of the licensees in their jurisdiction and to protect the public from physicians whose conduct is injurious to patients. A second correction can come through tort exposure.

State medical boards have been slow to recognize their responsibility to correct physicians who undertreat pain. Even in California, where the medical board has been remarkably progressive in adopting policy recognizing the importance of good pain management, the problem persists. Recently, the Medical Board of California was presented with a formal complaint, supported by an independent expert opinion, which indicated that the pain care provided to an elderly, terminally ill cancer patient was inadequate. Although the medical board determined that the physician had failed to provide adequate pain care, it did not pursue any action against the physician. Medical boards must become receptive to disciplining physician conduct that involves failure to provide adequate pain management.[70] Recognition of the need for such correction is now coming even from within the profession.[71] State legislatures can engage in the effort to create professional accountability for inadequate pain management by passing law that makes clear that failure to adequately treat pain is unprofessional conduct subject to disciplinary measures.[72] Medical boards should promulgate policies that require disciplinary action when there is failure to adequately prescribe, order, administer, or dispense controlled substances, including opioid analgesics, for the relief or modulation of pain in accordance with prevailing clinical practice guidelines.

Correction may also come from the tort system. Until recently, the tort system has not held physicians liable for failing to adequately treat the pain of their dying patients. However, we stand at the threshold of a new era, with real exposure for physicians, and health care facilities, in cases in which pain management is inadequate. Tort liability would be made easier if the safe-harbor laws were amended to include an explicit private cause of action for failure to treat pain. Even absent an explicit private cause of action, liability may be founded on more conventional theories of medical negligence or creative application of other statutes, such as those governing elder abuse.

In 2001 a case was tried before a state court jury in California in which the sole claim was failure of the physician to adequately treat the pain of an elderly man dying of a painful form of lung cancer. The physician was ignorant of the great body of authoritative literature governing pain management, had not bothered to stay current with the many developments in the field since graduating from medical school, and used outmoded and discredited pain management strategy, and as a result the patient suffered unnecessarily during his final week of life. The jury hearing the case determined that the physician's conduct was reckless and awarded the family $1.5 million for the patient's pain and suffering under the state elder-abuse statute. Such verdicts reverberate in the medical community and apply a strong prompt to correct such behavior.

Expanding Choice at the End of Life

Public opinion strongly favors permitting competent dying patients the right to choose a humane hastened death by obtaining a lethal dose of medications from their physician that can be self-administered for this purpose. The U.S. Supreme Court has encouraged the states to serve as a laboratory for the nation on this complex issue, and the data emerging from Oregon provide a wealth of valuable information on how a legalized practice of assisted dying works. Some religious organizations and right-to-life activists continue to obstruct and seek to nullify legislative reform, though even staunch opponents of the practice of assisted dying now argue that continued opposition cannot be justified in light of the Oregon experience.[73] As Ronald Dworkin has so eloquently observed, "Making someone die in a way that others approve, but he believes a horrifying contradiction of his life, is a devastating, odious form of tyranny."[74]

Excellence in end-of-life care requires that the pernicious problem of inadequate pain management be addressed. Increased correction by state medical boards is one part of the solution. There is also a role for correction through the tort system, and amendments to safe-harbor legislation to explicitly provide for such actions would facilitate this form of correction. In addition, mandatory minimum education for both physicians in training in the medical school curriculum and for physicians in practice through continuing medical education requirements could raise the floor of clinician knowledge in this arena. Improving pain care may serve to reduce the number of dying patients who seek a hastened death. Permitting the option of a humane hastened death brings with it measurable improvements in pain and symptom management, very likely thereby reducing the number of dying patients who would choose to hasten death while providing comfort to all in the knowledge that if their dying process becomes intolerable, there is a humane option for a peaceful death.

Notes

1. See, for example, M. Webb, *The Good Death: The New American Search to Reshape the End of Life* (New York, Bantam Books, 1997), chaps. 1–3.

2. F. Newport, "Public Historically Supports a Terminally Ill Patient's Right to Die," Gallup News Service, October 30, 2003; J.G. Bachman, K.H. Alchser, D.J. Doukas, R. L. Lichtenstein, A.D. Corning, and H. Brody, "Attitudes of Michigan Physicians and the Public toward Legalizing Physician-Assisted Suicide and Voluntary Euthanasia," *New England Journal of Medicine* 334 (1996): 303–9; M.A. Lee, H.D. Nelson, V.P. Tilden, L. Ganzini, T.A. Schmidt, and S.W. Tolle, "Legalizing Assisted Suicide—Views of Physicians in Oregon," *New England Journal of Medicine* 334 (1996): 310–15; J.S. Cohen, S.D. Fihn, E.J. Boyko, A.R. Jonsen, and R.W. Wood, "Attitudes Toward Assisted Suicide and Euthanasia Among Physicians in Washington State," *New England Journal of Medicine* 331 (1994): 89–94.

3. See K.L. Tucker and D.J. Burman, "Physician Aid in Dying: A Humane Option, a Constitutionally Protected Choice," *Seattle University Law Review* 18 (1995): 495–508, 495 n. 1.

4. See, for example, A.L. Back, J.I. Wallace, H.E. Starks, and R.A. Pearlman, "Physician-Assisted Suicide and Euthanasia in Washington State: Patient Requests and Physician Responses," *Journal of the American Medical Association* 275 (1996): 919–25; R. Knox, "1 in 5 Doctors Say They Assisted a Patient's Death, Survey Finds," *Boston Globe,* February 28, 1992, 5; S. Heilig, R. Brody, F.S. Marcus, L. Shavelson, and P.C. Sussman, "Physician-

Hastened Death, Advisory Guidelines for the San Francisco Bay Area from the Bay Area Network of Ethics Committees," *Western Journal of Medicine* 166 (1997): 370–78.

5. *Washington v. Glucksberg,* 521 U.S. 702 (1997); *Vacco v. Quill,* 521 U.S. 793 (1997).

6. See *Compassion in Dying v. Washington,* 79 F.3d 790 (9th Cir. 1996) (en banc), *rev'd sub nom. Washington v. Glucksberg,* 521 U.S. 702 (1997); *Vacco v. Quill,* 521 U.S. 793 (1997).

7. *Glucksberg,* 117 S. Ct. at 2293.

8. Ibid., at 2269.

9. Ibid., at 2275 n. 24.

10. Ibid., at 2303.

11. Ibid.

12. Ibid., at 2303, 2312. The available data indicate that though most patients will be able to get relief with palliative care, some patients have intractable pain that cannot be relieved short of sedation to an unconscious state. See, for example, A. Jacox, D.B. Carr, and R. Payne, "New Clinical-Practice Guidelines for the Management of Pain in Patients with Cancer," *New England Journal of Medicine* 330 (1994): 651–55; Webb, *Good Death,* chap. 4.

13. *Glucksberg,* 117 S. Ct. at 2303.

14. Ibid., at 2303; see also 2312.

15. Ibid., at 2311.

16. Ibid.

17. Ibid.

18. Jacox, Carr, and Payne, "New Clinical-Practice Guidelines for the Management of Pain in Patients with Cancer"; B. Rich, "A Prescription for the Pain: The Emerging Standard of Care for Pain Management," *Wm. Mitchell Law Review* 26 (2000): 1–91; R.S. Shapiro, "Health Care Providers' Liability Exposure for Inappropriate Pain Management," *Law, Medicine and Ethics* 24 (1996): 360–64, 363; D. Joranson, "State Medical Board Guidelines for Treatment of Intractable Pain," *American Pain Society Bulletin* 5, no. 3 (1995): 1–5, 2; M.J. Field and C.K. Cassel, eds., *Approaching Death: Improving Care at the End of Life* (Washington, D.C.: National Academy Press, 1997), 191, 197.

19. See, for example, R.A. Burt, "The Supreme Court Speaks: Not Assisted Suicide but a Constitutional Right to Palliative Care," *New England Journal of Medicine* 337 (1997): 1234–36.

20. *Glucksberg,* 117 S. Ct. at 2304.

21. Ibid. Stevens further stated (at 2305) that "a decision upholding a general statutory prohibition of assisted suicide does not mean that every possible application of the statute would be valid."

22. Ibid., at 2293.

23. Ibid., at 2275.

24. Ibid., at 2293.

25. Ibid., at 2303.

26. At least one justice has explicitly indicated that he would be inclined to intervene with judicial relief if legislative foot-dragging occurs (*Glucksberg,* 117 S. Ct. at 2293).

27. Oregon Death with Dignity Act, *Oregon Revised Statutes,* secs. 127.800–127.995 (1995).

28. *Lee v. Oregon,* 891 F. Supp. 1429 (D. Or. 1995), vacated, 107 F.3d 1382 (9th Cir. 1997).

29. Ibid., at 1386.

30. Ibid., at 1390.

31. D. Garrow, "The Oregon Trail," *New York Times,* November 6, 1997, A31; K. Murphy, "Voters in Oregon Soundly Endorse Assisted Suicide," *Los Angeles Times,* November 5, 1997, 1.

32. See, generally, T. Egan, "Threat from Washington Has Chilling Effect on Oregon Law Allowing Assisted Suicide," *New York Times,* November 19, 1997, A12.

33. In an opinion letter issued June 5, 1998, Reno stated that "the Department has reviewed the issue thoroughly and has concluded that adverse action against a physician who has assisted in a suicide in full compliance with the Oregon Act would not be authorized by the CSA." Reno concluded that "there is no evidence that Congress, in the CSA, intended to displace the states as the primary regulators of the medical profession, or to override a state's determination as to what constitutes legitimate medical practice in the absence of a federal law prohibiting that practice." (On file with author.)

34. Lethal Drug Abuse Prevention Act of 1998 (H.R. 4006, June 5; S. 2151, June 9); Pain Relief Promotion Act of 1999 (H.R. 2260; June 17; S. 1272, June 23).

35. M. Angell, "Caring for the Dying, Congressional Mischief," editorial, *New England Journal of Medicine* 341 (1999): 1923–25; D. Orentlicher and A.L. Caplan, "The Pain Relief Promotion Act of 1999, A Serious Threat to Palliative Care," editorial, *Journal of the American Medical Association* 283 (2000): 255–58.

36. AG Order No. 2534-2001, "Dispensing of Controlled Substances to Assist Suicide."

37. *Oregon v. Ashcroft,* 192 F . Supp. 2d 1077, 1092 (D. Or. 2002). This decision was appealed to the Ninth Circuit Court of Appeals and in a decision issued on May 26, 2004; the appellate court, employing similar analysis, reached the same conclusion and continued the injunction against the Ashcroft Directive. 2004 WL 1162238 C.A. 9 (OR.), May 26, 2004 (Case No. 02-35587).

38. A.E. Chin, K. Hedberg, G.K. Higginson, and D.W. Fleming, "Legalized Physician-Assisted Suicide in Oregon—The First Year's Experience," *New England Journal of Medicine* 340 (1999): 577–83; A.D. Sullivan, K. Hedberg, and D.W. Fleming, "Legalized Physician-Assisted Suicide in Oregon—The Second Year," *New England Journal of Medicine* 342 (2000): 598–604; A.D. Sullivan, K. Hedberg, and D. Hopkins, "Legalized Physician-Assisted Suicide in Oregon, 1998–2000," *New England Journal of Medicine* 344 (2001): 605–7; K. Hedberg, D. Hopkins, and K. Southwick, "Legalized Physician-Assisted Suicide in Oregon, 2001," *New England Journal of Medicine* 346 (2002): 450–52; K. Hedberg, D. Hopkins, and M. Kohn, "Five Years of Legal Physician-Assisted Suicide in Oregon," *New England Journal of Medicine* 348 (2003): 961–64.; "Sixth Annual Report on Oregon's Death with Dignity Act," available at www.dhs.state.or.us/publichealth/chs/pas/ar-index.cfm (accessed May 26, 2004).

39. Ibid.

40. Ibid. See also L. Ganzini, H.D. Nelson, M.A. Lee, D.F. Kraemer, T.A. Schmidt, and M.A. Delorit, "Oregon Physicians' Attitudes about and Experiences with End-of-Life Care Since Passage of the Oregon Death with Dignity Act," *Journal of the American Medical Association* 285 (2001): 2363–69.

41. See, for example, Jacox et al., *supra* note 18 at 651 (the pain associated with cancer is frequently undertreated); see generally Ben Rich, "A Prescription for the Pain: The Emerging Standard of Care for Inappropriate Pain Management," *Journal of Law, Medicine and Ethics* 360, 363 (1966): 24 (identifying legal penalties, especially disciplinary action, as one of the most important reasons health care professionals undertreat pain); see also Field and Cassel, *Approaching Death*, 191, 197; Jerome Groopman, "Separating Death from Agony," *New York Times*, November 9, 2001, A27 ("Nothing could be further from the truth than Mr. Ashcroft's statement that a federal drug agency could readily discern the 'important medical, ethical and legal distinctions between intentionally causing a patient's death and providing sufficient dosages of pain medication necessary to eliminate or alleviate pain.' In fact, it is medically impossible to dissociate intentionally ameliorating a dying patient's agony from intentionally shortening the time left to live").

42. J.N. Eule, "Judicial Review of Direct Democracy," *Yale Law Journal* 99 (1990): 1503–90, 1509 n. 22; see also D.B. Magley, "Direct Legislation: Voting on Ballot Propositions in the United States," in *Direct Legislation: Voting on Ballot Propositions in the United States* (Baltimore: Johns Hopkins University Press, 1984): 38–39.

43. See, for example, J. Daar, "Direct Democracy and Bioethical Choices: Voting Life and Death at the Ballot Box," *University of Michigan Journal of Law Reform* 28 (1995): 799–859; see also D.B. Magley, "Governing by Initiative: Let the Voters Decide? An Assessment of the Initiative and Referendum Process," *University of Colorado Law Review* 66 (1995): 13–46, 18.

44. Although legislators are reluctant to take on socially divisive issues such as assisted dying, the growing public support for the practice, particularly in the wake of the Oregon experience with a carefully regulated practice, is making legislators increasingly willing to address this matter. In Hawaii's 2002 legislative session, an assisted-dying bill modeled on the Oregon bill came very close to passage.

45. See, for example, F.G. Miller, T.E. Quill, H. Brody, J.C. Fletcher, L.O. Gostin, and D.E. Meier, "Regulating Physician-Assisted Death," *New England Journal of Medicine* 331 (1994): 119–23.

46. It is noteworthy that even staunch opponents of assisted suicide have begun to publicly acknowledge that continued opposition to such laws cannot be justified in light of the Oregon experience. See, for example, D. Lee, "Physician-Assisted Suicide: A Conservative Critique of Intervention," *Hastings Center Report* 33, no. 1 (2003): 17–19.

47. See, generally, W.J. Brennan Jr., "State Constitutions and the Protection of Individual Rights," *Harvard Law Review* 90 (1977): 489–504; J. Friesen, *State Constitutional Law: Litigating Individual Rights, Claims and Defenses* (New York: M. Bender, 1992), chap. 2; R.F. Williams, "State Constitutional Law: Teaching and Scholarship," *Journal of Legal Education* 41 (1991): 243–49.

48. L.M. Vanzi, "Freedom at Home: State Constitutions and Medicaid Funding for Abortions," *New Mexico Law Review* 26 (1996): 433–54; *Maher v. Roe*, 432 U.S. 464 (1977); *Harris v. McRae*, 448 U.S. 297 (1980).

49. See, for example, *Gryczan v. State*, 942 P.2d 112 (Mont. 1997); *Bowers v. Hardwick*, 478 U.S. 186 (1986). *Bowers* was overturned by the U.S. Supreme Court in 2003, in *Lawrence v. Texas*, 123 S. Ct. 2472.

50. *American Academy of Pediatrics v. Lungren*, 940 P.2d 797, 808–9 (Cal. 1997).

51. R.F. Williams, "In the Glare of the Supreme Court: Continuing Methodology and Legitimacy Problems in Independent State Constitutional Rights Adjudication," *Notre Dame Law Review* 72 (1997): 1015–64, 1017.

52. *Krischer v. McIver*, 697 So.2d 97 (Fla. 1997); *Sampson v. Alaska*, 31 P.3d 88 (2001).

53. Lee, "Physician-Assisted Suicide."

54. The *Glucksberg* and *Quill* cases have been widely credited with focusing attention and efforts on improving the care of the dying. See, for example, Field and Cassel, *Approaching Death*, 206.

55. Joranson, "State Medical Board Guidelines for Treatment of Intractable Pain"; Field and Cassel, *Approaching Death*.

56. American Medical Association, Council on Ethical and Judicial Affairs, *Code of Medical Ethics* (Chicago: American Medical Association, 1996), 4.

57. See, for example, World Health Organization, *Cancer Pain Relief* (Geneva: World Health Organization, 1986); American Pain Society, Quality of Care Committee, "Quality Improvement Guidelines for the Treatment of Acute Pain and Cancer Pain," *Journal of the American Medical Association* 274 (1995): 1874–80; W.T. McGivney and G.M. Crooks, "The Care of Patients with Severe Chronic Pain in Terminal Illness," *Journal of the American Medical Association* 251 (1984): 1182–88; Agency for Health Care Policy and Research, "Acute Pain Management: Operative or Medical Procedures and Trauma Clinical Practice Guideline," Publication 92-0032 (1992), www.ahcpr.gov/clinic/medtep.acute.htm (accessed December 1, 2003); "Clinical Practice Guideline No. 9: Management of Cancer Pain," Publication 94-0592 (1994); available at www.hospice patients.org/clinicalpracticeguidelines1994.html (accessed May 27, 2004); "Model Guidelines for the Use of Controlled Substances for the Treatment of Pain," *Federation Bulletin: The Journal of Medical Licensure and Discipline* 85, no. 2 (1998): 84–89; Joint Commission on Accreditation of Healthcare Organizations, *Comprehensive Accreditation Manual for Hospitals: The Official Handbook*, www.jcaho.org/standard/pm_ac.html (accessed May 26, 2004).

58. *Vacco v. Quill*, 117 S. Ct. 2293 (1997); *Washington v. Glucksberg*, 117 S. Ct. 2258 (1997).

59. SUPPORT Principal Investigators, "A Controlled Trial to Improve Care for Seriously Ill, Hospitalized Patients: The Study to Understand Prognoses and Preferences for Outcomes and Risks of Treatments (SUPPORT)," *Journal of the American Medical Association* 274 (1995): 1591–98, 1594. Rich, "Prescription for the Pain."

60. Jacox, Carr, and Payne, "New Clinical-Practice Guidelines for the Management of Pain in Patients with Cancer"; American Pain Society, "Treatment of Pain at the End

of Life: A Position Statement from the American Pain Society," www.ampainsoc.org/advocacy/treatment/htm (accessed May 30, 2000).

61. New York Public Health Council, *Breaking Down the Barriers to Effective Pain Management, Recommendations to Improve the Assessment and Treatment of Pain in New York State, Report to the Commissioner of Health* (Albany: New York State Department of Health, 1998); Field and Cassel, *Approaching Death;* Joranson, "State Medical Board Guidelines for Treatment of Intractable Pain," 2; Shapiro, "Health Care Providers' Liability Exposure for Inappropriate Pain Management."

62. See, for example, *Hoover v. Agency for Health Care Administration,* 676 So.2d 1380 (1996); *Hollabaugh v. Arkansas State Medical Board,* 861 S.W.2d 317 (1993).

63. See, for example, J. Groopman, "Separating Death from Agony," *New York Times,* November 9, 2001, A27.

64. Rich, "Prescription for the Pain"; see also G. Hellen, "Professional Education in Palliative and End-of-Life Care for Physicians, Nurses, and Social Workers," in *Improving Palliative Care for Cancer,* edited by K.M. Foley and H. Gelbrand (Washington, D.C.: National Academy Press, 2001), 277–310.

65. General Assembly of North Carolina, 2003 sess., S. 145 (filed February 20, 2003).

66. Rich, "Prescription for the Pain," 40–41; Hellen, "Professional Education in Palliative and End-of-Life Care for Physicians, Nurses, and Social Workers."

67. *California Business and Professional Code,* sec. 2190.5 (West 2002); West Virginia Code Annals 30-1-7a (Michie 2001).

68. "The Pain Relief Act," *Journal of Law, Medicine and Ethics* 24 (1996): 317–18.

69. K.L. Tucker, "Improving Pain Care: A Safe Harbor Is Not Enough," *Health Lawyer* 11, no. 4 (1999): 15–16.

70. K.L. Tucker, "Medical Board Corrective Action with Physicians Who Fail to Provide Adequate Pain Care," *Journal of Medical Licensure and Discipline* 87 (2001): 130–31. As this chapter goes to press, only two state medical boards have disciplined physicians for failure to treat pain adequately: the Oregon board disciplined a physician in 1999 and reportedly disciplined the same physician again in 2002. In the Matter of the Accusation Against Eugene B. Whitney, M.D., Case No. 12 2002 13376, the Medical Board of California filed alleging inadequate treatment of pain on March 13, 2003. A "Stipulation for Public Reprimand" was decided on December 15, 2003. (Dr. Whitney received a Public Reprimand and was ordered to undergo an assessment of knowledge and skills, complete a minimum of 40 hours of Continuing Medical Education in pain management/palliative care, and complete a physician/patient communication course.)

71. See, for example, D.E. Weissman, "Care Near the End of Life: What Is Unprofessional Behavior?" *Journal of Palliative Medicine* 6 (2003): 1–3.

72. A proposal under consideration for the 2004 legislative session in New York would require mandatory education of medical students in the subjects of pain management and palliative care as well as mandatory continuing medical education of licensed physicians in these subjects. Pending proposed legislation S 6312 and A 10407.

73. Lee, "Physician-Assisted Suicide."

74. R. Dworkin, *Life's Dominion* (New York: Knopf, 1993), 217.

19

Physician-Assisted Suicide

Shifting the Focus from Means to Ends

Alan Meisel, J.D.

The United States Supreme Court has decided that state laws making as- sisted suicide a crime do not violate the U.S. Constitution, even when the person rendering assistance is a licensed physician, as long as the person to whom the assistance is rendered is terminally ill and competent and has volun- tarily requested the assistance.[1] Regardless of the Court's decisions, efforts to extend legalization of physician-assisted suicide are no more likely to end than is the practice of assisted suicide, or actively hastening death, or physician aid- in-dying, or whatever else one wishes to call it. Indeed, the Supreme Court ex- pressly left the door open for further debate and development of the law.

One method of legalization is the enactment of citizen legislative initiatives, such as that in Oregon, in other states. Another is by the action of state legisla- tures, as almost happened in Hawaii in 2002. Neither of these methods is likely to lead to widespread legalization in the short run. Physician-assisted suicide, like abortion, may be too controversial an issue to be addressed by elected leg- islators, whatever their personal views on the subject. Another possible forum for legalization efforts is state courts, which over the past two decades have been the vehicle for the legalization of *passively* hastening death. State courts could decide to legalize physician-assisted suicide through state constitutional claims, which has already been attempted (though without success) in Florida and Alaska, or by the use of common-law reasoning.

This chapter returns to legal basics to analyze the applicability of state homi- cide laws to physician-assisted suicide. Thus far, the legalization of *passively* hastening death has relied significantly on distinguishing it from *actively* has- tening death (including, but not limited to, physician-assisted suicide).

For more than twenty years our society has permitted doctors to end the lives of terminally ill patients under the aegis of sanitizing phrases like "forgoing life-sustaining treatment." If this practice is legally acceptable—as indeed it is if done in compliance with the guidelines established by all state courts or legislatures—it is a major hypocrisy to continue to distinguish among the *means* of hastening death. "Actively hastening death" is in truth no different from "passively hastening death." Given this fact, we have only two choices: criminalize forgoing life-sustaining treatment—which is clearly unacceptable—or decriminalize physician-assisted suicide. Public debate should be focused not on the means of hastening death, but on the safeguards that should be in place, regardless of the means by which death is hastened.

Passively hastening death by withholding or withdrawing life-sustaining medical treatment satisfies all of the elements of the crimes of homicide or assisted suicide. Nonetheless, it is not illegal because it represents an exercise of an individual's fundamental right to self-determination. Actively hastening death is an exercise of the same right, and it too is legitimated by the giving or withholding of consent. Moreover, any argument of any substance that can be made against actively hastening death can be made equally against passively hastening death. We do not accept such arguments in the case of the latter, and we should not accept them in the case of the former.

The Bright Line between Actively and Passively Hastening Death

Hastening the death of a dying person is not a new phenomenon. Historical accounts of it are widespread—and not merely in practices of our barbarian forebears. There is evidence that aid in dying has been practiced continually throughout modern history by physicians and nonphysicians alike.

Physician aid in dying in some forms has been accepted in American law for a quarter century, since the celebrated case of Karen Ann Quinlan in 1976.[2] *Quinlan* was the first case in which a U.S. appellate court ruled on the request of close family members to permit the termination of life support for a patient in a persistent vegetative state. *Quinlan* spawned similar cases in about half the states and a variety of legislation in all states, which recognize the legal right to withhold or withdraw life-sustaining medical treatment. This agglomeration of case and statutory law has given rise to a well-accepted legal consensus, which rests on three fundamental points:

1. There is a legal right, variously referred to as self-determination, autonomy, or privacy, that vests in competent individuals the right to refuse medical treatment, even if death results.

2. Persons who have lost decision-making capacity have a right to have their family decide to have medical treatment withheld or withdrawn even if death results.

3. There is a "bright line" between forgoing treatment that "passively" results in death through the withholding or withdrawing of treatment and more "active" means of hastening death, such as assisted suicide and active euthanasia.

To be sure, *Quinlan* and the cases and legislation flowing from it deal with a particular kind of hastening death, implemented by the withholding or withdrawing of life-sustaining medical treatment, which is characterized as "passively hastening death." Both the case law and the legislation comprising the consensus about end-of-life decision making acknowledge a clear awareness of the distinction between passively and actively hastening death. In fact, it is fair to say that it has been the bedrock of the consensus. Without the distinction, it is doubtful that *Quinlan* would have been decided as it was or that the legal consensus about forgoing life-sustaining treatment to which *Quinlan* gave birth could have evolved as it has.

Despite the pronouncements of courts and legislatures, however, there never was any logical or moral line between the two; the bright line was never more than semantic. As the former chief justice of the Florida Supreme Court explained in a dissenting opinion in a case rejecting a right to physician-assisted suicide, "The notion of 'dying by natural causes' contrasts neatly with the word 'suicide,' suggesting two categories readily distinguishable from one another. How nice it would be if today's reality were so simple. No doubt there once was a time when, for all practical purposes, the distinction was clear enough to all." The line between actively and passively hastening death, if it was ever bright, has forever been eroded, he continued, by the "technology [that has] crept into medicine. . . . Dying no longer falls into the neat categories our ancestors knew. In today's world, we demean the hard reality of terminal illness to say otherwise."[3]

Yet for two decades courts and legislatures have created and maintained the fiction that there is a difference—a determinative difference—between passively and actively hastening death. Doing so has served a useful political purpose: that of making passively hastening death acceptable to legislatures, to the medical profession, to the public, and not least important, to the courts themselves. If the withholding or withdrawing of life-sustaining medical treatment had been viewed as "killing" a patient, it would have been far more difficult—probably impossible—for the practice of passively hastening death ever to have achieved legitimacy. As courts embarked on the legitimation of passively hastening death, they recognized that legalization met a symbolic, and perhaps a real, need to make and emphasize the distinction between passively and actively hastening death—especially when more florid synonyms are used for the latter—in order to preserve the fundamental societal prohibition on the killing of innocent human beings.

The most fundamental way in which courts did this was to proclaim not merely a significant difference but a *legally determinative* difference between actively and passively hastening death. Specifically, they concluded that passively hastening death does not meet the requirements of the criminal offenses of homicide or assisted suicide, but actively hastening death does. To reach this conclusion, courts have had to engage in a number of sleights of hand.

Judicial Distinctions between Passively and Actively Hastening Death

From *Quinlan* to the present, the primary motivation for seeking judicial review in cases involving end-of-life decision making has been the fear of criminal liability. Those seeking dispensation have usually not been disappointed. The courts have steadfastly hewed to the position that withholding or withdrawing life-sustaining treatment does not subject the participants—either those who make the decision or those who actually withhold or withdraw the treatment—to criminal liability. In a complementary fashion, they have also—usually in dictum, simply because so few cases of actively hastening death have been the subject of judicial review—consistently characterized actively hastening death as criminal.

The courts have achieved this dual effort by employing three sometimes overlapping stratagems, any one of which, in effect, negates one or more essential elements of a crime: act, intent, or causation. Passively hastening death is held not to be a crime because

- death results from an *omission* rather than an act
- the *intent* necessary to support a crime is lacking
- passively hastening death is not the *cause* of the patient's death

(The fourth element of a crime is some specified consequence, which depends upon the particular crime and which, in this case, is the death of a human being.) In addition, a small number of courts have taken a fourth tack; they have concluded that there is also no criminal liability because the patient has a *legal right* to refuse treatment.

Act and Omission

The first argument begins with the assertion that the forgoing of treatment is an *omission* to treat, not an act. The locution sometimes used is that when treatment is forgone, we are merely allowing the patient to die, not killing him or her.[4] This argument is founded on the assumption that acts are culpable but omissions are not. The conclusion is then drawn that passively hastening death by forgoing life-sustaining treatment is not culpable, but actively hastening death is.

There are at least three problems with this approach, any one of which is fatal to the claim: that liability cannot be imposed for an omission, that forgoing treatment is always accomplished by an omission rather than an act, and that to classify behavior as either an act or an omission is a straightforward matter. The more general problem of the three is that the assertion about the nature of criminal liability is flat-out wrong; liability may be imposed for an omission if the party who omitted to act was under a duty to carry out the act.[5] Although as a general rule a physician has no duty to undertake to treat a patient, once there is an agreement to do so, an obligation arises to continue to provide treatment until the relationship is terminated in any one of a number of legally acceptable ways. In the treatment of those who are terminally ill, what excuses a physician from the obligation to provide treatment is the patient's consent for the physician to forgo treatment or, if the patient lacks decision-making capacity, the permission of a person legally authorized (a surrogate) to act on behalf of the patient.

The second problem with the argument is that sometimes, forgoing life-sustaining treatment *is* accomplished by an act. There are two ways in which treatment may be forgone. One, "withholding" treatment, is readily and uncontroversially denominated an omission. However, the other way—and the one almost universally involved in the reported legal cases—is by "withdrawing" treatment. In this case, someone has performed an act that leads to the patient's death. Indeed, physician-assisted suicide may be more passive than the withdrawal of treatment. As contemplated by the Oregon Death with Dignity

Act, the physician's "act" is the writing of a prescription, which on an active-passive scale, is arguably more passive than removing a patient from a ventilator, a common form of "withdrawing" treatment.

The third problem is the difficulty in characterizing *any* behavior as an act or as an omission. The New Jersey Supreme Court addressed this problem in the *Conroy* case, in which it observed that "characterizing conduct as active or passive is often an elusive notion, even outside the context of medical decision-making. Saint Anselm of Canterbury was fond of citing the trickiness of the distinction between 'to do' (facere) and 'not to do' (non facere). In answer to the question 'What's he doing?' we say 'He's just sitting there' (positive), really meaning something negative: 'He's not doing anything at all.'"[6]

The distinction is particularly nebulous, however, in the context of decisions whether to withhold or withdraw life-sustaining treatment.[7] That the very same treatment can be forgone for the very same patient either by withholding (omitting to act) or by withdrawing (acting) suggests that the legal consequences should not depend on such slim semantic distinction.

Take the case of a patient who is being kept alive by a feeding tube, as has so often been the situation in litigated cases, including the *Conroy* case. When a decision is made to forgo tube-feeding, there are two general ways to accomplish it. One is to take the feeding tube out; the other is to leave it in but not introduce any further fluids or nourishment through the tube. The conventional analysis is that in the former, death is brought about by an act; in the latter by an omission. But should legal—or moral—culpability turn on such hair-splitting distinctions that have no practical difference?

Thus the New Jersey Supreme Court concluded in *Conroy* that "merely determining whether what was done involved a fatal act or omission does not establish whether it was morally acceptable. . . . [In fact,] active steps to terminate life-sustaining interventions may be permitted, indeed required, by the patient's authority to forego therapy even when such steps lead to death."[8] Other courts have uniformly concluded that it makes no difference whether life-sustaining medical treatment—whether the use of feeding tubes or other forms of treatment—is forgone by withholding treatment or forgone by withdrawing treatment. The fact that one involves an act and one involves an omission is deemed to be of no legal significance. Both are legally permissible forms of forgoing life-sustaining medical treatment.

Although this solves one problem—the preclusion of liability for passively hastening death by the withdrawal of treatment—it creates another. By equating withdrawing with withholding, "acts of withdrawing" attain the same legal status as omissions. Why some acts (those involved in passively hastening death) are omissions but others (those involved in actively hastening death) are not is never satisfactorily explained. Is it because that kind of an act "causes" the patient's death, whereas the kind of an act involved in forgoing treatment does not? That explanation holds no water, either.

Intent

Some courts have distinguished passively and actively hastening death on the basis of there being a different intent in each, and they have justified non-liability for the former on the absence of the kind of intent necessary to constitute a crime.[9] It is conventionally reasoned that in cases of suicide (a form of *actively* hastening death), the individual's intent is to bring about death. By contrast, forgoing life-sustaining treatment (passively hastening death) does not constitute suicide because the patient's wish is not to end his or her life. Rather, the patient's intent is said to be the relief of suffering.[10] Under this explanation, because death from forgoing life-sustaining treatment is not suicide, the physician who has withheld or withdrawn treatment has not aided suicide and therefore is not subject to criminal liability. By contrast, actively hastening death is said to be quite different because the intent is unabashedly to cause the patient's death.

On closer analysis, these stock explanations do not hold. The intent-based explanations of why there is no liability for a patient's death from forgoing treatment—and of the purported distinction between passively and actively hastening death based on differential intent—are unsupportable.[11] For there to be criminal liability, there must be proof of a requisite mental element, traditionally referred to as *mens rea*.[12] This requirement has been replaced by the concept of culpability. Under the Model Penal Code, the basis of modern U.S. criminal law, the general requirement of culpability is that there be evidence that the actor acted "purposely, knowingly, recklessly or negligently."[13] The courts have taken the position that when life-sustaining medical treatment is forgone, there is no criminal liability for assisted suicide, homicide, or related crimes because the physician's *purpose* was not to cause death but to relieve suffering.

This explanation suffers from two defects. First, it overlooks the fact that culpability may be established in other ways. Second, it confuses intent with motive. According to the Model Penal Code, culpability may also be established by showing that the actor acted "knowingly." That is, one may be criminally liable, even absent a *purpose* to cause death, if one knew that one's conduct would cause death.[14] The assertion that the physician's intent is to relieve suffering is certainly credible in such situations. However, the existence of a nonblameworthy intent (the intent to relieve suffering) does not eliminate the possibility of the actor's simultaneously possessing a blameworthy intent (the intent to cause death), and in law the existence of the former does not cancel the effect of the latter.

One possible way out of this trouble is to claim that the actor's intent was to relieve suffering but that this intent could be accomplished only by causing death; that is, that death is not intended but is the unintended consequence of another, intended consequence. This, in effect, constitutes the invocation of the doctrine of double effect. Although seemingly approved by the United States Supreme Court,[15] the logic of double effect skirts the edges of accepted principles of intent and causation in criminal (and tort) law.[16]

Another difficulty with the argument that forgoing life-sustaining treatment does not invoke criminal sanctions because the actor's intent is not blameworthy is that it confuses intent with motive. Prosser, the legendary torts scholar, tells us that "'intent' is the word commonly used to describe the purpose to bring about stated physical consequences; the more remote objective which inspires the act and the intent is called 'motive.'"[17]

If a patient's suffering or a patient's own evaluation of his quality of life is such that he wishes to end his life, then it is correct to say that his motive—what motivates him to end his life or to authorize another to do so—is to relieve suffering. However, his legally relevant *intent* is still to cause death because that is the *consequence* he seeks to achieve. The same is true of homicide. Although a physician may be motivated to end a patient's suffering—and the patient's surrogate may authorize the physician to forgo life-sustaining treatment motivated by the same concern—the *intent,* as far as the law is concerned, is still to bring about the patient's death. Thus although we might not wish to call a death resulting from forgoing life-sustaining treatment a suicide or homicide, it is impossible in law to avoid this result simply by saying that the intent to bring about death is absent.

A final problem with the effort to distinguish passively and actively hastening death on the basis of differential intent is that whatever one can say about the intent in the former is true in the latter as well. If we assume that my arguments about intent are incorrect—that when treatment is forgone, there is *no* intent to cause death but rather an intent to relieve suffering and that this intent is insufficient to support criminal liability—then precisely the same could be said of intent in the case of *actively* hastening death. We can just as readily say that when a terminally ill patient in great pain takes an overdose of medication (either provided by a physician or obtained by some other means), the patient is merely intending to relieve suffering. Death is the incidental by-product of this effort, as it is in forgoing treatment, and thus the patient's death is not a suicide, and the person who provides the patient with the means of "relieving suffering" is not assisting suicide. In fact, by this argument, homicide would not be committed if someone other than the patient were to administer a lethal medication to the patient at the patient's request in order to relieve the patient's suffering, a conclusion which is plainly false in law.

Causation

The third stratagem used by courts to avoid characterizing the passive hastening of death as unlawful killing is to claim that when life-sustaining medical treatment is withheld or withdrawn, death results from natural causes rather than from the actions of the physician or other health care professional who withdraws or withholds treatment.[18] Because the conduct of the physician is said not to be the legal cause of death, there is no criminal liability. Other ways commonly used to express this same line of reasoning are that when treatment is withheld or withdrawn, the patient dies a natural death and that we are letting nature take its course; both locutions are intended to signify that Mother Nature, who is beyond prosecution, is the causal agent of death rather than the health care professionals who withhold or withdraw treatment.[19]

By contrast, courts conclude that when a physician engages in conduct that *actively* hastens death, the physician's conduct is the cause of death.[20] Causation may be clearer in instances of actively hastening death than in instances of passively hastening death, but this does not end the inquiry. It should merely invite us to probe deeper in the latter situations, which courts have been steadfastly unwilling to do.

There are several accepted tests of causation traditionally applied in criminal law. Under any of them, explanations as to why the physician who passively hastens death is not the cause of the death, yet the physician who actively hastens death is, do not wash.[21] The primary test accepted by the Model Penal Code is the "sine qua non" test. Under this test, to escape liability, we must be able to say that the defendant's conduct is not the sine qua non of the patient's death, that is, it is not the condition without which the patient would not have died.[22] When life-sustaining treatment is withheld or withdrawn, this test is clearly met if, had treatment not been withheld or withdrawn, the patient would not have died, at least not then and there, and it is well established that shortening the life of one who is close to death is still criminally culpable.[23]

A second test of causation is the "natural and probable consequences" test. Under this test, an actor's conduct is said to be the legally responsible cause of a result if the result is the natural and probable consequence of the actor's conduct.[24] If a patient is being maintained by some form of life support, it is because there is reasonable medical certainty that if that treatment is not administered, the patient will die. Thus if life-sustaining treatment is withdrawn, death is the natural and probable consequence of the withdrawal, and there would be no difficulty making a prima facie showing that this test of causation is met.

In situations in which life-sustaining medical treatment is withheld rather than withdrawn, as a practical matter it may be more difficult to establish that if the patient dies, not initiating the treatment causes the patient's death. Conceptually, however, if the treatment in question is truly "life-sustaining" treatment, then *ex hypothesis* the failure to administer it is the cause of the patient's death. In any event, these are questions of fact. What is important for present purposes is that in some situations of withholding of treatment, in accordance with this test the physician who withholds the intervention could be held to have caused the death. Thus we cannot make the blanket statement that withholding of treatment could never be the legal cause of death.

Sometimes a test of causation based on foreseeability is employed in adjudicating criminal liability. This test is not significantly different from the natural and probable consequences test,[25] and the analysis for present purposes is similar. So again, if a patient is being kept alive by a life-sustaining medical treatment, and the entire course of treatment or an essential ingredient of it is discontinued, it is reasonably foreseeable that the patient will die. Thus if such treatment is terminated, at least a prima facie case of causation in accordance with this test will easily be made.

The same is true of the other important test of causation used in criminal law, the "substantial factor" test,[26] used when there is more than one factual cause contributing to the result in question. Under this test, a person who terminates life support could be excluded as the legal cause of a patient's death only if termination were not a substantial factor in bringing about death, which clearly cannot be the case. In all instances of withdrawing life-sustaining treatment, the patient would not have died, at least not then and there, had treatment been continued. In other words, any time the sine qua non test is met, the substantial factor test is also met (though the converse is not always true).

Summary

Even when we recognize, as we must, that the concept of legal causation is ultimately a mix of factual and policy considerations about whom we want to hold responsible for what, to deny that there is legal causation in passively hastening death yet to find it in actively hastening death requires more than the mere assertion that causation is different in the two types of hastening death. Of course, these two types of hastening death are factually different; the question is whether those facts ought to make a difference with respect to the ultimate issue of culpability. To answer that question, we must be able to point to important, relevant differences between passively and actively hastening death. Perhaps there are some, but they are not to be found in the realm of legal causation, as they are not in the nature of the act or intent.

Legal Right

If it is the case, as I claim, that all of the elements of homicide or assisted suicide are met when life-sustaining treatment is withheld or withdrawn—act, intent, causation, and result—how could it be that criminal liability still does not ensue? In the case law adjudicating the legality of passively hastening death, the answer that has generally been given in determining that there is no criminal liability is that one or more of the elements of a crime cannot be established.

Some courts have added another and more forthright reason for refusing to brand passively hastening death as criminal: There is no criminal liability for passively hastening death because, in the words of one court, "the decision and its implementation are authorized under the common law."[27] Courts have in effect—though not always in these terms—concluded that it does not matter whether the elements of a crime have been satisfied when life-sustaining treatment is forgone. There is no criminal liability for passively hastening death because there is a *legal right* to have life-sustaining medical treatment withheld or withdrawn. Of course, there is no liability for doing something one has a right to do, but that begs the question of whether one has a legal right to do it. What these courts seem to be saying is that although one might be able to make a prima facie case based on each of the elements of assisted suicide or criminal homicide when life-sustaining medical treatment is withheld or withdrawn, nonetheless the conduct in question cannot constitute the basis for the imposition of criminal liability because there is a defense based on law to such charges.

Consent as Legitimating Actively Hastening Death

I have argued that actively and passively hastening death are on an equal footing before the law and that each ought to be treated as prima facie criminal because in each the elements of act, intent, and causation are met. Yet we do not treat passively hastening death as criminal when there is legally valid consent. I now want to turn to a consideration of whether we ought to treat actively hastening death similarly.

Passively hastening death is criminally nonculpable, when it *is* nonculpable, because the patient (or someone with legal authority to speak for the patient) gives consent to that over which the patient has legal dominion—that is, a valid right to control. The substantive right implemented by giving (or withholding) consent is the right to be let alone[28] (based on the common law, or the Constitution,[29] or both), which is itself derivative of a broader common-law right to be free from unwanted invasions of one's bodily and psychic integrity. In his concurring opinion in the Supreme Court cases, Justice Breyer said he "would use words roughly like a 'right to die with dignity'" to describe this right. He continued, "Irrespective of the exact words used, at its core would lie personal control over the manner of death, professional medical assistance, and the avoidance of unnecessary and severe physical suffering—combined."[30]

Opponents of legalization claim that actively hastening death does not implicate the right to be let alone. Their claim is that by its nature actively hastening death requires that there be some invasion of the patient's bodily and psychic integrity—the opposite of letting the patient alone.[31] Thus at bottom, they contend, the individual interests implicated in passively hastening death and actively hastening death are not only different, they are polar opposites.

Sometimes this argument is put in terms of the difference between a negative and a positive right. In passively hastening death, a negative right is said to be involved: a right to be free *from* unwanted interference with one's bodily integrity. By contrast, in actively hastening death, a positive right is said to be at stake: the patient is claiming entitlement against another to have something done *for* him. Positive rights are strongly disfavored by the common law[32] and by the Constitution,[33] and generally a positive right can be conferred only by statute. Thus if actively hastening death is to be legalized, it must be achieved by statutory enactment, as in Oregon.

This argument betrays a fundamental misunderstanding of what is at stake in the debate about actively and passively hastening death. First, to put it somewhat concretely, dying is at stake in both situations, or as Judge Reinhardt repeatedly penned in the *Compassion in Dying* case, "determining the time and manner of one's death."[34] As Justices Brennan and Stevens[35] and Breyer[36] have recognized, human dignity is as stake.

Second, this objection to actively hastening death—and the correlative attempt to distinguish it from passively hastening death—views the underlying right at stake in the "passive" cases too narrowly. What is involved is not merely a right to be free from unwanted bodily and psychic invasions; it is "a right to *determine* what shall be done with [one's] body," as Justice Cardozo put it generations ago.[37] The familiar locutions—such as the right to refuse treatment— are used simply because of the medical context in which the broader right has traditionally been made manifest.

Finally, the nature of the right involved in actively hastening death can just as surely be characterized as a negative right as that implicated in the "passive" cases.[38] What is fundamentally at stake in the legalization of actively hastening death, as it has been in the legalization of passively hastening death, is the *preclusion of state-imposed penalization of the conduct in question.* For example, in *Quinlan*—the first appellate case of passively hastening death—what the patient's guardian wanted was a decree that the power of the state, as manifested through the criminal process, would not be exacted against the physician whom the guardian sought to authorize to passively hasten death.

This is precisely what patients and physicians seek in cases attempting to legalize physician-assisted suicide. Proponents of physician-assisted suicide have not sought, nor should they be accorded, the right to compel physicians (or anyone else) to actively hasten death, even with a patient's consent. That would be a claim for a disfavored positive right. Instead, they seek to preclude the imposition by the state of penalties on a physician who willingly complies with the voluntarily made request of a competent patient to actively hasten that patient's death.

The analogy to abortion helps to illuminate this point. The litigation to establish a woman's right to choose abortion has sought not merely an abstract right to terminate a pregnancy. It would be an empty right if what had been sought and granted were merely the right of a woman to have an abortion without being subjected to criminal prosecution for so doing. Indeed, such a limited right would completely undercut the harm sought to be prevented—namely, the right not to have to subject oneself to dangerous self-performed measures to terminate a pregnancy. The right sought was to have a physician perform the operation without his or her being subject to prosecution.

The same is true in actively hastening death. Although some patients can actively hasten their own deaths, some—perhaps many—cannot. The right to actively hasten death, if there is to be one, is hardly a robust right if terminally ill people are denied the right to enlist the assistance of another.

The analogy to abortion is again useful. A woman can attempt to perform an abortion on herself, and she might even be successful. A terminally ill person can attempt to end his own life through a variety of means. In both cases, however, there are two kinds of risks in doing so. The first is that the effort will not succeed, and the second is that the person may incur a range of physical and psychic harms in the process of not succeeding. Then, of course, there are terminally ill people who lack the physical ability to even begin to arrange their own deaths and of necessity must rely on the assistance of another. The fundamental interest at stake in both actively and passively hastening death is the right to decide the time and manner of one's death and to procure the assistance necessary to transform that right into reality, *free from state interference.*[39]

The Need for Protections, Regardless of the Means

The battle over the legalization of actively hastening death turns out largely to be a battle over means, not ends. By this, I mean that there is little disagreement that it is humane to permit competent patients to end terminal suffering, indignity, dependence, and demoralization if they genuinely and steadfastly wish to do so. As long as that is guaranteed, virtually everyone accepts—certainly all legal authorities accept—that death sooner, rather than later, is permissible if that is the patient's will. Indeed, to deny competent patients the right to dispense with the indignities of a prolonged terminal illness is indisputably inhumane. As the former chief justice of the Florida Supreme Court observed, society has no interest in saving a life "when there is nothing of life to save but a final convulsion of agony."[40] For more than a quarter century, it has been legally acceptable to effectuate this result by one means—forgoing life-sustaining treatment—but not by another—so-called active interventions.

In some instances—what proportion may be impossible to gauge—people near the end of life cannot achieve their desired objective of hastening death by passive means because they are not dependent on any form of medical treatment that is prolonging the process of dying. To deny them the only form of relief available to them is no less inhumane than to deny patients on life support the right to terminate it.

Nonetheless, it is hard to deny that there are dangers lurking in the legalization of actively hastening death. They have been recited over and over in public debates, in legislative hearings, and in litigation. My purpose is not to attempt to refute these arguments. They must be taken seriously, and for argument's sake, at the very least, I grant their validity. However, what has been mostly overlooked is that these dangers also inhere in the now widely accepted—and legally acceptable—practice of forgoing life-sustaining treatment. Yet there is no evidence that, nor is there any abstract reason why, these arguments should be thought to be more compelling in the context of *actively* hastening death than they are in the context of *passively* hastening death. Virtually any argument that can be made against actively hastening death can be leveled with equal vigor against passively hastening death.

To take just few of the more prominent ones: It has been said that patients will be pressured into physician-assisted suicide.[41] However, physicians can subtly or heavy-handedly pressure patients into forgoing life-sustaining treatment by telling them that it is useless, painful, and expensive, or in myriad other ways. The claim is made that the lack of access to health care can cause patients to despair of getting the treatment they need and want, and they may reluctantly request or accede to a suggestion that they hasten their deaths through physician-assisted suicide.[42] However, patients dependent on life support might, for the same reasons, request or accede to a suggestion that they forgo life-sustaining treatment.

Physician-assisted suicide is said to be at odds with the ethics of the medical profession.[43] However, forgoing treatment was once at odds—or said to be at odds—with the ethics of the medical profession, and one of the factors in its acceptance by the medical profession was its legalization. It is feared that physicians will become hardened to the plight of the terminally ill by the knowledge that there is an easy way out for the patient—*easy* for the physicians, that is; but this is equally true of forgoing life-sustaining treatment. Family members will suffer severe loss when a terminally ill patient dies from assisted suicide; but they will suffer too if the patient chooses to forgo treatment or wishes to forgo treatment and is not allowed to do so. Finally, predictions that terminally ill patients should be prohibited from controlling the circumstances of their own deaths because the practice would be subject to widespread abuse applies equally to hastening death by forgoing life-sustaining treatment; and in the latter case, these fears have proved to be unfounded.

The debate about the legalization of actively hastening death has diverted public attention from the true problem. What we need to be concerned about —and where the public debate ought to be focused—is not the dangers of legalization of actively hastening death but the dangers of legalization of hastening death by whatever means—active or passive. To gain public confidence, both in passively and actively hastening death, the focus of our efforts should be on ensuring voluntary and informed consent.

Implications for Public Policy

I have attempted to show several things. First, the arguments that courts have put forth for two decades to justify the criminal nonculpability of passively hastening death are fundamentally unsound. Under the basic principles of criminal law, withholding or withdrawing life-sustaining treatment qualifies as homicide or assisted suicide. Nonetheless, these practices do not invoke criminal sanctions if there is legally adequate consent, and they should not.

Second, once the stock legal arguments used to justify passively hastening death are shown to be spurious, the purported legal distinctions between actively and passively hastening death begin to fade. They fade further when the distinction between active and passive is itself further probed, for at core, what is being sought in both cases is the *preclusion of state-imposed penalization* of the conduct in question.

Although there are sound, indeed strong, arguments against the legitimation of actively hastening death, these same arguments can be made with equal force against passively hastening death.[44] Yet they are not made, or when made they are rejected, despite the risks posed by the practice of passively hastening death. The focus of public policy needs to shift from the means by which death is hastened to the provision of adequate safeguards regardless of the means.

Notes

This chapter is adapted from "Physician-Assisted Suicide: A Roadmap for State Courts," *Fordham Urban Law Journal* 24 (1997): 801–41.

1. *Washington v. Glucksberg,* 521 U.S. 702 (1997); *Vacco v. Quill,* 521 U.S. 793 (1997).
2. *In re* Quinlan, 355 A.2d 647 (N.J. 1976).
3. *McIver v. Krischer,* 697 So.2d 97, 109 (Fla. 1997) (Kogan, C.J. concurring).

4. President's Commission for the Study of Ethical Problems in Medicine and Bio-medical and Behavioral Research, *Deciding to Forgo Life-Sustaining Treatment: Ethical, Medical and Legal Issues in Treatment Decisions* (Washington, D.C.: U.S. Government Printing Office, 1983), 64–66; *In re* Conroy, 486 A.2d 1209 (N.J. 1985), 1224.

5. W.R. LaFave and A.W. Scott Jr., *Substantive Criminal Law*, 2d ed. (St. Paul, Minn.: West Publishing, 1986), 202–3.

6. *In re* Conroy, 1234.

7. President's Commission for the Study of Ethical Problems, *Deciding to Forego Life-Sustaining Treatment*, 74.

8. *In re* Conroy, 1234.

9. *Superintendent of Belchertown State School v. Saikewicz*, 370 N.E.2d 417, 427 n. 11 (Mass. 1977).

10. *In re* Conroy, 1224.

11. *Compassion in Dying v. Washington*, 79 F.3d 790 (9th Cir. 1996), *rev'd sub nom. Washington v. Glucksberg*, 521 U.S. 702, 823 (1997).

12. American Law Institute, *Model Penal Code* (Philadelphia: American Law Institute, 1985), 230.

13. Ibid., sec. 2.02(1).

14. Ibid., sec. 2.02(b)(ii).

15. *Vacco v. Quill*, 808 n. 11.

16. W.C. Wilson and N.G. Smedira, "Ordering and Administration of Sedatives and Analgesics During the Withholding and Withdrawal of Life Support from Critically Ill Patients," *Journal of the American Medical Association* 267 (1992): 949–53, 949.

17. See D.B. Dobbs, R.E. Keeton, and D.G. Owen, eds., *Prosser and Keeton on the Law of Torts*, 5th ed. (St. Paul, Minn.: West Publishing, 1984), sec. 8, 35; LaFave and Scott, *Substantive Criminal Law*, 228.

18. *Rosebush v. Oakland County Prosecutor*, 491 N.W.2d 633 (Mich. Ct. App. 1992).

19. *Satz v. Perlmutter*, 362 So.2d 160, 162–63 (Fla. Dist. Ct. App. 1978).

20. *Vacco v. Quill*, 801.

21. *Compassion in Dying v. Washington*, 822–23.

22. American Law Institute, *Model Penal Code*, sec. 2.03(1)(a).

23. *Washington v. Glucksberg*, 714; *Barber v. Superior Court*, 195 Cal. Rptr. 484 (Ct. App. 1983).

24. R.M. Perkins and R.N. Boyce, *Criminal Law*, 3d ed. (Mineola, N.Y.: Foundation Press, 1982), 812–13.

25. Ibid., 812–13.

26. Ibid., 799–800.

27. *Rosebush v. Oakland County Prosecutor*, 641.

28. S.D. Warren and L.D. Brandeis, "The Right to Privacy," *Harvard Law Review* 4 (1890): 193–220.

29. *Olmstead v. United States*, 277 U.S. 438, 478 (1928) (Brandeis, J., dissenting).

30. *Washington v. Glucksberg*, 790.

31. *Washington v. Glucksberg*, 703.

32. Dobbs, Keeton, and Owen, *Prosser and Keeton on the Law of Torts,* 356–59, 373–85.

33. *DeShaney v. Winnebago County Department of Social Services,* 489 U.S. 189 (1989).

34. *Compassion in Dying v. Washington,* 793.

35. *Cruzan v. Director, Missouri Department of Health,* 497 U.S. 261 (1990).

36. *Washington v. Glucksberg,* 790.

37. *Schloendorff v. Society of New York Hospital,* 105 N.E. 92, 93 (N.Y. 1914).

38. *In re* Conroy, 1234.

39. J.E. Fleming, "Constitutional Tragedy in Dying: Responses to Some Common Arguments against the Constitutional Right to Die," *Fordham Urban Law Journal* 24 (1997): 881–88.

40. *McIver v. Krischer,* 109.

41. *Washington v. Glucksberg,* 730–31; *Compassion in Dying v. Washington,* 825.

42. *Compassion in Dying v. Washington,* 826.

43. *Washington v. Glucksberg,* 731; *Compassion in Dying v. Washington,* p. 827.

44. *Quill v. Vacco,* 80 F.3d 716, 730 (2d Cir. 1996), *rev'd,* 521 U.S. 793 (1997).

20

Choice in Dying

A Political and Constitutional Context

Sylvia A. Law, J.D.

This chapter seeks to place in historic perspective the current movement for compassion and patient choice at the end of life. While legal principles are important, the complex factors that shape individual consciousness, human relations, and social movement are also critical.

Since 1990 a vibrant movement for patient choice at the end of life has emerged in the United States. Two important developments promote this movement: first, advances in medicine and technology; second, the ongoing struggles for civil rights, respect, and choice on the part of racial minorities, women, gay people, and people with disabilities.

What Medicine Makes Possible

Until recent decades people rarely confronted questions about choice at the end of life. People died, and there was little that could be done to prolong the process. Beginning in the 1950s, medical science and technology began to be able to delay death and preserve base physical function. Since then, advances in the power to intervene, and to prolong dying, have come rapidly.

In 1968 doctors at Harvard Medical School proposed redefining death to include brain death as a supplement to heart and lung death.[1] Today, every state recognizes brain death as the legal and functional equivalent of the irreversible cessation of the heart or lungs. As we have developed our capacity to save life through organ transplants, powerful humanitarian reasons support recognition that dead is dead, whether it is the brain or the heart that cannot be revived.

In 1976, in the Karen Ann Quinlan case, the law recognized the "persistent vegetative state," in which people who are not brain dead are nonetheless extremely unlikely to regain consciousness.[2] The common law has always recognized that competent adults can refuse any medical treatment, even if death is a near certain consequence.[3] The Quinlan case extended the right to refuse treatment to people who are incompetent because they are in a persistent vegetative state. Today, in every state except New York and Missouri, the legal question asked is, "What would Karen Ann Quinlan want if she were able to express her own will?" If the evidence is that she would want the respirator or the feeding tube removed, that may be done. New York and Missouri demand more powerful evidence that the irreversibly unconscious patient would reject life support.[4]

These developments in medicine and technology have generated passionate debate. Technology can keep our physical bodies "alive" even when all hope for sentient humanity is gone. Millions of people have signed living wills and advance directives, and even more share their views about end-of-life care with loved ones. These developments also highlight the tension between our acknowledged right to refuse or end treatment, even if death is a certain consequence, and the fact that—except in Oregon—the law denies us the right to assistance in hastening death, however compelling the circumstances. In 1996 the federal Second Circuit Court of Appeals held that this logical inconsistency demanded that the law allow doctors to help hasten death so that all terminally ill people are treated equally to those who are dependent upon machines and can insist that they be turned off.[5]

Rights, Respect, and Choice

The movement for choice at the end of life is not simply the product of developments in medicine and technology. It is also an outgrowth of the liberation movements for people of color, women, gay people, and people with disabilities. Many events laid the foundation for the liberation movements of the 1970s. Following World War II, our collective human understanding of the atrocities authorized by the "law" of Hitler and Stalin led us, including the Supreme Court, to recognize fundamental human rights of equality, personal liberty, and privacy.[6] The African American civil rights movement of the 1960s heightened consciousness about the complexity of equality, the pervasive ways in which black experience was hidden and devalued, and the power of collective actions by common people. The war in Vietnam produced deep skepticism about official views of reality. Women noted and protested irrational limits on their capacities and opportunities. The movements against the war and in support of civil rights for black people and women suggested that ordinary people, acting collectively, could change strongly entrenched public policy.

These liberation movements grew through common and mutually reinforcing processes. By talking about their own experiences, people came to understand the dynamics that had for so long prevented them from asserting even straightforward claims to equal treatment or the right to control their own bodies and lives. Simultaneously with the rise of feminist consciousness, gay men began to resist police harassment. People who had previously acquiesced to public condemnation of their sexuality affirmed their self-worth. People with disabilities protested that they were being categorized, segregated, and condemned in ways that were cruel and irrational.[7]

The movement for compassion and choice in dying dates not from the 1960s or 1970s but rather from 1990. In that year the Supreme Court decided the *Cruzan* case, and Congress passed the Patient Self-Determination Act, which requires hospitals to inform patients of their right to sign an advance directive demanding or refusing treatment at the end of life.[8] Dr. Jack Kevorkian helped Janet Adkins, a patient from Oregon with Alzheimer's disease, die in the back of his rusty Volkswagen van.[9] Derek Humphry, founder of the Hemlock Society, published his suicide manual *Final Exit,* which within a few months topped the *New York Times* best-seller list.[10] Dr. Timothy Quill helped Patricia Diane Trumball die and described the experience in the *New England Journal of Medicine.*[11]

Just as feminism depended on consciousness raising (that is, on small groups of people sharing experience in honest ways), so too the movement for choice at the end of life seeks to promote frank exploration of feelings about complex choices. Compassion in Dying is the national organization that trains and supports volunteers to help dying people and their families engage in these difficult conversations.[12] Although people like Humphry and Kevorkian brought death out of the closet, they did so in ways that did not promote the kind of honest, collective personal exploration necessary to authentic individual choice. By contrast, through its trained volunteers, Compassion in Dying provides a means by which people confronting complex issues at the end of life can explore alternatives, deal with conflicting feelings, communicate, connect, and act. After the click of understanding, and the empowerment of collective consciousness raising, every liberation movement confronts the fact that liberty and equality—for blacks, women, gay people, those who are disabled, and those who are dying—is denied by the law. Liberty is denied not simply because internalized false consciousness makes people too shy to ask. It is denied because the law defines liberty and choice for these groups as a crime.

The battle to change the law can be fought locally by persuading prosecutors not to prosecute or by getting criminal sanctions repealed at the state level through legislation, referendums, or state constitutional decision. The law can be changed more grandly by getting the U.S. Supreme Court to recognize a fundamental, nationally protected, constitutional liberty.

Every liberation movement starts by challenging the law at the state and local levels. This grassroots work is exhausting, and liberation movements eventually turn to the Supreme Court, seeking recognition of a constitutionally protected right. The claims of liberty and choice for women, gay people, and people confronting death are similar. Control of reproduction, of adult consensual sexuality, and of the circumstances of death profoundly touch who we are and how we live. Each claim implicates deep and weighty individual interests in freedom of choice, however that choice is exercised. In each case, individuals have an important stake in avoiding shame and isolation.

On the other side, the public interests in criminalizing abortion, adult consensual sex, or physician-assisted death for adults who are terminally ill are vanishingly thin. The Oregon experience suggests that interests such as promotion of good pain care, the integrity of the medical profession, and the protection of vulnerable people all support legalized choice for terminally ill people. The only support for criminal prohibitions on choice is a particular concept of "morality."

In 1973 in *Roe v. Wade,* the Supreme Court affirmed, by a six-to-three majority, that the Constitution protects a woman's right to reproductive choice.[13] In 1992 the Court reaffirmed that right in *Casey,* five to four.[14] In 1986, in *Bowers v. Hardwick,* the Court (again five to four) rejected the claim that the Constitution prevents the criminal prosecution of consenting adults who engage in homosexual conduct.[15] In 1997, this time unanimously, the Court rejected Compassion in Dying's claim that the Constitution protects competent, terminally ill patients who seek physician aid in dying and affirmed that the state may subject doctors who provide such aid to criminal prosecution.[16]

It seems that these were huge victories for reproductive choice and huge losses for gay people and death with dignity. But sometimes winning is losing. *Roe v. Wade* unleashed a backlash unprecedented in modern American politics. The National Conference of Catholic Bishops organized a political campaign larger and better funded than any before or since. Understanding that Catholics are a minority, themselves divided, and cannot win politically by themselves, they recruited the fundamentalist Christian churches. Catholics are motivated by a theology that defines human life as beginning at conception and defines moral sex as necessarily open to the possibility of conception. Fundamentalists oppose abortion for slightly different reasons. They defend the patriarchal family as essential to God's plan and see the woman's right to choose as inconsistent with man's dominion over her. The key move politically, however, was made by Phyllis Shlafley, a longtime, effective leader of the Republican Party. She understood that the "anticommunism" of the 1950s was the core moral, non-economic appeal of the Republican Party. Republicans needed a new moral issue, and Shlafley persuaded them that "traditional family values" and opposition to abortion could play that role. Today, the Republican Party is a more powerful voice against reproductive choice than the Catholic Church.[17]

The constitutional right to reproductive choice prevailed in *Roe, Casey,* and even in the 2001 "partial birth abortion" case.[18] In 1980, however, the Supreme Court upheld exclusion of payment for abortion from the otherwise comprehensive Medicaid program for the poor.[19] Since then, it has approved onerous waiting periods and biased informed-consent requirements and allowed to stand state laws that require young people seeking abortion to obtain consent from both parents, even if a parent is abusive or absent.[20] Today there is no abortion provider in 89 percent of the counties in the United States.[21]

If abortion underscores that a constitutional victory can be defeated on the ground, then *Hardwick,* the gay rights case, may illustrate that losing can be transformed into victory. Had the Supreme Court recognized the constitutional liberty of homosexual people in 1986, we could have expected a backlash perhaps even more furious than the one triggered by *Roe.* Press reaction to the Supreme Court's decision in *Hardwick* was uniformly critical of the Court.[22] Since that decision, criminal prosecutions of gay people have virtually disappeared. There have been modest but steady improvements in the civil rights of gay people in relation to employment, domestic partner benefits, and in more general cultural values. In 2003 the Supreme Court acknowledged this changing social reality by overruling *Bowers v. Hardwick* and recognizing that criminal condemnation of homosexual acts "demeans the lives of homosexual persons."[23] It remains to be seen what sort of cultural backlash the decision will produce.

In sum, in the law, sometimes winning can be losing and losing can be winning. Certainly, our experience with reproductive choice shows that winning at the federal constitutional level is not enough by itself.

Change Outside the Law

Another lesson of the earlier movements for human liberation is that the most important changes often come outside of the law. Take childbirth, for example. Until the 1970s, standard medical practice dictated that a woman in labor be sedated and restrained, that she be given an episiotomy, and that the baby be removed from the unconscious mother by forceps. Friends and family were kept out of the delivery room. In the 1970s, women challenged these practices. Physician-controlled childbirth was often injurious both to women and to infants. Furthermore, the standard procedures failed to acknowledge that birth is a social and spiritual experience as well as a medical event. Although problems remain, childbirth in this country has been transformed. Virtually none of this transformation has been accomplished through the law, and absolutely none through the constitutional law. Rather, the change came about because women became informed and empowered. They questioned their doctors and picked services that would best meet their needs. The market responded.[24]

Movement for choice in dying is now generating a similar transformation. It has empowered people to question physicians about their approaches to pain and to death. It has encouraged the informed use of advance directives and powers of attorney. It has improved pain care through work with medical educators, professional associations, accrediting bodies, federal funders, medical licensing boards, and dramatic tort recoveries such as the *Bergman* case in California, in which a doctor was held liable for grossly inadequate treatment of his patient's pain.[25] It is proving more difficult to transform consciousness and practice in relation to death than in relation to birth, but huge strides have been made. Win or lose in the courts, the biggest changes come in human consciousness and on the ground.

When the Supreme Court rejected Compassion in Dying's constitutional claim in 1997, a central reason given was that no state had ever legalized physician-assisted dying and we knew very little about whether the practice would lead to involuntary euthanasia of the most vulnerable people. The Court rarely recognizes a constitutional right that no state has embraced. When the Court recognized the right to use contraception in *Griswold v. Connecticut* in 1965, every state except Connecticut had already done so.[26] Similarly, by the time of *Roe*, most states had legalized abortion, and New York was providing free abortions in its public hospitals to women from other states. While Supreme Court recognition of a constitutional right sounds like a grand affirmation of liberty, most often it is a mopping-up operation to bring the outliers into the consensus that has already been reached in the states.

In 1997, when the Court rejected Compassion in Dying's constitutional claim, we did not know what would happen under the Oregon Death with Dignity Act. We did not know that the law, and the practice it legally recognized, would be humane and compassionate and would not lead to the abuse of vulnerable people.[27]

Shortly after the Oregon law went into effect, an official in the federal Drug Enforcement Administration sought to invoke the federal Controlled Substances Act to threaten Oregon doctors with loss of federal prescribing privileges if they provided dying patients services authorized by the state law. Janet Reno, President Bill Clinton's attorney general, ruled that this was not a legitimate use of the federal regulations. Reno found that the Controlled Substances Act addresses the illicit use of addictive drugs and does not apply to the Oregon's Death with Dignity Act. John Ashcroft, then a Republican senator from Missouri, proposed legislation to amend the Controlled Substances Act to overrule Oregon's Death with Dignity Act. His proposal was soundly rejected by the Senate. Then, in the midst of our post–September 11 crisis, Ashcroft adopted the regulations that Reno had previously rejected as not authorized by the statue.[28] The U.S. District Court for Oregon found that Ashcroft's actions were not authorized by the federal statute, and the Ninth Circuit affirmed.[29] If upheld, the Ashcroft directive is likely to have an adverse impact on palliative care, wholly apart from situations in which people seek to hasten death. Even if the federal courts eventually hold that Ashcroft's regulations were unauthorized, Congress could probably prohibit states from adopting laws like Oregon's Death with Dignity Act.

Choice at end of life is also an issue of class. Educated people with money have always been able to get abortions and to live comfortable, if discrete, lives as homosexuals. So too with death. John H. Pickering, senior counsel to the firm of Wilmer, Cutler and Pickering and senior adviser to the American Bar Association's Commission on Legal Problems of the Elderly, offered a ringing defense of bans on physician-assisted dying, relying on the need to protect the vulnerable. Quite curiously, and with admirable candor, he added, "At the same time I selfishly reserve my right to do in private what my family, my doctor and pastor and I, in loving consultation, voluntarily agree is best."[30] The compassion in dying movement defends for all the rights that Pickering asserts for himself.

The movement for choice at the end of life is part of a great cultural war. The post–World War II generation who have lived their lives making choices about relationships, sexuality, reproduction, and childbirth are not likely suddenly to say, "Well, now that I am dying, the state can tell me how." But history is never inevitable.

Notes

1. "A Definition of Irreversible Coma: Report of the Ad Hoc Committee of the Harvard Medical School to Examine the Definition of Brain Death," *Journal of the American Medical Association* 205 (1968): 337–40, 337.

2. *In re* Quinlan, 355 A.2d 647 (N.J. 1976), *cert. denied,* 429 U.S. 922 (1976).

3. See, for example, *Lane v. Candura,* 376 N.E.2d 1232 (Mass. App. Ct. 1978).

4. R.E. Rosenblatt, S.A. Law, and S. Rosenbaum, eds., *Law and the American Health Care System* (Westbury, N.Y.: Foundation Press, 1997).

5. *Quill v. Vacco,* 80 F.3d 716 (2d Cir. 1996), *rev'd,* 521 U.S. 793 (1997).

6. *Skinner v. Oklahoma ex rel. Williamson,* 316 U.S. 535 (1942).

7. See discussion in *Cleburne v. Cleburne Living Center, Inc.,* 473 U.S. 432 (1985).

8. *Cruzan v. Director, Missouri Department of Health,* 497 U.S. 261 (1990); Patient Self-Determination Act of 1990, *U.S. Code* 42, sec. 1395cc (2000).

9. *People ex rel. Oakland County Prosecuting Attorney v. Kevorkian,* 534 N.W.2d 172, 173 (Mich. Ct. App. 1995).

10. A. Solomon, "A Death of One's Own," *New Yorker,* May 22, 1995, 54–64, 59.

11. T.E. Quill, "Death and Dignity: A Case of Individualized Decision Making," *New England Journal of Medicine* 205 (1991): 691–94.

12. The Compassion in Dying website is found at http://www.compassionindying.org.

13. *Roe v. Wade,* 410 U.S. 133 (1973).

14. *Planned Parenthood of Southeastern Pennsylvania v. Casey,* 505 U.S. 833 (1992).

15. *Bowers v. Hardwick,* 478 U.S. 186 (1986).

16. *Washington v. Glucksberg,* 521 U.S. 702 (1997).

17. S.A. Law, "Tort Liability and the Availability of Contraceptive Drugs and Devices in the United States," *N.Y.U. Review of Law and Social Change* 23 (2003): 339–401, 398.

18. *Stenberg v. Carhart,* 530 U.S. 914 (2001).

19. *Harris v. McRae,* 448 U.S. 297 (1980).

20. *Planned Parenthood of Southeastern Pennsylvania v. Casey.*

21. S.K. Henshaw, "Factors Hindering Access to Abortion Services," *Family Planning Perspectives* 27 (1995): 54–64, 54.

22. S.A. Law, "Homosexuality and the Social Meaning of Gender," *Wisconsin Law Review* 1988 (1988): 187–235.

23. *Lawrence v. Texas,* 123 S. Ct. at 2484 (2003).

24. Rosenblatt, Law, and Rosenbaum, *Law and the American Health Care System,* 1270.

25. *Bergman v. Chin,* No. H205732-1 (Cal. Super. Ct. June 13, 2001).

26. *Griswold v. Connecticut,* 381 U.S. 479 (1965).

27. *Fifth Annual Report on Oregon's Death with Dignity Act (2002),* available at www.dhs.state.or.us/publichealth/chs/pas.cfm (accessed December 8, 2003).

28. See *Oregon v. Ashcroft,* 192 F. Supp. 2d 1077, 1082 (D. Or. 2002), aff'd 2004 U.S. App. LEXIS 10349 (9th Cir. 2004).

29. Ibid.

30. Cited in S.A. Law, "Physician Assisted Death: An Essay on Rights and Remedies," *Maryland Law Review* 55 (1996): 292–342, 314.

21

Hastening Death

The Seven Deadly Sins of the Status Quo

Charles H. Baron, A.B., LL.B., Ph.D.

The law regarding end-of-life treatment is at an awkward and dangerous stage. In response to modern medicine's capacity to prolong life beyond the point some patients can bear, U.S. courts, beginning with *Quinlan*,[1] have effected a series of compromises in the law of homicide and assisted suicide. The compromises have left us feeling fairly secure as to the handling of the most common and pressing end-of-life dilemmas. However, they rely on a complicated, fictional conceptual framework that will not bear close scrutiny. Under current law, positive acts, like switching off a ventilator, are treated as mere "omissions to act." (At least when physicians take such action for consenting, terminally ill patients. Turning off a ventilator would clearly be treated as an "action" if you and I went into an ICU and did it on a drunken spree.) Physicians' acts in hastening death with pain medication are considered not to be acts of homicide if, and only if, the physician who prescribes the medication is thinking (while prescribing) that he or she is primarily trying to suppress pain and only incidentally shortening life. (That such acts are homicide, however, if the secret intention at the moment of prescription is to shorten the life of the suffering patient is reminiscent of the regime of birth control before *Griswold v. Connecticut.*[2] In those days, packs of condoms bore the legend, "For prevention of disease only." Whether someone using a condom was committing a crime or not depended upon whether he or she secretly harbored a forbidden intention to avoid pregnancy at the time of use.)

The present conceptual framework finds defenders in those who seek "bright line" distinctions between what is to be forbidden and what is to be permitted in ending the lives of terminally ill patients. Kamisar and Coleman, for example, argue that we must cling to current boundary concepts to avoid sliding down a slippery slope to invidiously discriminatory involuntary euthanasia.[3] However, there is little evidence that current concepts mark clear boundaries for those in practice. Foley, among others, has pointed out the difficulty physicians have in understanding and applying current criteria for deciding what is lawful and what is not;[4] and experience over the years since *Quinlan* shows that grabbing at bright-line distinctions doesn't keep us from sliding down slippery slopes. *Quinlan*'s recognition of the right of a patient in a persistent vegetative state to refuse (by proxy) an indefinite existence on a ventilator, for example, seems to have become today's right of any competent patient to hasten death by refusing to eat or to drink.[5] Advocates of a bright-line distinction are continually forced to look for new stopping points. Kamisar, who used to argue that respect for human life would be unalterably undermined if laws regarding homicide and assisted suicide were interpreted to allow patients to refuse life-prolonging treatment, now takes only a rearguard position opposing exceptions for physician-assisted suicide and active euthanasia.[6]

Attempting to cling to bright-line distinctions does not seem to offer us much protection, and it comes at significant cost. In the case of the line purportedly drawn against physician-assisted suicide, we have created at least the following seven costly and dangerous problems that I shall call the "seven deadly sins of the status quo":

- inhumanity
- paternalism
- utilitarianism
- hypocrisy
- lawlessness
- injustice
- deadly risk of error and abuse

Inhumanity

Denying physician-assisted suicide as an option to terminally ill patients means enforced suffering for many patients. If hastening of death is available only to those who can obtain it through refusal of life-prolonging treatment, such as cardiopulmonary resuscitation or artificial ventilation, then patients who do not need such treatment are required to soldier on. (Ironically, the opposite may be true for terminally ill patients who require temporary life support or an intervention to correct a life-threatening complication. They may feel forced into refusing treatment prematurely for fear that an option to refuse may not come later, at a time when they might dearly want it.) Of course, recent years have seen efforts to expand the concept of "refusal of treatment" to include refusal to drink or eat—an option that is available to any patient at any time. Even assuming that the law recognizes such a right to dehydrate or starve oneself to death, it hardly provides the humane option (for the patient or the patient's loved ones) afforded by a system of physician-assisted suicide that might provide a swift, painless, and dignified death at a time of the patient's choosing and in the company of his or her friends and family.

Paternalism

In denying legality to physician-assisted suicide, we are currently granting society the power to tell dying patients, "You must continue to suffer because it is good for you." Some members of our society believe, as Callahan does, that suffering at the end of life may serve some important goal for the dying person. "Our duty," he says, "is to enhance one another's good and welfare, and the relief of suffering will ordinarily be an important way to accomplish that. But not always. What we need to know is whether the suffering exists because without it some other human good cannot be attained; and that is exactly the case with the suffering caused by living out one's moral duties or ideals for a life."[7] Adherents of such a view may base their paternalism on avowedly religious grounds. In some religious systems, suicide is forbidden under all circumstances —even if it is to avoid unbearable suffering while facing imminent death from a terminal disease. Certainly, those who wish to follow such religious precepts by bravely bearing a long and painful dying process should have the right to do so—whether or not society believes it is good for them. On the other hand, why shouldn't those who are not so committed have the same right to decide what is best for themselves? Imagine a legislature dominated by Jehovah's Witnesses: Would we tolerate its members' forbidding those of us who are not adherents of their religion the right to a life-saving blood transfusion because they believed it to be proscribed in the Bible?

Of course, Jehovah's Witnesses have typically been victims, rather than practitioners, of medical paternalism. In the 1960s and early 1970s, blood transfusions were often forced on them "for their own good." Doctors who believed that rejecting life-saving treatment on such religious grounds was irrational got the legal system to support them in that judgment.[8] American physicians were at the peak of their power to decide what was best for their patients. In a 1961 article in the *Journal of the American Medical Association,* Oken reports that oncologists regularly refused to tell patients the truth about their condition. "Most people do not want to know," was a typical reason given for not being honest. "Knowledge of cancer is 'a death sentence,' 'a Buchenwald,' and 'torture.' Telling is 'the cruelest thing in the world,' 'awful,' and 'hitting the patient with a baseball bat.'" However, study after study had demonstrated that the vast majority of cancer patients actually wanted to be told the truth. How to explain the discrepancy? Oken concludes,

> Avoidance of telling reflects the psychological problems of the doctor. If any group is constantly bombarded with the awful fact of death it is doctors— the same group which has such strong needs to conquer it. . . . Situations of this kind, associated with intense charges of unpleasant emotions, call forth a variety of psychological defenses which reduce the intensity of feelings to manageable proportions. Among such defenses are those which involve the avoidance, negation, or denial of the existence of some unpleasant fact, and acting as if it were not real.[9]

Similarly, those physicians who today oppose legalization of physician-assisted suicide may be concerned more with their own feelings than with their patients' welfare. Solomon has documented the fact that physicians tend to avoid methods of hastening death that leave them feeling directly responsible for "killing" the patient.[10] They prefer ending life-prolonging treatment over assisting suicide and, still more, favor not starting such treatment over stopping it once it's begun. "Among the motivations for entering medicine," Oken observes, "the wish to conquer suffering and death stands high on the list. Practicing physicians are not the kind of persons who can sit quietly by while nature pursues its course."[11] The law no longer allows the physician's needs to outweigh those of the patient when it comes to sitting quietly by "while nature pursues its course." The law should not allow them to trump those of the patient as regards legalization of the practice of physician-assisted suicide.

Utilitarianism

The most common form of argument made in support of the status quo essentially tells dying patients, "You must continue to suffer because it is good for *us.*" Dying patients' interests, it is said, must be sacrificed for the public good. One variant is the claim that keeping physician-assisted suicide illegal helps motivate the health care system to improve delivery of palliative care. Reducing patient suffering by allowing physicians to hasten death makes it too easy, this argument contends, for society to escape its obligation to render dying more comfortable. Foley and Hendin, for example, endorse "the World Health Organization recommendation that governments not consider the legalization of physician-assisted suicide and euthanasia until they have demonstrated the full availability and practice of palliative care for all citizens."[12] It is hard not to sympathize with any strategy for improving the delivery of palliative care; but what evidence is there that forcing individual patients to undergo unnecessarily prolonged lives will succeed in doing that? Indeed, empirical evidence from the Oregon experiment would seem to demonstrate just the opposite—that delivery of palliative care improves when physician-assisted suicide is an option.[13]

Most troubling, this strategy conscripts suffering patients as cannon fodder—and for what is likely to be a very long campaign. ("I'm sorry, Mr. Smith. Letting you end your life early to avoid your personal suffering is too easy an out for the health care delivery system. We can't let anyone do that until the system has demonstrated to our satisfaction that there is 'full availability and practice of palliative care for all citizens.'") If winning the palliative care battle in this way really makes sense and has moral validity, why aren't we denying patients the right to refuse life-prolonging treatment in situations in which better palliative care might have prevented them from throwing in the towel? This would put at stake the suffering of many thousands more patients each year and would presumably apply that much more pressure on "the system."

A willingness to sacrifice the interests of individual dying patients for those of society as a whole is also at the heart of every form of "slippery-slope" argument made in support of the status quo. Opponents of physician-assisted suicide warn us that the price of too much compassion for a particular suffering, terminally ill patient may be abuse of other patients and a general undermining of respect for human life. These seem to be empirical claims—appeals to laws of cause and effect. However, it is sometimes hard to know exactly what is being predicted. That doctors or relatives will not fully understand how to use the criteria for determining when it is all right, and when not, to assist a suffering patient to end his life? That they will make mistakes in determining the relevant facts? That they will cheat (out of self-interest, on the basis of prejudice, and the like)? Or is it a more global claim that the bonds of civilization will be generally cast aside once our society no longer enshrines as an absolute principle the sanctity of human life?

Whatever the precise import of the claims, they are serious and deserve to be taken seriously. They were, of course, taken seriously by the U.S. courts that gradually fashioned what has become the right to refuse life-prolonging treatment. At each stage, the courts recognized that respect for the rights of individual suffering patients required more than merely giving in to fear of the unknown. Taking tentative steps, the courts promulgated substantive standards and procedural protections that were designed to mitigate the risk of slippery-slope problems while freeing palliative care practitioners to act with greater respect for patient autonomy and increased compassion for the plight of the terminally ill.[14]

Would legalizing physician-assisted suicide make the risks any greater or more intractable? The patient who is considering a hastened death by refusal of life support is no less vulnerable to depression, coercion, prejudice, financial pressure, ineffective communication, mental incompetence, failure of adequate palliative care, impatience of medical personnel, or mistaken prognosis or diagnosis than the patient who is considering a hastened death by physician-assisted suicide. Indeed, as to some of these risks, legalization of refusal of treatment would seem more dangerous than legalization of physician-assisted suicide. Is a vulnerable patient more likely to succumb to a request that she commit suicide or to the statement, "You know, Mrs. Jones, maybe we've put you through enough. Maybe it's time to think of giving up?" Are impatient or prejudiced medical personnel more likely to be tempted to cut financial and emotional costs by means of physician-assisted suicide or by terminating life-prolonging treatment that they can claim has become "medically inappropriate"? Ironically, there may be less slippery-slope basis for denying patients the option of physician-assisted suicide than for denying them the right to refuse treatment. At the very least, there is no more.

Hypocrisy

A major vice of the current regime is its corrupting influence on the health care professions. An air of hypocrisy currently surrounds the practice of palliative care. Despite the illegality of physician-assisted suicide and euthanasia, many health care professionals admit to engaging in one or the other practice when they feel circumstances require it. "Don't worry," they will say in private (almost with a wink), "such steps are being taken when they need to be. Everyone knows that they are. The law doesn't need to get involved here. Better to leave all this to the individual physician's clinical judgment." Although the American Medical Association takes a public stand against physician-assisted suicide,[15] it seems opposed only to its legalization, not to its practice. Despite a number of articles reporting fairly widespread practice of physician-assisted suicide—some of them published in the pages of its own journal[16]—the association has not taken steps to find out who these physicians are in order to have them disciplined. Indeed, it has not even expressed shock to find that the practice is going on. Rather than being concerned with protecting society and patients from the evils of assisted suicide, the American Medical Association appears concerned to protect its members from the evils of legalization—the bad public relations or increased legal oversight that might result from an admission that doctors sometimes take positive steps to terminate the lives of suffering patients.[17]

Lawlessness

Physicians are not the only ones taking the law into their own hands. Mercy killings by family members are regularly reported in the press; many more most likely go unreported and undetected. Prosecutions are often dropped, grand juries do not indict, and trial juries acquit. When there are convictions, they are usually followed by light sentences. As a particularly striking example, consider the case of Vernal "Bob" Ohlrich of Nebraska. In October 1998, when Mr. Ohlrich was seventy-six, he responded to his seventy-four-year-old wife's pleas for relief from the pain she suffered while being treated for colon cancer by entering her hospital room with a gun and killing her with one shot to the head. Mr. Ohlrich then turned the gun on himself, but it misfired. He was charged with first-degree murder but avoided trial by agreeing to plead to manslaughter. In a bizarre twist, the state pathologist who autopsied Mrs. Ohlrich reported her to have been free of cancer at the time of her death. The prosecutor accepted the results of the autopsy but, noting that Mrs. Ohlrich had once been diagnosed with cancer and was in pain at the time of her death, recommended that Mr. Ohlrich serve only a short term in prison.[18] In July 1999 Mr. Ohlrich was sentenced to two years in a correctional facility. (The maximum penalty for manslaughter in Nebraska is twenty years in prison and a $25,000 fine.) A year later, he was paroled.[19]

Mr. Ohlrich fared better than sixty-six-year-old Dietrich "Whitey" Brandt of Pennsylvania, who was sentenced to life imprisonment for beating his sixty-five-year-old wife to death with a two-foot-long oxygen tank in answer to her prayers for death to end her suffering from asthma, congestive heart failure, and diabetes.[20] Mr. Ohlrich did not do as well, however, as forty-two-year-old Susan Scheufler of New York. She smothered her fifty-five-year-old terminally ill husband with a pillow on his deathbed. The Rensselaer County district attorney refused to prosecute.[21] Overall, mercy killings receive increasingly lenient treatment. Back in 1985, when seventy-five-year-old Roswell Gilbert shot to death his seventy-three-year-old wife to end her suffering from Alzheimer's disease and osteoporosis, the State of Florida convicted him of first-degree murder and sent him to prison for life. In 1990 the governor pardoned him.[22] By 1998 a Florida court felt it could acquit seventy-two-year-old Justina Rivero of attempted murder (on grounds of insanity) for having laced her Alzheimer's-afflicted husband's food with rat poison.[23] In that same year, a Florida prosecutor refused even to bring charges against seventy-one-year-old Elaine McIlroy after she confessed three times to three different police departments that she had assisted the suicide of her seventy-five-year-old, leukemia-suffering husband by sprinkling the contents of Seconal tablets over his chocolate ice cream. Florida judges and prosecutors expressed decreased willingness to pursue such cases because they viewed them more compassionately than they previously had and because of "lack of evidence, uncooperative family members, and juries' reluctance to convict defendants."[24]

Injustice

Manifestly, those who break the law to end the suffering of patients and loved ones cannot expect equal treatment under law. Whether they will be sentenced to life in prison or left completely alone will depend on the luck of their draw of police officers, emergency medical personnel, public prosecutors, grand juries, trial juries, and judges—each of whom will have the chance to exercise his or her discretion for or against leniency. Similarly, terminally ill patients cannot expect just treatment under such a system. Although physician-assisted suicide is technically illegal in almost all American jurisdictions, it most likely takes place in all of them. Whether it will be available, however, to any given patient will depend (everywhere but Oregon) less on the merit of that patient's case than on his or her ability to find an empathetic and courageous physician who feels safe with the patient, the patient's family, and the patient's attending medical personnel. In this respect, the present regime regarding physician-assisted suicide is much like that regarding abortion before *Roe v. Wade*. In the 1960s and the early 1970s, women with the right connections found physicians to provide them with professional help; those without were abandoned to the often grotesque ministrations of amateurs. Today, it is the terminally ill patient—unable to obtain physician assistance in suicide—who may be forced to resort to a gunshot to the head or rat poison sprinkled on dessert.

Deadly Risk of Error and Abuse

Maintaining the present legal regime unduly heightens the risk of deadly mistakes and abuse in the treatment of terminally ill patients. In the face of increasing sympathy for the plight of suffering patients, the legal system largely looks the other way when physicians—and even family members—assist in suicide. Of course, persons providing assistance have to keep in mind that there is always the chance that they could be caught and punished, and some argue that the threat of punishment provides a check against abuse sufficient to ensure that assistance in suicide and euthanasia will be employed in only the most compelling and meritorious cases.[25] In the 1970s some commentators similarly argued that the threat of criminal punishment was enough to regulate decisions to withdraw life-prolonging treatment from terminally ill patients.[26] However, we have wisely abandoned the "slow codes" and secret do-not-resuscitate orders of days gone by in favor of open procedures for permitting patients to die without undergoing last-ditch efforts at resuscitation. Post hoc criminal review is a very rough tool for regulating such sensitive decisions— especially when both the life of the patient and the freedom and reputation of the actor are at stake. Criminal review comes too late to rectify any errors, such as the apparent error involved in diagnosing colon cancer as the source of Mrs. Ohlrich's pain, and at a time when patients can no longer be interviewed as to whether steps were taken on the basis of their competent, informed, and voluntary consent.

Leaving regulation to the possibility of post hoc criminal review also discourages honest communication among health care professionals and between professionals and their patients.[27] It inhibits helpful professional consultations and the development of medical protocols. Fear of open discussion creates the possibility that physician's orders or patient's wishes will be misread.[28] Making matters worse, the chilling effect of post hoc criminal review extends beyond the realm of technically illegal practices such as physician-assisted suicide. Among other things, physicians' fear of appearing after the fact to have intentionally hastened a patient's death with morphine, as Foley points out, is a leading cause of undertreatment of pain in terminally ill patients.[29]

The risk of deadly mistakes and abuse in the treatment of terminally ill patients is exacerbated in yet another way by the current regime. In attempting to maintain a bright-line distinction between physician-assisted suicide and refusal of life-prolonging treatment, the regime does not treat decisions opting for the latter as seriously as it should. Today, we recognize not only the right of

Jehovah's Witnesses and others to refuse treatment on the ground that the treatment itself is offensive to them and the right of patients or their proxies to decide that, on balance, the patient would prefer to die relatively comfortably without chemotherapy than live a somewhat extended uncomfortable life with chemotherapy, but also the right of a patient who has decided that life no longer has any meaning for him or her to end that life by refusing life-prolonging treatment. In *Brophy v. New England Sinai Hospital, Inc.,* for example, Brophy's exercise of his right to refuse life support was not based on any objection to artificial nutrition or hydration; it was based on his frequently expressed preference to have his life terminated by any means if he were ever to end up in a persistent vegetative state. It just happened that ending artificial nutrition and hydration was a convenient, if not the most merciful, way to accomplish that end.[30]

Such decisions to die raise the same issues of patient autonomy and compassion toward suffering patients that are raised by physician-assisted suicide, and they face all the same risks of abuse and mistake. Yet the present regime categorizes them as mere determinations to "let nature take its course." Coleman, for one, sees the danger in this and calls on us to work with the organization Not Dead Yet "to minimize the damage resulting from professional, cultural, and economic factors in the context of refusal of treatment." (Indeed, all of the cases of abuse of the disabled that she points to are cases involving refusal of treatment.) She herself, however, is so caught up in the effort to retain "the *relatively* 'bright line' distinction between passive measures that cause death and active measures that cause death" that she treats the problem of abuse of passive euthanasia as a lesser priority.[31]

Moving Forward

In 1691 the Virginia Colony passed a law forbidding freed slaves from continuing to reside within its boundaries.[32] The society could not abide the presence of living counterexamples to its racist theories of the black man's inability to become civilized and to live with whites in anything but a state of servitude. Today, in similar fashion, U.S. Attorney General John Ashcroft and other foes of legalization of physician-assisted suicide feel they must do all they can to terminate the Oregon experiment. It is a living contradiction of their claims that progressing beyond the current regime will inevitably lead to unchecked abuse and invidious discrimination. As legal experiments go, the Oregon law has been extraordinarily successful. Over time, problems will doubtless surface, and changes will have to be made to correct them. Nevertheless, the five-year Oregon experience demonstrates that there is no longer need to fear the unknown. Whether through common-law development in the courts or by legislative action, it is time to move on to the next stage in making laws that show greater respect for patient autonomy and increased compassion for the plight of the terminally ill.

Notes

1. *In re* Quinlan, 70 N.J. 10, 355 A.2d 647 (1976).

2. *Griswold v. Connecticut,* 381 U.S. 479 (1965).

3. Y. Kamisar, "The Rise and Fall of the 'Right' to Assisted Suicide," in *The Case against Assisted Suicide: For the Right to End-of-Life Care,* edited by K. Foley and H. Hendin (Baltimore: Johns Hopkins University Press, 2002), 69–93; D. Coleman, "Not Dead Yet," in *The Case against Assisted Suicide: For the Right to End-of-Life Care,* edited by K. Foley and H. Hendin (Baltimore: Johns Hopkins University Press, 2002), 213–37.

4. K. Foley, "Compassionate Care, Not Assisted Suicide," in *The Case against Assisted Suicide: For the Right to End-of-Life Care,* edited by K. Foley and H. Hendin (Baltimore: Johns Hopkins University Press, 2002), 293–309, 304.

5. R. McStay, "Terminal Sedation: Palliative Care for Intractable Pain, Post *Glucksberg* and *Quill,*" *American Journal of Law and Medicine* 29 (2003): 45–76, 57.

6. Y. Kamisar, "Some Non-Religious Views against Proposed 'Mercy-Killing' Legislation," *Minnesota Law Review* 42 (1958): 969–1042, 977, 1031; Kamisar, "Rise and Fall of the 'Right' to Assisted Suicide," 72–74.

7. D. Callahan, "Reason, Self-Determination, and Physician-Assisted Suicide," in *The Case against Assisted Suicide: For the Right to End-of-Life Care,* edited by K. Foley and H. Hendin (Baltimore: Johns Hopkins University Press, 2002), 52–68, 56.

8. *Raleigh Fitkin-Paul Morgan Memorial Hospital v. Anderson,* 42 NJ 10, 355 A.2d 647 (1076).

9. D. Oken, "What to Tell Cancer Patients: A Study of Medical Attitudes," *Journal of the American Medical Association* 175 (1961): 1120–28, 1120, 1125, 1127.

10. M.Z. Solomon, L. O'Donnell, B. Jennings, V. Guilfoy, S.M. Wolf, K. Nolan, R. Jackson, D. Koch-Weser, and S. Donnelley, "Decisions Near the End of Life: Professional Views on Life-Sustaining Treatments," *American Journal of Public Health* 83 (1993): 14–23

11. Oken, "What to Tell Cancer Patients," 1126.

12. K. Foley and H. Hendin, "A Medical, Ethical, Legal, and Psychosocial Perspective," introduction to *The Case against Assisted Suicide: For the Right to End-of-Life Care,* edited by K. Foley and H. Hendin (Baltimore: Johns Hopkins University Press, 2002), 1–14, 2.

13. L. Ganzini, H.D. Nelson, M.A. Lee, D.F. Kraemer, T.A. Schmidt, and M.A. Delorit, "Oregon Physicians' Attitudes about and Experiences with End-of-Life Care Since Passage

of the Oregon Death with Dignity Act," *Journal of the American Medical Association* 285 (2001): 2363–69.

14. C.H. Baron, "Medicine and Human Rights: Emerging Substantive Standards and Procedural Protections for Medical Decision Making within the American Family," *Family Law Quarterly* 17 (1983): 1–40.

15. P.R. Muskin, "The Request to Die: Role for a Psychodynamic Perspective on Physician-Assisted Suicide," *Journal of the American Medical Association* 279 (1998): 323–28; T.E. Quill, B. Lo, and D.W. Brock, "Palliative Options of Last Resort: A Comparison of Voluntarily Stopping Eating and Drinking, Terminal Sedation, Physician-Assisted Suicide, and Voluntary Active Euthanasia," *Journal of the American Medical Association* 278 (1997): 2099–104.

16. A.L. Back, J.I. Wallace, H.E. Starks, and R.A. Pearlman, "Physician-Assisted Suicide and Euthanasia in Washington State: Patient Requests and Physician Responses," *Journal of the American Medical Association* 275 (1996): 919–25; S.H. Miles, "Physicians and Their Patients' Suicides," *Journal of the American Medical Association* 271 (1994): 1786–88.

17. A.M. Capron, "The Right to Die: Progress and Peril," *Euthanasia Review* 2 (1987): 41–59; S.M. Wolf, "Holding the Line on Euthanasia," *Hastings Center Report* 19, Suppl. no. 1 (1999): 13–15.

18. D. Hendee, "Deshler Man Calls Plea Right Thing 'For the Kids,'" *Omaha (Neb.) World Herald*, February 8, 1999, 9; D. Hendee, "Accuracy of Slaying Victim's Autopsy Questioned," *Omaha (Neb.) World Herald*, February 10, 1999, 19.

19. D. Hendee, "Deshler Man Sentenced to Prison in Wife's Death," *Omaha (Neb.) World Herald*, July 3, 1999, 1; R. Tysver, "Deshler Man Who Shot Ill Wife Wins Parole," *Omaha (Neb.) World Herald*, August 30, 2000, 1.

20. T. Gibb, "He Calls it Mercy, Jury Says Murder," *Pittsburgh Post-Gazette*, February 18, 1999, C1.

21. C. Woodruff, "A Final Breath Cloaked in Doubt," *Albany (N.Y.) Times Union*, January 17, 1999, A1.

22. M. Billington and B. Walsh, "Freedom for Gilbert Quick Clemency in Murder Case Stuns Family," *Fort Lauderdale (Fla.) Sun-Sentinel*, August 2, 1990, 1A.

23. N. Sterghos and D. Lade, "Judge Rules Wife Insane, She Tried to Kill Husband and Herself," *Fort Lauderdale (Fla.) Sun-Sentinel*, December 19, 1999, 1B.

24. S.P. Freedberg, "Murder or Mercy?" *St. Petersburg (Fla.) Times*, January 31, 1999, A1.

25. G.J. Annas, "Physician-Assisted Suicide—Michigan's Temporary Solution," *Ohio Northern University Law Review* 20 (1994): 561–70, 566.

26. R.A. Burt, "Conversation with Silent Patients," in *Genetics and the Law II*, edited by A. Milunsky and G.J. Annas (New York: Plenum, 1980), 159–74, 159.

27. Back et al., "Physician-Assisted Suicide and Euthanasia in Washington State."

28. D.A. Asch, "The Role of Critical Care Nurses in Euthanasia and Assisted Suicide," *New England Journal of Medicine* 334 (1996): 1374–79, 1376.

29. Foley, "Compassionate Care, Not Assisted Suicide."

30. *Brophy v. New England Sinai Hospital, Inc.*, 398 Mass. 417, 497 N.E.2d 626 (1986).

31. Coleman, "Not Dead Yet," 229 (emphasis in original).

32. A.L. Higginbotham and F.M. Higginbotham, "'Yearning to Breathe Free': Legal Barriers Against and Options in Favor of Liberty in Antebellum Virginia," *New York University Law Review* 68 (1993): 1213–71, 1256–57.

CONCLUSION

Excellent Palliative Care as the Standard, Physician-Assisted Dying as a Last Resort

Timothy E. Quill, M.D., and Margaret P. Battin, Ph.D.

To understand the role of physician-assisted death as a last-resort option restricted to dying patients for whom palliative care or hospice has become
ineffective or unacceptable, one must understand how frequently and under
what circumstances that occurs. If al! such cases are the result of inadequately
delivered palliative care, then the best answer would be to improve the standard of care and make the problem disappear. Most experts in pain management believe that 95 to 98 percent of pain among those who are terminally ill
can be adequately relieved using modern pain management,[1] which is a remarkable track record—unless you are unfortunate enough to be in the 2 to 5 percent for whom it is unsuccessful. However, among hospice patients who were
asked about their pain level one week before their death, 5 to 35 percent rated
their pain as "severe" or "unbearable."[2] An additional 25 percent reported their
shortness of breath to be "unbearable" one week before death.[3] This says nothing of the physical symptoms that are harder to relieve, such as nausea, vomiting, confusion, and open wounds, including pressure sores, which many patients
experience.[4]

Of course, dying patients do not have the luxury of cleanly separating their
physical suffering from their psychological, spiritual, and existential suffering.[5]
These common physical symptoms are only part of the puzzle of suffering at
the end of life. We now know from Oregon that many patients who contemplate ending their own lives under the Death with Dignity Act have these physical symptoms but also report that tiredness with the process of dying, feeling
out of control, and lack of meaning are frequently the most important reasons
for requesting a hastened death.[6] We also know that dying patients who con-

sider hastening their deaths have trouble envisioning a meaningful future and that they score high on hopelessness scales.[7] Some patients who consider ending their lives under these circumstances are clinically depressed, but others are not, and none of these patients evaluated by a psychiatrist under the Death with Dignity Act was found to have distorted judgment from depression.[8] The reality faced by dying patients and their families in terms of suffering, even in the best of hospice programs, is much more complex than is ordinarily acknowledged. Eighty-five percent of the 171 patients who died with the assistance of a physician under the Oregon law were simultaneously enrolled in a hospice program,[9] so for them the dichotomous choice "palliative care or physician-assisted death" was clearly insufficient.

What are the effects of current prohibitions against access to physician-assisted death? Practices of last resort, such as physician-assisted suicide, that are illegal outside of Oregon are difficult to study because clinicians and family members could be criminally liable if they openly admitted to having participated. In reality, U.S. policy outside of Oregon would more aptly be characterized as "don't ask, don't tell," as the medical and legal professions have shown little enthusiasm about actively pursuing such cases through either legal or professional channels. Empirical studies on the illegal practice of physician-assisted death suggest that it accounts for a small percentage of overall deaths everywhere it has been studied, although in select populations, such as AIDS patients in San Francisco before the introduction of protease inhibitors, the practice may have accounted for almost 50 percent of deaths.[10]

If the "don't ask, don't tell" policy is working reasonably well, why not just leave it alone? The answer to this question is that it is not working well, for several reasons. First, access to the option of physician-assisted death is uneven and unpredictable, probably depending more on the physician's values and willingness to take a risk on the patient's behalf than on the patient's values and clinical circumstances.[11] Second, explicit conversation carries some risk, so patients, families, and their medical providers may communicate tacitly, with a wink and a nod instead of forthright conversation, with the concomitant potential for dangerous, possibly lethal misunderstandings in this delicate area.[12] Third, there would be no guarantee of adequate palliative care being in place before last-resort options were considered, so it would be more likely that a hastened death would be implemented in the absence of standard of care for the dying. Empirical data potentially comparing open, legal access to physician-assisted death to secret, illegal practice in many localities—including the United States outside of Oregon, Australia, Belgium, Denmark, Italy, the Netherlands, Sweden, and Switzerland—are now becoming available.[13] Of course, empirical data will not resolve the associated ethical or religious questions, but they will help to resolve some of the more secular issues around relative harm and benefit from legalization of assisted dying.

One of the positive outcomes of the debate about legalization of physician-assisted suicide is that other last-resort options have been considered—and, in some cases, legitimated.[14] There is growing acknowledgment that some patients experience unacceptable levels of suffering toward the end of their terminal illness, even though they are receiving state-of-the-art palliative care, and that some of these patients are capable of making rational decisions to hasten death (that is, they are not all clinically depressed or delirious).[15] For example, patients are allowed to discontinue life support as part of their right to bodily integrity, even when their desire is to die sooner rather than later. Patients who may have been taking a lesser amount of opioids for their pain so as to maintain alertness at one point in their illness may at a later stage request or accept more risk of sedation to achieve better pain relief as death approaches.

Two new options of last resort, voluntarily stopping eating and drinking and terminal sedation, have now been recognized as legally acceptable and are beginning to be more completely discussed from ethical and religious perspectives.[16] Voluntary cessation of eating and drinking involves a conscious choice to hasten death by a severely ill person who is still capable of eating and drinking. It is viewed ethically by many as a variant of the right to refuse treatment, as part of an individual's right to bodily integrity. Terminal sedation, which involves sedating the patient to unconsciousness (to allow an escape from suffering) and then withholding or withdrawing hydration and nutrition, is generally reserved for imminently dying patients whose physical suffering is severe and otherwise unrelievable. Sedation to the point of unconsciousness is viewed by many as aggressive symptom palliation with the intent to relieve suffering (therefore consistent with the doctrine of double effect), and the withdrawal of life-sustaining nutrition and hydration as part of the right to bodily integrity. Of course, either or both of these acts could be used intentionally to hasten a wished-for death and therefore be consistent with physician-assisted suicide or even voluntary active euthanasia, which makes these practices problematic for some clinicians and patients even if they are legally permissible.

Becoming more explicit about the acceptability of these last-resort practices has been an important contribution to enhancing end-of-life options for many patients. It acknowledges that tough cases of unacceptable suffering exist, and it reinforces clinicians' obligation to respond to suffering.[17] Additional options can be offered to patients who otherwise would have no acceptable possibilities. For patients who are morally opposed to physician-assisted suicide yet nonetheless find themselves in intolerable clinical circumstances, these alternative last-resort practices may provide acceptable options to allow them to live (and die) on their own terms.

The possibility of a predictable escape from suffering if it becomes overwhelming is important to many patients,[18] especially those who have witnessed bad deaths in loved ones toward whom the medical profession was unable or unwilling to be responsive. This fear is probably the driving force behind the desire for legalization of physician-assisted suicide. Patients will speak about this when asked questions like, "As you look to your future, what are your biggest fears?" or "What kinds of deaths (good or bad) have you seen among your family or friends?"[19] Having this conversation relatively early on in a patient's potentially terminal illness lets the patient know that the clinician is not afraid of the dying process and provides opportunity to educate the patient about all the advances palliative care has made in terms of addressing pain and other symptoms. Some patients, however, may push the family or their medical providers further by asking questions like, "If my pain becomes intolerable, will you help me die?" Sometimes this will be a general exploration of the extent of commitment not to abandon,[20] but at other times it may include explicit exploration of what last-resort options can be supported. We know from the Netherlands that only about one in nine patients who explore the option of physician-assisted dying actually dies in this way. Patients who know that their doctor is a committed medical partner, and that acceptable medical options are available to address their fears and concerns, will then have the freedom to spend their time and energy on other more vital matters as they are dying. Those without this knowledge and commitment are left to wonder fearfully how their final weeks and months might unfold.

Usually, even when a physician has promised to be responsive in helping a patient die, careful delivery of palliative care and then hospice is sufficient to facilitate an acceptable, if not always ideal, death. Anecdotal evidence suggests that many patients try to protect their physicians and family members from legal risk even at the cost of their own suffering. Yet there will be cases in which suffering becomes severe and unacceptable, and a patient becomes ready to die sooner rather than later and is willing to ask for help. All such patients should be assessed in a similar way to ensure that all reasonable palliative care options have been considered, no matter which last-resort options are also being contemplated.[21] Have pain or other physical symptoms been adequately addressed?

Has the patient become depressed in a way that is distorting his judgment? Has a family or spiritual crisis developed?[22] If a careful assessment finds none of those elements present, is the request genuine and in proportion to the degree of the patient's suffering? Here the safeguards and second opinions of an open process become invaluable.[23] Whether the physician is considering stopping life support (legal) or providing medication that can be taken as an overdose (in the United States, illegal outside of Oregon), he or she must recognize that the patient is likely to die as a result of this decision, so it should be approached with the utmost care and caution. As always, safeguards for any of these last-resort practices must balance invasiveness and safety.

Once the assessment has been carried out to ensure that all reasonable palliative care alternatives that the patient is willing to accept have been considered and that the patient is clear about the request and the implications for him- or herself and the family, then a decision must be made about methods. The method chosen should be the least invasive and risky for the particular patient, taking into account his or her values and clinical circumstances. If the method includes physician participation, the physician's values must be taken into account, as well. If a physician is unwilling to participate in a legally accepted option for which the patient otherwise would qualify and which he or she desires, then the physician is obligated to offer to transfer the patient's care to a qualified physician with different views and values. The physician must not entrap patients by seeming to promise a physician-assisted death but then reneging on this promise.[24] If a physician is aware of all the last-resort options and is opposed to granting a request for assisted suicide by a particular patient, the physician might explore those options that he or she *can* support to see whether common ground can be found. Clearly, physicians should attempt to extend themselves to remain responsive to such suffering patients and their families, but that should not include violating fundamental personal moral values for either the physician or the patient. On the other hand, it is imperative that we now recognize that the patient's fundamental moral values may include physician-assisted suicide and that this option, for those who are dying, should be part of recognized law.

Although issues around legal access to physician-assisted death remain complex and controversial, we support the following conclusions based on the information presented in the preceding chapters:

• Excellent palliative care must be the standard of care for those who are severely ill and dying. It can address, and sufficiently relieve, most but not all suffering that accompanies the dying process.

• Strong philosophical, ethical, and religious principles—especially autonomy, mercy, and nonabandonment—support access to physician-assisted death as a last resort for those circumstances in which suffering becomes intolerable to a dying patient who has access to palliative care.

• When conflicts about values exist in end-of-life care, it is the patient's values that count most (it is his or her death, after all), followed by those of the family (who have to make sense of the decisions that have been made) and then those of the health care providers (if it involves their participation). In areas in which there is no societal consensus about permissible versus impermissible actions, patients, families, and their health care providers should be given as much leeway and support as possible as they face these difficult decisions.

• Traditional distinctions between killing and letting die, or between actively and passively assisting death remain controversial, and are not conceptually helpful by themselves in distinguishing between acceptable and unacceptable methods of assisting death.

• Patients' motivations for seeking physician-assisted death come from multiple sources, including illness-related symptoms and loss of function, desire for control and loss of sense of self, and fears about future losses. The first step in evaluating any request should be to fully explore its underlying meaning and the reason it is emerging at a particular point in time, in the context of this individual patient's personal values and culture.

• Patients requesting a physician-assisted death should be carefully evaluated for depression and other medical disorders that could be interfering with their decision-making capacity, but it should not be assumed that they lack capacity simply because they are asking questions about a practice that many disagree with or find uncomfortable to talk about. The clinical challenge is to learn to talk openly with such patients about their suffering and how they see their future and to respond as constructively and compassionately as possible.

• Although relatively few patients actually receive physician-assisted suicide, knowing about it as a possibility (as well as knowing about other last-resort options, such as stopping life-sustaining therapy, terminal sedation, or stopping eating and drinking) is important to many who fear hard death and need to know that they could have some choice in the process.

• Physician-assisted suicide should be viewed in the context of other last-resort options in which death is hastened, including discontinuing life-sustaining therapy, terminal sedation, and cessation of eating and drinking. The challenge clinically is to respond appropriately to the particular patient's clinical circumstances in light of his or her values and those of the family and the physician.

• As presented in detail in part 3 of this volume, six years of data from Oregon and three comprehensive studies spanning sixteen years from the Netherlands provide strong empirical evidence that a legally tolerated practice of physician-assisted death can be controlled. In both settings, physician-assisted death comprises only a small percentage of all deaths, which has been stable over time (Oregon less than 1 percent and the Netherlands about 3 percent); and, as the articles from the Netherlands have clearly shown, there has been no pattern of widespread abuse. In Oregon, as noted earlier, 85 percent of patients who died under the Oregon Death with Dignity Act were simultaneously enrolled in hospice programs, showing the potential compatibility of the two approaches. Furthermore, improvements in end-of-life care since implementation of the Death with Dignity Act have included the highest rate of at-home deaths in the nation; high use of prescribed opioids; high referral rates to hospice programs; comprehensive, statewide do-not-resuscitate policies; and a high level of public awareness of end-of-life options.

For those who do not reject the practice of physician-assisted death as a last resort on moral grounds, the main empirical question is whether an open, legally regulated practice is safer and better for patients than the more secretive, arbitrary practice that is currently present in the rest of the country. The experience from Oregon attests to the potential compatibility of improvements in palliative care and limited legal access to physician-assisted death. Whether Oregon's experience will be replicated in the rest of the country depends on how and when similar legislation is passed in other states. For those of us who believe these practices are not only compatible but complementary, the data from Oregon are reassuring and motivating.

In our opinion, physician-assisted death should represent a small but critical piece of a larger puzzle of improving end-of-life care for all dying persons. In the absence of universal medical insurance coverage, the first step in working with patients who are nearing death, whether or not they are exploring the possibility of an assisted death, is to ensure they have access to the best medical care possible. We must all join together in working toward improvements in palliative care and hospice, in hopes of making them accessible to all seriously ill patients.

Should we wait to consider the option of legal access to a physician-assisted death until we have solved the problem of universal access? In the interest of fairness to those patients who are suffering intolerably in the face of excellent palliative care and are requesting this kind of assistance now, the answer should be a resounding no. We do not withhold expensive, marginally effective treatments for the few who might possibly benefit from them because so many lack coverage. Similarly, we do not prevent patients from stopping potentially effective treatment because they may be intentionally seeking to hasten their death or because others might not have access to effective treatment. Working with patients who are considering stopping life supports can and should be challenging, as they will most likely die as a result of that decision. But that does not mean that we should not listen carefully to their requests and do our best to respond. The same is true for patients who seek aid from their physicians in dying. The best protection we can offer is not absolute prohibition but rather to require full disclosure, second opinions to ensure the adequacy of palliative care and the careful assessment of patient decision-making capacity, involvement of experienced clinicians, and open documentation for study and review.

Vulnerable patients are asking us to listen to their requests with an open mind and heart and to keep their values and priorities at the center of the decision-making process. After all, this is a process driven by the experiences of dying patients and their families. Patients who begin to experience a bad death need access to experienced palliative care consultants who can make sure everything possible is being done to address their suffering, and make it tolerable. They need committed medical partners who will help them explore all potential alternatives but also address the reality that sometimes death is not the enemy. People who are terminally ill do not have a choice about whether to die, but they are asking for some choice and control over *how* they die. For many, potential access to a physician-assisted death allows reassurance that there could be an escape that they may never need. For a few who reach a point at which continued living becomes unacceptable and personhood is rapidly disintegrating, open access to a physician-assisted death can be vital to maintaining dignity and meaning at death.

Notes

1. K.M. Foley, "Physician-Assisted Suicide and Euthanasia," *Pain Forum* 4 (1995): 163–78; R.L. Kane, L. Bernstein, J. Wales, and R. Rothenberg, "Hospice Effectiveness in Controlling Pain," *Journal of the American Medical Association* 253 (1985): 2683–86.

2. G.A. Kasting, "The Nonnecessity of Euthanasia," in *Physician-Assisted Death*, edited by J.D. Humber, R.F. Almeder, and G.A. Kasting (Totowa, N.J.: Humana, 1993), 25–43; B. Ventafridda, C. Ripamonti, F. DeConno, M. Tamburini, and B.R. Cassileth, "Symptom Prevalence and Control During Cancer Patients' Last Days of Life," *Journal of Palliative Care* 6 (1990): 7–11; N. Coyle, J. Adelhardt, K.M. Foley, and R.K. Portenoy, "Character of Terminal Illness in the Advanced Cancer Patient: Pain and Other Symptoms

During the Last Four Weeks of Life," *Journal of Pain and Symptom Management* 5 (1990): 83–93.

3. J. Ingham and R. Portenoy, "Symptom Assessment," in *Pain and Palliative Care*, edited by N.I. Cherny and K.M. Foley, *Hematology Clinics of North America* 5 (1996): 21–39.

4. Kasting, "Nonnecessity of Euthanasia"; S. Donnelly and D. Walsh, "The Symptoms of Advanced Cancer," *Seminars in Oncology* 22 (1995): 67–72.

5. E.J. Cassell, *The Nature of Suffering and the Goals of Medicine* (New York: Oxford University Press, 1991); T.E. Quill, *Caring for Patients at the End of Life: Facing an Uncertain Future Together* (New York: Oxford University Press, 2001).

6. A.E. Chin, K. Hedberg, G.K. Higginson, and D.W. Fleming, "Legalized Physician-Assisted Suicide in Oregon—The First Year's Experience," *New England Journal of Medicine* 340 (1999): 577–83; A.D. Sullivan, K. Hedberg, and D.W. Fleming, "Legalized Physician-Assisted Suicide in Oregon—The Second Year," *New England Journal of Medicine* 342 (2000): 598–604; A.D. Sullivan, K. Hedberg, and D. Hopkins, "Legalized Physician-Assisted Suicide in Oregon, 1998–2000," *New England Journal of Medicine* 344 (2001): 605–7. Sixth Annual Report of data from the Oregon Death with Dignity Act available at www.ohd.hr.state.or.us/chs/pas/ar-index.cfm (last accessed May 29, 2004).

7. W. Breitbart, B. Rosenfeld, H. Pessin, M. Kaim, J. Funesti-Esch, M. Galretta, C.J. Nelson, and R. Bresica, "Depression, Hopelessness, and Desire for Hastened Death in Terminally Ill Patients with Cancer," *Journal of the American Medical Association* 284 (2000): 2907–11.

8. H.M. Chochinov, K.G. Wilson, M. Enns, and S. Lander, "Prevalence of Depression in the Terminally Ill: Effects of Diagnostic Criteria and Symptom Threshold Judgments," *American Journal of Psychiatry* 151 (1994): 537–40; S.D. Block, "Assessing and Managing Depression in the Terminally Ill Patient," *Annals of Internal Medicine* 132 (2000): 209–18; Linda Ganzini, professor of psychiatry, Portland VA Medical Center, personal communication, July 2004.

9. Sullivan, Hedberg, and Fleming, "Legalized Physician-Assisted Suicide in Oregon—The Second Year."

10. D.E. Meier, C. Emmons, S. Wallenstein, T.E. Quill, R.S. Morrison, and C.K. Cassel, "A National Survey of Physician-Assisted Suicide and Euthanasia in the United States," *New England Journal of Medicine* 338 (1998): 1193–1201; A.L. Back, J.I. Wallace, H.E. Starks, and R.A. Pearlman, "Physician-Assisted Suicide and Euthanasia in Washington State: Patient Requests and Physician Responses," *Journal of the American Medical Association* 275 (1996): 919–25; L.R. Slome, T.F. Mitchell, E. Charlebois, J.M. Benevedes, and D.I. Abrams, "Physician-Assisted Suicide and Patients with Human Immunodeficiency Virus Disease," *New England Journal of Medicine* 336 (1997): 417–21.

11. D.T. Watts, T. Howell, and B.A. Priefer, "Geriatricians' Attitudes toward Assisting Suicide in Dementia Patients," *Journal of the American Geriatric Society* 40 (1992): 878–85; L. Slome, J. Moulton, C. Huffine, R. Gorter, and D. Abrams, "Physicians' Attitudes Toward Assisted Suicide in AIDS," *Journal of Acquired Immune Deficiency Syndromes* 5 (1992): 712–18; P.R. Duberstein, Y. Conwell, C. Cox, C.A. Podgorski, R.S. Glazer, and

E.D. Caine, "Attitudes toward Self-Determined Death: A Survey of Primary Care Physicians," *Journal of the American Geriatric Society* 43 (1995): 395–400; F.Y. Huang and L.L. Emanuel, "Physician Aid in Dying and the Relief of Patients' Suffering: Physicians' Attitudes Regarding Patients' Suffering and End-of-Life Decisions," *Journal of Clinical Ethics* 6 (1995): 62–67; J.G. Bachman, K.H. Alchser, D.J. Doukas, R.L. Lichtenstein, A.D. Corning, and H. Brody, "Attitudes of Michigan Physicians and the Public toward Legalizing Physician-Assisted Suicide and Voluntary Euthanasia," *New England Journal of Medicine* 334 (1996): 303–9; R. Shapiro, A.R. Derse, M. Gottlieb, D. Scheidermayer, and M. Olson, "Willingness to Perform Euthanasia: A Survey of Physician Attitudes," *Archives of Internal Medicine* 154 (1994): 575–84; J.S. Cohen, S.D. Fihn, E.J. Boyko, A.R. Jonsen, and R.W. Wood, "Attitudes toward Assisted Suicide and Euthanasia among Physicians in Washington State," *New England Journal of Medicine* 331 (1994): 89–94.

12. R.S. Magnusson, *Angels of Death: Exploring the Euthanasia Underground* (New Haven: Yale University Press, 2002).

13. A. van der Heide, L. Deliens, K. Faisst, T. Nilstun, M. Norup, E. Paci, G. van der Wal, and P.J. van der Maas, on behalf of the EURELD consortium, "End-of-Life Decision-Making in Six European Countries: Descriptive Study," *Lancet* 362 (2003): 345–50.

14. T.E. Quill, B. Lo, and D.W. Brock, "Palliative Options of Last Resort: A Comparison of Voluntarily Stopping Eating and Drinking, Terminal Sedation, Physician-Assisted Suicide, and Voluntary Active Euthanasia," *Journal of the American Medical Association* 278 (1997): 2099–104; T.E. Quill, B. Coombs Lee, and S. Nunn, "Palliative Treatments of Last Resort: Choosing the Least Harmful Alternative," *Annals of Internal Medicine* 132 (2000): 488–93.

15. T.E. Quill, D.E. Meier, S.D. Block, and J.A. Billings, "The Debate over Physician-Assisted Suicide: Empirical Data and Convergent Views," *Annals of Internal Medicine* 128 (1998): 552–58; Chochinov et al., "Prevalence of Depression in the Terminally Ill"; S.D. Block and J.A. Billings, "Patient Requests to Hasten Death: Evaluation and Management in Terminal Care," *Archives of Internal Medicine* 154 (1994): 2039–47.

16. *Vacco v. Quill*, 521 U.S. 793 (1997); *Washington v. Glucksberg*, 521 U.S. 702 (1997); T.E. Quill and I. Byock, "Responding to Intractable Terminal Suffering: The Role of Terminal Sedation and Voluntary Refusal of Food and Fluids," *Annals of Internal Medicine* 132 (2000): 408–14; L.A. Jansen and D.P. Sulmasy, "Sedation, Alimentation, Hydration, and Equivocation: Careful Conversation about Care at the End of Life," *Annals of Internal Medicine* 136 (2002): 845–49.

17. T.E. Quill and C.K. Cassel, "Nonabandonment: A Central Obligation for Physicians," *Annals of Internal Medicine* 122 (1995): 368–74.

18. Block and Billings, "Patient Requests to Hasten Death"; T.E. Quill, "Doctor, I Want to Die. Will You Help Me?" *Journal of the American Medical Association* 270 (1993): 870–73.

19. B. Lo, T.E. Quill, and J. Tulsky, "End-of-Life Care Consensus Panel. Discussing Palliative Care with Patients," *Annals of Internal Medicine* 130 (1999): 744–49.

20. Quill and Cassel, "Nonabandonment."

21. Block and Billings, "Patient Requests to Hasten Death"; Quill, "Doctor, I Want to Die. Will You Help Me?"

22. M.P. Battin, *The Least Worst Death: Essays in Bioethics on the End of Life* (New York: Oxford University Press, 1994).

23. T.E. Quill, C.K. Cassel, and D.E. Meier, "Care of the Hopelessly Ill: Proposed Clinical Criteria for Physician-Assisted Suicide," *New England Journal of Medicine* 327 (1992): 1380–84.

24. L.L. Emanuel, "Facing Requests for Physician-Assisted Suicide: Toward a Practical and Principled Clinical Skill Set," *Journal of the American Medical Association* 280 (1998): 643–47.

Index

abortion, analogy to, 57, 155, 203, 270, 282, 294–95, 303–4
acquired immune deficiency syndrome (AIDS), 59, 61, 106, 107, 133, 141, 174, 190, 195–96, 324
act versus omission, 286–88, 309, 318, 328. *See also* death, hastening of: active versus passive means
ADA. *See* Americans with Disabilities Act
Adkins, Janet, 302
advance directives, 160, 215, 301
aid in dying. *See* physician-assisted dying
AIDS. *See* acquired immune deficiency syndrome
ALS. *See* amyotrophic lateral sclerosis
AMA. *See* American Medical Association
ambivalence, patient. *See under* request to die
American Medical Association (AMA), 30, 34, 272, 314–15
American Paralysis Association, 57
American Society of Law, Medicine, and Ethics (ASLME), 273
Americans with Disabilities Act (ADA), 56, 63, 64
amyotrophic lateral sclerosis (ALS), 172, 174, 175, 192–94, 217, 218
Angell, Lester W., 19
Angell, Marcia, 8
Ashcroft, John, 19, 57, 61, 155, 166, 249, 268, 272, 306, 318

Asking to Die, 228, 233
ASLME. *See* American Society of Law, Medicine, and Ethics
assisted suicide. *See* physician-assisted dying
Australia, 209
autonomy, 7, 8, 20, 22, 23, 39, 40, 43, 44, 62, 63, 131, 141, 177, 199, 221, 272; as absolute right, 48, 52; and coercion, 40, 41; compromised by illness, 41, 42; concept of, 9; and control, 22, 39, 44–45; and dependence, 20, 41, 42, 43–44; extreme, 43, 45; as ideal, 39, 42–43, 52; maximizing, 44, 47, 52; of medical professionals, 40, 51, 139; principle of, 39–41, 44, 47–48, 50, 51, 52, 139, 209, 328; reproductive, 50; and self-centeredness, 43, 45–46. *See also* freedom; self-determination
AUTONOMY, Inc., 58–60, 72

Back, Anthony L., 3, 9
Barnett, Erin H., 186, 187
Baron, Charles, 10
Batavia, Andrew, v, 9
Beauchamp, Tom L., 9
Belgium, 130, 209
Bergman v. Chin, 305
Billings, J.A., 114
Block, Susan, 114
Borst-Eilers, Els, 10
Bouvia, Elizabeth, 65, 66–67
Bowers v. Hardwick, 303, 304

Bradbury, Bill, 245
Brandt, Dietrich, 315
breathing difficulties, 15, 18, 32, 83, 140, 185, 192, 193, 218; respiratory depression, 18, 140
Brennan, Justice William, 294
Breyer, Justice Stephen, 266, 293, 294
Brock, Dan, 9
Brongersma, Edward, 226
Brophy v. New England Sinai Hospital, Inc., 318
Buddhism, 25, 26, 31

California Medical Board, 274
California Supreme Court, 270
Callahan, Daniel, 44–45, 51, 311
capacity, decision-making. *See* competence in decision making
care: of others, 34; of self, 34; virtues of, 24
Casey v. Planned Parenthood, 303, 304
Cassel, Christine, 8, 30, 34
Cassell, Eric, 9, 175
Catholic Church, 246, 252, 253, 258–59, 260, 270, 304
causation, 119–20, 122–25, 127, 285, 290–92; foreseeability test, 291; natural and probable consequences test, 291; *sine qua non* test 290–91, 292; substantial factor test, 291
Cayetano, Ben, 253
Christianity, 9, 58, 150–60; and biblical literalism, 154–57; fundamentalist, 304. *See also* Catholic Church
coercion, 40, 41, 42, 43, 55, 62, 63, 186, 187, 198
Coleman, Diane, 309
comfort care. *See* palliative care
compassion, 49–50, 70, 76, 318
Compassion in Dying, 10, 58, 184, 185, 190–99, 264, 302, 303; client services, 192–94; data on aid in dying, 194–95
Compassion in Dying v. Washington, 294
competence in decision making: assessment of, 32, 99, 185, 186, 328; influences on, 2, 4, 41; and self-administration of lethal dose, 134, 275; and terminal sedation, 133, 208. *See also* informed consent; request to die, motivations for
confidentiality. *See* privacy
Conroy, Claire. *See In re* Conroy

control of dying, 3, 8, 9, 22, 92, 93–94, 98, 177, 199, 227, 228
Controlled Substances Act (CSA) (1970), 61, 166, 268, 272, 273, 306
Cruzan v. Director, Missouri Department of Health, 64, 302. *See also* right to die; withholding and withdrawing treatment
CSA. *See* Controlled Substances Act
culpability, 288–89, 293, 297

Daneault, Serge, 85
DEA. *See* Drug Enforcement Administration
death: acceptance of, 227; communication about, 105, 113, 224, 228, 312, 328; definition of, 300; as "enemy of our humanity" (St. Paul), 158; as "friend" or "brother," 158; medicalization of, 49, 51; perceptions of, 15, 16; ritualized, 111
death, hastening of: active versus passive means, 137–39, 143, 144, 282–97 (*see also* killing: versus letting die); and consent, 293–95; duty not to hasten death, 140; duty to relieve suffering, 126; and end-of-life care, 190, 325; and homicide, 282–83, 285, 289, 292–93, 297, 309; methods of, 9, 10, 131–44, 325; moral justifications for, 118–21, 124, 127–28, 130, 131; permissibility of, 126–27, 135, 144, 266; technical competence in, 110–11
death with dignity, state initiatives: California (Proposition 161), 251, 254, 258, 260; Hawaii (House Bill 2487), 253–54, 255, 258, 260, 282; Maine (Question 1), 253, 254, 255, 258–59, 260; Michigan (Proposal B), 252–53, 254, 258, 260; Oregon (Measure 16), 251–52; Oregon (Measure 51), 252; Washington (Initiative 119), 250–51, 254, 258, 260. *See also* Death with Dignity Act (Hawaii); Death with Dignity Act (Oregon)
Death with Dignity Act (Hawaii), 253–54
Death with Dignity Act (Oregon), 5, 6, 10, 15, 21, 33, 61, 102, 108, 113, 165–78, 184, 188, 196–98, 245, 261–67, 282, 286–87, 306, 323; cases, 165, 168, 171–72, 184–88; and Catholic Church, 252, 253, 258–59, 260, 270; data collection required under, 188; data on, 167–68, 170–78, 269, 271; history of, 165–67, 245–52, 256–61; as mechanism for protecting

physicians, 294, 297; and nonresident requests, 177; procedural requirements of, 165, 167, 177, 185, 196, 256, 257; reporting requirements, 167; sponsorship of, 257; surveys on, 167, 169–78

death with dignity movement, 254; and organized medicine, 254, 258, 270

Death with Dignity National Center, 59

decision making, surrogate, 28, 191, 284, 286

dehydration, 68, 131–32, 141

Denmark, 209

depression: and suicide, 174, 227; among terminally ill, 174, 227; treatment of, at end of life, 226. *See also under* request to die, motivations for

dignity, 20, 28, 103, 132, 133, 155, 159, 207, 221, 293, 294, 330

Diocese of Newark, N.J. (Episcopal), 151

disability, 9, 56, 318; and assistance in dying, 70–71, 222; community, 56, 61–62, 72; and discrimination, 63

disability rights movement, 59, 63, 64; and AIDS, 59; distrust of medical profession, 63; and independent living movement, 63, 67; and quality of life, 63, 64, 66; and religious conservatism, 57; and right-to-life movement, 57; and self-determination, 63–64; views about physician-assisted dying, 56–60, 61, 62, 71–71

doctor-patient relationship, 46, 232; boundaries in, 34, 108–10, 114; and communication about physician-assisted dying, 3, 9, 98, 102–15, 197, 224, 232; continuity in, 28; as contract, 34; as covenant, 24, 34; as "medical friendship," 233; mutuality in, 233; nature of, 77, 199, 232–33; and obligation to prevent harm, 77, 99; in physician-assisted dying, 232–33; pressures on, 24; and referral for physician-assisted dying, 197, 327; as therapeutic alliance, 114; trust and distrust in, 21–23, 25, 34, 63, 57, 70; and vulnerability, 29, 31, 110, 141. *See also* medicine: moral character of

double effect, doctrine of, 135–37, 139, 140, 143, 144, 289, 325. *See also* killing: versus letting die

Drug Enforcement Administration (DEA), 166, 249, 267, 306

due process, 265. *See also Vacco v. Quill; Washington v. Glucksberg*

Dworkin, Ronald, 275–76

dying. *See* death; physician-assisted dying

Edwards, Randall, 245

empathy, 28, 29

end-of-life care, 3, 10, 22; barriers to effective, 317; inadequacies in, 2; integrated with physician-assisted dying, 190–99, 238–39; schism regarding, 21, 23, 238. *See also* hospice; palliative care

equal protection and request to die, 63, 64, 265, 267. *See also* Fourteenth Amendment; *Vacco v. Quill; Washington v. Glucksberg*

ethics of medicine, 36, 296; duty not to hasten death, 140; duty to relieve suffering, 140. *See also* doctor-patient relationship; medicine: moral character of

euthanasia, 55, 71; characteristics of patients requesting, 206; definition of, 205, 208; as last resort, 203, 213–14; and Nazism, 59, 63; nonvoluntary, 63, 64, 207–9; passive, 150; practice of, 202–15; as social policy, 202–7, 251, 254, 256; voluntary, 10, 55, 134, 202, 325. *See also* Netherlands, euthanasia in

false dichotomy, 1, 3

Florida Supreme Court, 60, 284, 295

Foley, Kathleen, 2, 21, 184, 185, 187, 188, 222, 226, 310, 313, 317

force majeure, 204, 205

Fourteenth Amendment, 63, 265. *See also* due process; U.S. Court of Appeals for the Ninth Circuit; *Washington v. Glucksberg*

Francis of Assisi, Saint, 158

Free University (Amsterdam), 10

freedom, 2, 43, 45, 46. *See also* autonomy

Gallagher, Hugh G., 59

Ganzini, Linda, 9

geriatrics, 8

Gesser, Gina, 227

Gilbert, Roswell, 316

Glucksberg. See Washington v. Glucksberg

good, substantive notion of, 47–48, 52
Goodwin, Peter, 9
Gray, David, 59
grief, 115, 235
Griswold v. Connecticut, 305, 309
Gunderson, Martin, 8

Hall, Charles, 61
Halstead, Lauro, 60
Hamilton, N. Gregory, 187–88
harm principle, 47
Haverkate, Ilinka, 228, 237
healing, 35, 199. See also medicine: moral
    character of
health care, access to, 31, 222, 329
health care professionals: attitudes toward
    assisted suicide, 169, 171, 199; as gatekeepers,
    49. See also doctor-patient relationship;
    healing; medicine: moral character of
Hemlock Society, 70, 302
Hendin, Herbert, 2, 10, 21, 184, 185, 187, 188,
    222, 224, 225, 226, 227, 313
Hippocratic medicine, 125. See also medicine:
    moral character of
Hogan, Judge Michael, 166
Holocaust, 32
hope, 25, 26
hopelessness. See under request to die,
    motivations for
hospice, 6, 21, 25, 26, 28, 42, 51, 68, 76, 106, 168,
    170, 186, 188, 193, 197, 213, 214; access to, 2,
    171, 198; movement (international), 19, 22;
    and requests for physician-assisted dying,
    176, 324; and suffering, 87. See also palliative
    care
Humphry, Derek, 302. See also Hemlock
    Society
Hyde, Representative Henry, 152

informed consent, 45, 51, 137, 139, 142, 293,
    297, 304
In re Conroy, 287
In re Quinlan, 202, 283, 284, 285, 294, 309, 310
intent, 273, 285, 288–90, 292. See also double
    effect, doctrine of; killing: versus letting
    die
International Anti-Euthanasia Task Force, 185

Intractable Pain Treatment Acts, 274
Italy, 209

Jehovah's Witnesses, 311–12, 318
John, Saint, 160
Jones, Judge Robert, 166

Kaiser Permanente, 186, 197
Kamisar, Yale, 309, 310
Kass, Leon R., 21, 41, 43, 51
Kevorkian, Jack, 5, 185, 186, 252, 256, 302
killing: concept of, 7, 21, 119, 120; versus letting
    die, 9, 118, 119–24, 127–28, 137–38, 312, 328.
    See also act versus omission; death,
    hastening of: active versus passive means
Kimsma, Gerrit, 10
Kitzhaber, John, 245, 252
Kohlwes, Jeffrey, 113
Kübler-Ross, Elisabeth, 227
Kulongoski, Ted, 245

La Bohème, 16
Lain-Entralgo, Pedro, 233
Law, Sylvia, 10
Lee, Barbara Coombs, 9, 58, 59
Lethal Drug Abuse Prevention Act, 249
liberty: interest in controlling death, 118, 265,
    266, 267, 270, 271, 303; principle of, 6,
    127–28. See also right to die; Vacco v. Quill;
    Washington v. Glucksberg
life, sacredness of, 152–54, 157–59
life-sustaining treatment, 25, 42, 131, 141, 283,
    284; artificial nutrition and hydration, 131,
    132, 287, 318, 325; eating and drinking, 131–32,
    135, 136, 138, 139, 141, 142, 325, 328; right to
    refuse, 131, 284, 286, 292, 294, 301, 310, 314,
    325, 328. See also withholding and
    withdrawing treatment
Longmore, Paul, 63
Lost Weekend, The, 107
Lowell, James Russell, 157

Maguire, Peter, 112
managed care, 24, 42, 167, 177
Mayo, David, 8
McAfee, Larry, 65–66, 67
McIlroy, Elaine, 316

meaning, 22, 26, 29, 30, 35, 82–85, 173; of death, 4; existential, 2; of one's life, 25, 178, 215; of pain, 175; and symptoms, 83

Medicaid, 304

Medicare, 28

medical futility as justification for letting die, 120–22

medical necessity as justification for euthanasia. *See force majeure*

medicine: and conflicting obligations, 204, 205; moral character of, 124–25, 199; and principle of nonabandonment, 141; and professional integrity, 7, 223. *See also* health care professionals; nonabandonment

Meisel, Alan, 10

mercy, 7, 8, 18, 23, 328

mercy killing, 209, 251, 256, 315–16. *See also* euthanasia

Miles, Steven, 114

Mill, John Stuart, 47

Mills, Paul, 123

Model Penal Code, 288, 290

moral equivalence arguments. *See* act versus omission; death, hastening of: active versus passive means; killing: versus letting die

Morrison, Nancy, 123

Myers, Hardy, 245

National Conference of Catholic Bishops, 303

National Right-to-Life Committee, 57

Nazi Germany, 27, 59, 63, 64

Netherlands: Amsterdam Appellate Court, 226–27; culture of, 202–4, 213, 221–22; Dutch Hospital Association, 10; Dutch Parliament, 206; end-of-life care and palliative care in, 213–14, 223; Euthanasia Act, 211, 212, 229; Minister of Health, 10; Public Prosecution Service, 210, 211; Regional Euthanasia Evaluation Committees, 225, 229, 230, 236; Royal Dutch Medical Society, 204, 225, 235; Support Consultation Euthanasia the Netherlands (SCEN), 211, 213, 236; Supreme Court, 205, 206, 215, 226; Utrecht Academic Clinic, 235

Netherlands, euthanasia in: American criticism of, 221–23; assessment committees, 210; data on, 3, 5, 9, 10, 11, 206–10, 224, 229, 235, 237, 326, 329; due care criteria, 205, 211, 212–14; financial incentives for, 204, 213, 222; and *force majeure,* 204, 205; independent consultants, 213, 236; lethal injection, 230, 236; pain-control hotlines, 6; physician's emotional responses to, 236–38; practice of, 6, 63, 64, 70, 130, 206–15, 221–39, 256; procedural requirements for, 209–13, 224; regulation of, 55, 204–6, 211–13, 229; reporting of (notification procedure), 209–10, 215; transparency of, 212, 215. *See also* euthanasia

New Jersey Supreme Court, 287

nonabandonment, 7, 28, 112, 141, 218, 232; and medical ethics, 171; obligation of, 8, 24–36, 328; and suffering, 29

Not Dead Yet, 56–58, 59, 71–72, 318

Nuland, Sherwin, 45

O'Connor, Justice Sandra Day, 265–67

ODHS. *See* Oregon Department of Human Services

Ohlrich, Vernal, 315

Oken, Donald, 312

opioids, 3, 82, 136. *See also* pain

Oregon, physician-assisted dying in: data on, 3, 4, 5, 9, 165, 167–78, 245–46, 329; opponents of, 184–88, 198, 246, 318; and palliative care system, 170; as political litmus test, 246; and social cohesion, 170. *See also* Death with Dignity Act (Oregon)

Oregon Catholic Conference, 252

Oregon Death with Dignity Act. *See* Death with Dignity Act (Oregon)

Oregon Department of Human Services (ODHS), 167, 170, 175, 176, 177, 198

Oregon Health Division, 9, 188

Oregon Health and Science University, 9, 166, 186, 197

Oregon Hospice Association, 198

Oregon v. Ashcroft, 19

pain, 3, 18, 19, 23, 27, 28, 107, 266, 323; meaning of, 175; physiology of, 80–81; psychogenic, 81–82; and suffering, 76, 80, 84. *See also* palliative care pain, treatment of: accountability for, 274–75; and addiction, 16–18; barriers to, 16, 266, 271, 272; clinical education in, 273; constitutional right to adequate level of, 266, 271, 272; inadequate, 10, 16, 19, 130, 175, 266, 272, 274–75, 305, 317; and malingering, 81; medication for, 11; patient control over, 18, 19; and safe-harbor laws, 274, 275; and tort law, 275. See also opioids; palliative care

Pain Relief Act (ASLME model legislation), 273

Pain Relief Promotion Act (1999), 249

palliative care, 1, 5, 6, 8, 11, 15, 21, 26, 32, 33, 68, 79, 98, 130, 141, 143, 166, 225, 327; clinical training in, 77, 78, 87, 167; communication about, 102, 105; improvements in, 2, 23, 130, 313, 329; and life-prolonging treatment, 25; and suffering, 22, 79, 127, 130

paternalism, 42, 49, 51, 67, 311

patient-physician relationship. See doctor-patient relationship

Patient Self-Determination Act (1990), 45, 302

Paul, Saint, 158, 159

Pearlman, Robert A., 3, 9, 170

Pellegrino, Edmund D., 49, 51

persistent vegetative state, 283, 301, 310, 318

personal assistance services, 65–66, 71

physician-assisted dying: abuse of, 3, 5, 70, 142, 186, 198, 296, 313, 318; access to, 306, 324, 327; and advance directives, 98, 165; analogy to physician-assisted reproduction, 50; arguments against, 3–7, 21, 56, 62–63, 64–65, 134; autonomy argument for, 39–52, 63; cases of, 165, 168, 171–72, 184–88, 198; constitutionality of, 10, 60, 264–67, 268, 270–71, 305; data on, 3, 5, 9, 10, 11, 32, 99, 108, 113, 134–35, 167, 168–78, 206–10, 224, 229, 235, 237, 324–25; and disability rights, 56, 61–63; eligibility criteria, 191; emotional aspects of, 230–35, 236–38; failed attempts at, 67, 75, 111, 112, 134; family involvement in, 46, 109, 111, 112, 113, 115, 134, 191–92, 234; financial incentives for, 141, 167, 177, 188, 204, 213; and history of liberation movements, 10, 301–7; and homicide, 292–93, 297, 309; and hospice, 198, 324, 329; as impediment to

palliative care, 167, 176–77; and improved palliative care, 5, 6, 21–23, 87, 92, 97–98, 167, 215, 223, 269, 313, 329; integrated with end-of-life care, 190–99, 238–39, 328; as last resort, 6, 8, 11, 22, 130, 141, 203, 213–14, 323, 328; legalization of, as social policy, 2, 3, 4, 5, 7, 8, 9, 56, 69, 118, 160, 245, 249–55, 264–71, 293–94, 295–97, 306, 314; as legitimate medical practice, 196, 199, 205, 229; and lethal injection, 251, 254, 256; and lethal prescription, 15, 49, 51, 55, 61, 109, 114, 126, 127, 134, 165, 166, 167, 174, 175, 185, 193, 275; moral justifications for, 118, 124–28; and New York State law, 76, 135; and nonterminal conditions, 55, 63, 70, 143; nonvoluntary, 207–9, 223; oppression argument for, 63, 65–66, 67; permissibility of, 126–27; and personal assistance services, 65–69, 71; politics of, 10, 166, 245–61; procedural safeguards, 4, 5, 22–23, 49, 55, 79, 87, 135, 141–42, 165, 167, 188, 192, 197, 223–24, 283, 295–97, 327; right to, 10, 57, 60, 62, 63; as secret practice, 5, 11, 33, 64, 112, 134–35, 143, 188, 199, 257, 264, 314, 324, 329; and slippery-slope arguments, 3, 7, 64, 208, 209, 310, 313; and state law, 55, 60, 61, 165–67, 203, 250–60, 265, 267, 269, 273, 282, 284, 287, 303; surveys on, 102, 134–35, 167, 169, 245–49; in Switzerland, 130; and terminal illness, 2, 5, 9, 52, 55, 62, 63, 70, 143, 165; transparency of, 4, 197; voter initiatives on, 165–66. See also Netherlands, euthanasia in: practice of; request to die, motivations for

physician-assisted suicide. See physician-assisted dying

physician-patient relationship. See doctor-patient relationship

Physicians for Compassionate Care, 199

Pickering, John H., 306

prescription of lethal medication. See physician-assisted dying: and lethal injection

Preston, Thomas, 8

primary care, 8

privacy, 23, 60, 99, 131, 141, 199, 231, 270, 271, 284, 301

proportionality, 140, 144, 226
proxy decision making. *See* decision making, surrogate
Putnam, Constance, 6

quality of life, 25, 26, 33
Quill. See *Vacco v. Quill*
Quill, Timothy, 8, 30, 34, 302
Quinlan, Karen Ann, 202, 283. See also *In re* Quinlan

Rehnquist, Chief Justice William, 265
Reinhardt, Judge Stephen, 294
Reker, Gary, 227
religious conservatism, 57
Reno, Janet, 268, 306
request to die: evaluation of, 328; patient ambivalence, 218, 224, 226; patient characteristics, 171–78; and therapeutic alliance, 114
request to die, motivations for: burden on others, 114, 166, 168, 172, 213; desire for control, 9, 16, 93–94, 98, 103, 105, 107, 168, 173, 177–78, 195, 323; demoralization, 19; depression, 4, 92, 96, 98, 166, 172–73, 178, 185, 207, 228, 324; economic concerns, 166, 168, 171–72, 173; existential and meaning issues, 173, 177–78, 226, 323; fear, 22, 32, 92, 93–94, 97, 113, 114, 168, 172, 175–78, 195, 213, 225, 326; hopelessness, 96, 151, 175, 324; illness experiences, 92, 93–96, 168, 195; pain, 9, 93, 94, 95, 107, 113, 130, 151, 166, 167, 175, 178; physical symptoms, 173, 175–76, 178, 226; self-preservation, 2; suffering, 87, 98–99, 207; threat to sense of self, 92, 93–94, 96–97, 98, 130. *See also* pain; suffering
right to die, 57, 59, 60, 66, 67, 151, 160, 266, 293. *See also* life-sustaining treatment: right to refuse; withholding and withdrawing treatment
right to life, advocates for, 57, 61, 267, 275
right to refuse treatment. *See under* life-sustaining treatment
Rivero, Justina, 316
Rivlin, David, 65, 66–67

Roe v. Wade, 155, 246, 303, 304, 305
Ruvelson, Jane, 59

safe-harbor laws, 274, 275
Safranek, John P., 47–48
Salem, Tania, 48, 49, 51
Saunders, Cecily, 22. *See also* hospice
SCEN. *See* Support Consultation Euthanasia the Netherlands
Scheufler, Susan, 315
sedation, 22, 33, 68, 123, 132; and pain, 26, 27, 92, 107, 325; terminal, 3, 9, 11, 68, 126, 130, 132–35, 138, 139, 141, 142, 208, 325, 328. *See also* double effect, doctrine of
self-determination, 20, 21, 44, 198, 283, 284. *See also* autonomy
Shlafley, Phyllis, 304
Silveira, Maria J., 170
slavery, 318
slippery-slope arguments, 3, 7, 64, 208, 209, 310, 313
"slow code," 317
Smith, Gordon, 246
Smith, Wesley, 185
Solomon, Mildred, 312
Souter, Justice David, 266, 267
Spong, John Shelby, 9
Starks, Helene, 3, 9, 170
starvation, 68–69, 132
St Christopher's Hospice (London), 18
Stein, Michael, 60
Stevens, Justice John Paul, 266, 294
Stevens, Kenneth, 199
Study to Understand Prognosis and Preferences of Outcomes and Risks of Treatment (SUPPORT), 222
Stutsman, Eli, 10
suffering, 8, 9, 15, 21, 22, 23, 25, 26, 32, 98–99, 204, 218, 310, 311; and depression, 86; duty to relieve, 78, 140, 199, 204; exceptional cases of, 78; existential, 19, 20, 79; extremes of, 22, 25, 31, 32–33, 133, 225; inadequately treated, 78, 86, 225; individuality of, 79; and integrity of person, 84; and meaning, 22, 82–85, 311; nature of, 76, 79–86; and pain, 76, 80, 84,

suffering (*continued*)
323; relief of, as legal matter, 2; sources of, 75, 76, 79–86; subjectivity of, 19, 79. *See also* pain

suicide, 9, 27, 47, 50, 67, 69, 70, 107, 196, 288; biblical reference to, 154, 156; and depression, 2, 174; heroic, 2; medicalization of, 46, 49–51; prevention services, 63, 64, 66; rational, 2

SUPPORT. *See* Study to Understand Prognosis and Preferences of Outcomes and Risks of Treatment

Support Consultation Euthanasia the Netherlands (SCEN), 211, 213

Swarte, Nikkie, 235

Sweden, 209

Switzerland, 209

terminal dehydration, 68, 131–32, 141

terminal sedation. *See* sedation, terminal

Tribe, Lawrence, 10

Trumball, Patricia D., 302

Tucker, Kathryn, 10

United Cerebral Palsy, 57

U.S. Court of Appeals for the Ninth Circuit, 61, 166, 265, 267, 306. See also *Washington v. Glucksberg*

U.S. Court of Appeals for the Second Circuit, 301. See also *Vacco v. Quill*

U.S. Department of Justice, 61, 268

U.S. District Court (Oregon), 166

U.S. Supreme Court, 9, 10, 58, 60, 61, 131, 132, 135, 152, 265, 269, 270, 272, 275, 282, 302, 303, 304, 305. See also *Casey v. Planned Parenthood; Cruzan v. Director, Missouri*

Department of Health; Roe v. Wade; Vacco v. Quill; Washington v. Glucksberg

utilitarianism, 312

Vacco v. Quill, 9, 10, 58, 59, 60, 132–33, 264–67, 270, 271. *See also* U.S. Court of Appeals for the Second Circuit; *Washington v. Glucksberg*

values: of clinician, 30, 33, 35, 327, 328; of family, 328; of patient, 8, 11, 33, 40, 327, 328

van Delden, Hans, 10

van der Kloot Meijburg, Fritz, 217–20

van der Kloot Meijburg, Herman, 3, 10

van der Maas, P. J., 225

van der Wal, Gerrit, 224

van Leeuwen, Evert, 10

Visser, Jaap, 10

voluntariness, 41, 55, 132, 134, 139, 144, 223, 224. *See also* informed consent

Washington v. Glucksberg, 9, 10, 58, 59, 60, 132, 264–67, 270, 271. *See also* U.S. Court of Appeals for the Ninth Circuit; *Vacco v. Quill*

Webb, Susan, 60

WHO. *See* World Health Organization

withholding and withdrawing treatment, 3, 11, 66, 98, 119–24, 132, 283, 284, 286–97, 325; and criminal liability, 283, 285–97, 317; and culpability, 288; and decision-making capacity of patient, 284, 286; procedural safeguards, 141–43, 295–97, 314, 327. *See also* life-sustaining treatment: right to refuse; right to die

Wong, Paul, 227

World Health Organization (WHO), 313

Zylicz, Zbigniew, 45, 223, 227, 233